COVID-19 Pandemic, Crisis Responses and the Changing World

Simon X.B. Zhao · Johnston H.C. Wong ·
Charles Lowe · Edoardo Monaco · John Corbett
Editors

COVID-19 Pandemic, Crisis Responses and the Changing World

Perspectives in Humanities and Social Sciences

Springer

Editors
Simon X.B. Zhao
Division of Humanities and Social Sciences
BNU-HKBU United International College
Zhuhai, Guangdong, China

Charles Lowe
Division of Humanities and Social Sciences
BNU-HKBU United International College
Zhuhai, Guangdong, China

John Corbett
Division of Humanities and Social Sciences
BNU-HKBU United International College
Zhuhai, Guangdong, China

Johnston H.C. Wong
Social Work and Social Administration
(SWSA) Programme
Division of Humanities and Social Sciences
BNU-HKBU United International College
Zhuhai, Guangdong, China

Edoardo Monaco
Globalisation and Development (GAD)
Programme
Division of Humanities and Social Sciences
BNU-HKBU United International College
Zhuhai, Guangdong, China

ISBN 978-981-16-2429-2 ISBN 978-981-16-2430-8 (eBook)
https://doi.org/10.1007/978-981-16-2430-8

This Springer imprint is published by the registered company Springer Nature Singapore Pte Ltd.
The registered company address is: 152 Beach Road, #21-01/04 Gateway East, Singapore 189721, Singapore

Foreword

In the opening two decades of the twenty-first century, it became something of a cliché to echo the sociologist Zygmunt Bauman (2000) in describing the globalized, post-modern condition as 'light' or 'liquid'. The recent digital revolution had collapsed time and space, allowing instantaneous communication with practically all parts of the planet, and society was transformed. Liquid modernity was characterized by transnational flows: flows of capital from one financial center to the next, flows of migrant workers across borders, flows of ideas via the internet and social media, and flows of popular culture, first by disc and radio wave, and then by streaming services. In this new millennium, personal identities were fragmented and reassembled, and, for many, they were defined by the consumption of brand names. Everything was in flux, the 'gig' economy grew, and the consequent instability of the world gave rise to new forms of anxiety.

And then, on January 22, 2020, the WHO mission to China confirmed that the novel coronavirus COVID-19 was disseminated by human-to-human transmission, and liquid modernity froze. A new set of anxieties blossomed as cities and then whole nations went into lockdown. International travel shuddered to a halt. Businesses suspended their activities and watched their profits tumble. Citizens stayed at home, only venturing outdoors with a mask, keeping a safe distance between themselves and their neighbors.

Of course, under the layer of ice there was continued turbulence. The digital communications that had sparked the new era of globalization became even more vital to the continuing welfare of families, communities, and businesses. Members of families, whether separated by a few miles or many thousand miles, continued to communicate by social media, local authorities posted updates on changing regulations on websites, and enterprises such as restaurants and retailers moved their sales wholly online. In China and a few notable countries, the swift and strict application of uniform lockdown measures drastically reduced rates of contagion, and a measure of normality returned to daily life after only a few months. In others, notably the United States and Brazil, the response to the threat was slower and more chaotic. Some decried the pandemic as a hoax and saw instructions to wear a mask as an affront to their freedom to choose their own lifestyle. Others, more seriously, weighed the risk of infection versus the risk of economic ruin. There were demonstrations against public health restrictions, even riots. Meanwhile, millions were infected, and thousands died.

The pandemic, then, saw both discipline and irresponsibility, foresight and negligence. And there was also scientific brilliance. Very early in 2020, China shared the genetic code for the novel coronavirus, sparking an international race between multinational pharmaceutical giants to find a vaccine. By the end of the year, with unprecedented speed, the first vaccines were approved, offering the possibility of a gradual and general thaw. The question remains, a year after the first surge of the pandemic, with the rolling out of vaccines just beginning: will the world ever be the same? Or, as Aleksandra Borovitskaja (2020) has asked, will the Covid-19 crisis function as a 'cosmopolitan moment' (p. 3) that prompts a global rejection of the structures of inequality and exploitation that threaten our living environment and the continuing existence of our species?

This collection of articles marks an attempt by a group of scholars, largely at a single higher education institution in China, BNU-HKBU United International College, to address some of the possible consequences of the global pandemic that followed the outbreak of COVID-19. Our institution is a young liberal arts college, the first in China to use English as its medium of instruction, and consequently we have an energetic, largely youthful, and multinational faculty. Our colleagues found themselves locked down and many were stranded throughout the world during the peak of the pandemic; nevertheless, they strove to keep the university running, and also to respond constructively to the problems caused by the pandemic. Thus, the chapters in this volume, mainly from our colleagues in the humanities and social sciences, address aspects of the *experience* of the COVID-19 pandemic as it was endured by countries, businesses, educational institutions, and individuals at the height of the crisis. It is a series of varied snapshots of how the pandemic gripped different parts of the world, affecting different areas of the economy, society, the media and education, and impacting on different groups of people. It is also a record of how a community of scholars perceived the unfolding of this outbreak narrative, interpreted the developing plot, and assessed the possible consequences, even as the pandemic raged. I salute the vision of Professor Zhao Xiaobin and his editorial team, who instigated this volume and whose energy and enthusiasm sustained its development, and I congratulate the editors and all the contributors. Their insight affords a valuable historical perspective on a global crisis that has deeply affected us all.

Tang Tao
Chair Professor
President of BNU-HKBU
United International College
Zhuhai, China

References

Bauman, Z. (2000). *Liquid Modernity*. Cambridge: Polity Press.
Borovitskaja, A. (2020). Covid-19: Into the inferno. *Amsterdam Law Forum*, 12(3), 1–6.

Preface

This collection of essays in response to the COVID-19 crisis is an admittedly ambitious but necessary enterprise that has drawn upon the scholarly talents of members of BNU-HKBU United International College. It is increasingly recognized across the globe that the humanities and social sciences have a key role to play in addressing the 'grand challenges' of the twenty-first century, not only in disciplines such as history, languages, the arts, social sciences, the media and other cultural industries, but also in less obvious domains like technology, sustainable development, climate change, conflict resolution and healthcare. In the case of the COVID-19 pandemic it is, for example, incumbent upon social scientists and humanities scholars to add their voices to those who are urgently assessing the immediate impact of the health crisis on national, professional and other communities.

Thus, in the first part of the present volume, we have solicited contributions on global economics, politics and public health responses to COVID-19. Our contributors suggest that, in many cases, it is a simplification to suggest that the pandemic alone has transformed social life; rather it has accelerated deep-rooted processes that were already in train. For example, the rivalry between the United States and China and the general reconfiguration of global supply chains both predate the outbreak of COVID-19, but the pandemic has exacerbated national economic and political tensions, and further prompted multinational corporations to redistribute their supply chains, to the extent that it seems like we are indeed moving inexorably toward a fundamentally different world. Our contributors critically assess the implications for this new world order, turning their eyes upon such diverse topics as European integration and the lessons learned for sustainable healthcare in Greater China.

One of the great misconceptions about globalization, of course, is that the world has become homogenous. The comparative country reports in this volume show similarities but also many differences in regional responses to the COVID-19 outbreak. These studies may not encompass the world as a whole, but they offer a balance of perspectives from the Global North and South, coming as they do from East and South Asia, Africa and the Middle East, and North and South America. While certain recurring themes are evident in the country reports, they offer distinctive national experiences of the pandemic and consequently offer a range of perspectives on the successes and failures of governmental responses to the crisis. Priscilla Ward (2008) observes in her prescient study of outbreak narratives, 'The ever-present health threat [...] signals at once the (presumed) need for the power of the state to regulate its borders and protect its citizens and the limits of that power' (p. 58). Each state also needs to spin its actions so that they meet with popular approval. The responses to the threat of COVID-19, and the war of words against 'the Asian virus', and, latterly, 'the Brazilian variant' or 'the South African variant' demonstrate the populist tensions that all too easily arise when a disease that respects no borders infects the citizens of communities whose governments need to adopt a rhetorical as well as a practical stance toward it.

Viruses, then, are not just epidemiological phenomena; they are protagonists in narratives that transform the complex experience of pandemics into social dramas that have their own moral, educational, persuasive and aesthetic functions. The final part of this volume, accordingly, shifts from the social sciences toward the humanities and education. The chapters solicited here reflect on how this and earlier pandemics have been represented, in fields as diverse as literature, university public relations, health-care communication and translation, commercial marketing, and journalism. The contributors also consider the implications of changing working practices in the arts, commerce, media and education in response to the necessary and abrupt shift online.

The volume cannot, of course, be comprehensive in its treatment of such a broad range of topics as the new world order, national responses to the pandemic, and the impact of COVID-10 on business, education, culture and society. It aims, however, to gather a stimulating set of interventions that offer distinctive insights into the first great global health crisis of the twenty-first century. It is tempting, in the midst of such a crisis, to believe that the observations and emotions it provokes are new. Yet one need only look at an entry in *The Diary of Samuel Pepys* to realize that many of the sentiments we now feel were expressed with uncanny familiarity in the middle of the seventeenth century. In the final days of a pestilence that had severely afflicted London in the 1660s, Pepys wrote the following (pp. 191–2):

> 31st December 1665
>
> But now the plague has abated almost to nothing, and I [am] intending to get to London as fast as I can. [...] My whole family hath been well all this while, and all my friends I know of, saving my aunt Bell, who is dead, and some children of my cousin Sarah's, of the plague. But many of such as I know very well, dead; yet, to our great joy, the town fills apace, and shops begin to open again. Pray God continue the plague's decrease!

It is to be hoped that the present volume will give future commentators some sense of how this generation has dealt with its own health emergency, and that future crises may be better managed as a result. And, in conclusion, as the pandemic slowly recedes, we can only echo Pepys' final, fervent wish.

Chen Zhi
Chair Professor
Provost of BNU-HKBU
United International College
Zhuhai, China

References

Pepys, S. (1887). *The Diary of Samuel Pepys 1664–1665*. London, Paris, New York & Melbourne: Cassell & Company, Ltd.
Wald, P. (2008). *Contagious: Cultures, Carriers, and the Outbreak Narrative*. Durham and London: Duke University Press.

Acknowledgments

We are most thankful for the support of the Springer Nature team, who responded in a timely and supportive manner to our book proposal during the eventful summer of 2020. Gratitude also goes to our reviewers who, at various stages of this ambitious project, took the time to consider our manuscript, providing invaluable guidance and direction to our authors. We would like further to thank Dean Prof. Adrian Bailey whose leadership and vision helped fuel the project. Additionally, our heartfelt thanks goes out to Ms. Yang Aiying and Ms. Li Yifan who showed their dedication and commitment, offering much-needed administrative and editing support for our team. Last but not least, we gratefully acknowledge the contribution of the whole community at the Beijing Normal University—Hong Kong Baptist University United International College (BNU-HKBU UIC), and its Division of Humanities and Social Sciences (DHSS), which inspired this project, and supported the endeavor with remarkable enthusiasm through these challenging times.

—Editorial Team

Contents

Introduction

Edoardo Monaco

This volume represents an ambitious project aiming at capturing the intense impact that the ongoing COVID-19 pandemic has been exerting throughout the globe in a variety of domains across humanities and social sciences.

This undertaking does not aspire in any way to be exhaustive or definitive, as the events of the pandemic are still unfolding at the time of writing. It stems from the need to, at least, begin taking stock of global dynamics of vast proportions, which started manifesting themselves in 2020, but whose effects will inevitably reverberate across continents and disciplines for years to come.

The COVID-19 crisis has certainly been a truly extraordinary—although not entirely unpredictable, given the numerous scientific warnings over the years—event that has tested established notions and consolidated practices, and profoundly affected billions across the globe, with massive social implications, across economic, political, cultural domains. Lives have been endangered and lost, livelihoods have been threatened in both developed and developing nations, governance and business patterns have been severely tested and profoundly altered—possibly for good.

Yet, first and foremost, it's probably fair to say that the crisis has affected us all as a species, serving as a "wake up call", a stark reminder of our own very limitations and shortcomings. In particular, it has highlighted in the most humbling of manners the importance of striking a proper balance in our relationship with nature and its very forces—too often challenged, exploited, ignored in the name of unfettered growth and "progress".

If anything, the pandemic has reminded us of the highly multidimensional nature of real societal progress, which, to be truly sustainable, requires simultaneous achievements across domains, territories and generations—hence, across relevant dimensions of "time and space". For long—especially from the reconstruction of a

E. Monaco (✉)
Globalisation and Development (GAD) Programme, Division of Humanities and Social Sciences, BNU-HKBU United International College (UIC), Zhuhai, Guangdong, China
e-mail: emonaco@uic.edu.cn

S.X.B. Zhao et al. (eds.), *COVID-19 Pandemic, Crisis Responses and the Changing World*, https://doi.org/10.1007/978-981-16-2430-8_1

neo-liberalist world order at the end of World War II onwards—economic achievements have in fact been conceived as predominant and distinct from environmental or social ones, with the needs of present generations being prioritized to the potential detriment of future ones. This has inevitably led to the destruction of natural environments and to the shrinking of "wild" spaces for the sake of urban expansion, commercial agriculture and increased industrial output. Even the threat of highly resistant strains of viruses and bacteria was often denounced by the scientific community over the past decades in light of the growing incidence of zoonotic epidemics across the world, yet ultimately ignored.

Despite attempts to fence the crisis within specific borders, or to even brand it as one particular country's responsibility, the COVID-19 crisis has represented a truly global challenge—the likes of which the world had not seen since perhaps the first half of the twentieth century—ideally requiring, as such, a global response.

While successful examples of international cooperation at bilateral or regional levels have indeed been produced, the overall reality so far has shown a world that, as a whole, has been essentially unable to identify the origins of the crisis, devise containment measures and implement response mechanisms in a truly concerted, coordinated manner. This represents a major concern that transcends the current pandemic, given the increasingly global—and to some extent existential—nature of modern challenges, such as climate change, for instance.

Much of the response to the spread of COVID-19, in fact, has so far been left to national (or regional, as in the case of the EU) authorities who have had, in many cases, to fend for themselves in search for effective solutions and to leverage traditional diplomatic alliances for aid and assistance.

Strict lockdowns, mandatory use of personal protective equipment, restrictions of movement, compulsory quarantines and closures of borders appear to have produced remarkable public health effects in countries where they were proportioned to the actual capacity of the health care system, as well as accurately enforced and widely participated by both authorities and citizens alike. The very same measures appear to have encountered significant resistance in contexts where the inevitable trade-offs in terms of personal liberties and pursuit of economic activities were considered too burdensome—from political, cultural or merely financial points of view.

Thus far, the response to the crisis has therefore essentially consisted of a variety of national public governance initiatives which deserve to be assessed, given the diversity of both the factors that inspired them and of the results they produced.

This volume intends precisely to constitute an initial survey of this diverse range of approaches, measures, impacts, achievements and shortcomings across social sciences.

Many of the authors of this book are faculty members of the "United International College" of Beijing Normal University and Hong Kong Baptist University (BNU-HKBU UIC), an English-medium, liberal arts joint-venture located in Zhuhai, Guangdong Province, China—the country considered, initially, the very epicenter of the crisis and, soon after, a prominent example of successful containment and effective response.

Right from emergence of the COVID-19 menace, in January 2020, the activities of the college were severely affected, with students and teachers alike being forced to devise, in the shortest time possible, alternative solutions to keep pursuing their educational mission. Online platforms were swiftly established, allowing the college community to interact, share and communicate despite the tragic exponential growth of the surrounding public health threat.

In particular, the college's Division of Humanities and Social Sciences (DHSS) perceived very early on the need to allow faculty members from a variety of countries and backgrounds to share how the pandemic was affecting them, their context and their areas of expertise. A series of online lectures was therefore organized between April and June 2020: this enlightening and somewhat cathartic experience planted the seed for the present volume, which collects some of the contributions initially made in that very series.

The book is organized in three parts, the first of which deals with "Global Economics, Politics and Public Health Responses". In this section, authors have delved into the politico-economic governance side of the pandemic, mostly from a transnational perspective. Zhao Suiheng, Zhao Xiaobin and Zhang Zhen, for instance, have notably assessed the bilateral relations between the world's two largest economies—namely the USA and China—highlighting how their increasing "competition" was further exacerbated by the 2020 pandemic. The authors explore how Sino-American interactions have deteriorated in particular regard to intellectual property rights, technology transfers and South China Sea disputes. They also highlight how the Trump presidency has often insisted on labelling the pandemic as China's exclusive "responsibility", rather than engaging in constructive dialogue and seeking concerted solutions that would have benefitted both the USA and the world as a whole right from the early stages of the crisis. Lapses in global leadership are further assessed in the second chapter of the section, while in the third global supply chains—and China's role within them—are analyzed in the context of the COVID-19 pandemic to identify possible trends of "de-globalization", the likes of which were already observed in the aftermath of major natural disasters affecting manufacturing hubs in Thailand or Japan.

The chapter entitled "Actions Across Government and COVID-19: The Experience of Mainland China, Macao and Hong Kong" attempts to present a diversified, holistic "whole-of-government" approach as key to the ultimately successful containment of the crisis in Mainland China, in the Macao Special Administrative Region (SAR), as well as, albeit to a different extent, in the other Chinese "SAR", Hong Kong.

COVID-19 has also severely impacted Europe, where the "Union", at least initially, proved itself rather slow in reacting to the challenge in a truly cohesive manner. In the EU, in fact, the onset of the public health crisis inevitably added fuel to the ongoing fire of intra-union economic disparities and diverging views over the fiscal management of the regional block, still ailing from the 2008 financial crisis and struggling to identify a common strategy that would effectively balance rigor and inclusion across its diverse membership base. As discussed in the chapter "COVID-19 and the Political Economy of the European Union: New Crisis, Old

Concerns", existing problems of sovereign debt, deficit and sluggish growth especially among southern EU members states have only been exacerbated by the severe economic contraction and large public expenditures that COVID-19 brought about, setting the stage for a crucial debate on fiscal discipline and economic recovery in a time of emergency that may characterize European politics for years to come.

The composite global overview of impacts and responses across a series of pandemic hotspots that is initiated in the chapter "Government Emergency Responses During the COVID-19 Pandemic in the Context of Health Emergency and Disaster Risk Management: A Comparative Study" by Johnston H.C. Wong, is then developed in further detail in Part 2, which assesses a diverse range of countries across four continents, with particular regard to Asia.

The chapter "Experiences of and Responses to COVID-19 in East Asia: The Cases of Japan and Korea" looks at the unfolding of the COVID-19 crisis in Japan and Korea, and at the measures implemented to contain the number of cases especially across the older population—a particular concern to governments in both nations, yet more urgent in Japan, where the median age of males and females combined exceeds 48 years.

The city state of Singapore is then presented as a case of relatively successful containment of the crisis, with factors such as high trust in government, close coordination among concerned government entities, swift implementation of "circuit-breaker" lockdowns and high levels of community mobilization and engagement playing crucial roles. In a vast country like India, on the other hand, a large, highly diverse population prompts an analysis that transcends the mere epidemiological dimension of the pandemic: Nazrul Islam, in fact, engages in a timely study of the early socio-economic impact of the public health crisis in a context still plagued by various forms of poverty and inequality.

Africa features in this section of the volume with a chapter on Ghana: government as well as wider society's response—often relying exclusively on locally available resources—have yielded positive results in terms of reducing the mere public health impact of the pandemic in the country. Yet, as for India, broader socio-economic consequences have been registered, such as increased poverty and marginalization among the most vulnerable sections of the population, as well as severe disruptions to traditional patterns of social and cultural interaction.

The attention then shifts to the Americas: in their chapter on the United States, Charles Lowe and Benjamin Barber explore the extent to which the recurrent theme of American "exceptionalism"—combined with the Trump presidency, the anti-intellectualism typical of the constituency it represented and, in general, a growing distrust in both central government and mainstream media—may have informed the failure to provide adequate public safety measures and to produce an effective overall strategy to control the spreading of COVID-19 in the country. John Corbett, instead, presents the case of Brazil, where the *laissez-faire* attitude of President Jair Bolsonaro—a right-wing populist leader elected in 2018, who, not unlike Trump, often downplayed the dangers of COVID-19 with rather unscientific arguments—and of the federal government as a whole contributed to high rates of infection and mortality, in a national context of political fragmentation, slow economic growth and persisting inequalities. The chapter holistically assesses the role that humanities and social sciences can play in helping Brazil recover from the crisis and end a stalemate which, once again, seems to transcend the mere sphere of public health.

The third section is less geographically bound, yet still very diverse, as it contains a series of chapters assessing the early COVID-19 impact on a variety of social science domains: Jiang Mengying, for instance, investigates how translation services—and their providers—can actively and effectively contribute to international crisis management. Ge Song looks at the phenomenon of online exhibitions as a timely tool to promote cross-cultural engagement and understanding during a pandemic. Lessons from the journalistic coverage of the COVID-19 crisis in the USA are drawn by Jesse Owen Hearns-Branaman, who laments in particular the lack of experienced medical reporters, the inaccurate reporting of statistics as well as the distracting "fact-checking loops" that many outlets fell victim of in response to the (mis)information coming from the Trump administration. Jesse Owen Hearns-Branaman also co-authors a chapter with Johnny Bliss, whom he interviews to learn how his long experience as a travel journalist has evolved over the years, amid new technologies, changing cultural trends, restrictions to physical travel and new forms of "exploration".

Benjamin Barber looks at the sheer complexity of human nature and its range of its responses to traumatic events through the prism of literature, as he embarks in a timely and evocative review of Boccaccio's "Decameron" and Albert Camus' "The Plague", while Edith M. Y. Yan instead examines recent trends and methodologies of online teaching and learning in higher education—another landscape profoundly transformed by the pandemic.

The role that public relations and advertising play at a time of severe uncertainty is then assessed in a series of chapters, the first of which, by Lan Xiaomeng, looks at how corporations can chart their way out of the pandemic in a manner that aptly inspires solidarity, trust and optimism, but also positively contributes to social values and political debate, thus effectively managing "postmodernist" tides. The second, by Lim Chai Lee, focuses more specifically on relevant trends in media consumption and on the advertising strategies that major brands may adopt amid COVID-19 so as to engage new types of consumers, accelerate the digital outreach and in general actively respond to an increasingly widespread expectation for "empathy" and participation. Qian Hong and Zhang Jia, then, employ a multimodal approach to present a specific case study of university image building against the backdrop of the pandemic, focused on the very "United International College" of Beijing Normal University and Hong Kong Baptist University (BNU-HKBU UIC) in Zhuhai, Guangdong Province, China, that cradled the present book project and its particular use of a locally-prominent social media platform, "WeChat". This very same platform is also central to Jiaqi Liang and Xiaying Xu's assessment of the "native advertising" phenomenon, which the pandemic appears to have significantly promoted.

A conclusion chapter by Charles Lowe will then summarise the "journey" across borders and disciplines that this volume is pleased to take the reader on, at a time in which challenges are steep, yet opportunities for a brighter, safer, more sustainable future remain well within reach of an aware, conscious, proactive global community.

Global Economics, Politics and Public Health Responses

US-China Rivalry and Its Implications for the Post-Pandemic World

Suisheng Zhao, Simon X.B. Zhao, and Zhen Zhang

Abstract The COVID-19 pandemic has exacerbated the tension and underscores the importance of cooperation between the United States and China on shared interests even as they compete ferociously on almost all fronts. While a duopoly with China and the United States working in tandem is unlikely because of their increasingly competitive relationship, a large-scale conflict shall be extremely costly as neither is strong enough to prevail. Under above background, this paper describes the grim nature of the current Sino-US relations and the expected trend of Sino-US rivalry in the post-pandemic era. We expect that both United States and China can mutually prevent deeper and larger conflicts from happening, as well as maintain rational economic and political interactions under an integrated and effective global governance mechanism.

1 Introduction: The Unprecedented Deterioration in Sino-US Relations

In December 2019, when China and the United States signed the first phase of a trade agreement, many people believed that US-China rivalry had come to an end. However, after the outbreak of the COVID-19 pandemic, the situation changed completely as the two countries criticized each other furiously; the Trump administration started attacking China on almost all fronts, affecting bilateral relations. In 2020 July, the United States forcibly closing the Chinese Consulate in Houston in July. In response,

S. Zhao (✉)
Director, Center for China-US Cooperation, Josef Korbel School of International Studies, University of Denver, Denver, CO, USA
e-mail: Suisheng.Zhao@du.edu; szhao@du.edu

S. X.B. Zhao · Z. Zhang
Division of Humanities and Social Sciences, Beijing Normal University-Hong Baptist University United International College, Zhuhai, Guangdong, China
e-mail: sxzhao@uic.edu.cn

Z. Zhang
e-mail: 1730007013@alumni.uic.edu.cn

S.X.B. Zhao et al. (eds.), *COVID-19 Pandemic, Crisis Responses and the Changing World*, https://doi.org/10.1007/978-981-16-2430-8_2

China also closed the U.S. Consulate in Chengdu. In September, the U.S. Government once again put forward a number of restrictions on Chinese diplomatic officials, which evoked serious protests from the Chinese Foreign Ministry. On July 24, 2020, U.S. Secretary of State Mike Pompeo delivered a speech titled "Communist China and the Free World's Future" at the Nixon Library in California where he declared that the U.S. Policy of "engagement" with China over the past 41 years had failed, and called on the United States to unite with other partners in the "free world" against China (Pompeo 2020). This speech was full of hostility towards China and indicated an atmosphere conducive to declaration of war. It was compared by the international community with the "Sinews of Peace" Speech delivered by the former British Prime Minister Winston Churchill in 1946, regarded as a sign that Sino-US relations are approaching the US-Soviet Cold War pattern in the eyes of many scholars of international relations.

Looking at the deterioration in Sino-US relations since Donald Trump took office, this worry is not illogical. Since the United States imposed tariffs on China in 2018 and vigorously suppressed Huawei, ZTE and other Chinese high-tech firms like Byte Dance and Tencent, and even 13 universities in China, economic, trade and political relations between China and the United States have begun to decline at an unprecedented pace. With the outbreak of the COVID-19 pandemic, a new round of Sino-US rivalry had been launched, and the future of Sino-US relations once again faces new uncertainties.

This chapter describes the grim nature of current Sino-US relations and expected trend of Sino-US rivalry in the post pandemic era (that is, to mutually prevent deeper and larger conflicts from happening, as well as to maintain normal economic and political interactions under the current global governance mechanism), with quantitative data and qualitative details. This chapter also shows that for China and the United States, complete decoupling is totally unrealistic. Peace should be the most important characteristic of the relationship between these two great powers.

This chapter is divided into five parts. First there is a discussion of what we shall describe as the "Thucydides Trap" and the future of Sino-US relations, and a digest of perspectives from various scholars and politicians, from both China and the United States, on the US-China rivalry and its implications after the outbreak of the COVID-19. Then we provide a historical review of Sino-US relations over the past 41 years, which might be considered the "good old days" in the eyes of the Chinese and American people. After this brief review, this chapter illustrates recent changes and conflicts in Sino-US relations in areas such as trade, economy, geopolitics, military, the pandemic issue, and ideology. At the same time, the shaken foundations of Sino-US relations and the outbreak of the accumulation of contradictory positions between China and the United States are explained. Finally, the possible future development of Sino-US relations is described, with particular attention given to the potential for starting a "New Cold War," the need to avoid further escalation, and the efforts required to recover a basic pattern of coordination for these two great powers.

2 The "Thucydides Trap": Competition for Power and Cultural Confrontation

Since the unprecedented deterioration of Sino-US relations after Donald Trump took office in 2017, scholars of political relations between China and the United States have had different views on the future of interaction. Among them, Allison and Mearsheimer, hold a pessimistic attitude, while Nye and Ikenberry insist that there is still a huge space available for the avoidance of war and the maintenance of peaceful development. We turn to a summary of their viewpoints as well as others concerning recent changes and the surging conflicts between China and the United States following the outbreak of the COVID-19 pandemic.

The "Thucydides Trap" describes a recurring situation whereby a new rising power will inevitably challenge the existing power, and the existing power will inevitably respond to this threat, so that war becomes inevitable. This theory originates from Thucydides, the ancient Greek historian who believed that when a rising power competes with the existing ruling power, the ensuing mutual antagonism inexorably leads to war. Thucydides' book *The History of the Peloponnesian War*, relates the circumstances that gave rise to armed conflict between Athens, a rising polis, and Sparta, a traditional powerful polis, as the two were contenders for political dominance on the Aegean Sea. This unavoidable conflict was the earliest case of the "Thucydides Trap".

Graham Allison (2017), founder of Harvard Kennedy School, published *Destined for War: Can America and China Escape Thucydides Trap?* In this book, he listed 16 cases of challengers and defenders in history. Among them, 13 cases ended in war, and only 3 cases ended in peace. Consequently he concludes: "War between the U.S. and China is more likely than is being recognized at the moment. Indeed, judging by the historical record, war is more likely than not" (Allison 2015).

However, political and academic commentators in the United States and China have taken varying positions on the likelihood of these two nations falling into a "Thucydides Trap." For example, former U.S. Secretary of State Henry Kissinger (2018) believes that although in 12 of the 16 cases cited by Ellison there was a war, the two cases since the end of the WWII went on to have peaceful outcomes. Most recent experience indicates that the "Thucydides Trap" is not a satisfactory model for contemporary relations between great powers.

Even so, the "Thucydides Trap' may still be valid for reasons that go beyond economic and strategic dominance. Samuel Huntington's "Clash of Civilizations" Theory considers that the root of international conflicts in the future will be mainly cultural rather than economic, and that the core of international politics will be a competition between Western Civilization and Non-Western Civilizations (Huntington 1997). Like Huntington, Wang (2020) argues that the reason for the aggravation of current conflicts between China and the United States lies in the difference between their cultures, values, political systems, and concepts of development. These "soft level" differences and contradictions are also important factors that could still lead the two countries to fall into the "Thucydides Trap" and may eventually lead to war.

3 Arguments Between Realism and Liberalism: War or Peace in the Future

Mearsheimer (2018) emphasized that international politics, especially Sino-US competition, is basically a zero-sum game, in his book *The Tragedy of Great Power Politics*, while Nye (2019) believes there is a risk that policy makers and citizens of China and the United States will expect the worst from each other, a situation which they need to avoid. On the one hand, this phenomenon is caused by the long-term accumulation of resentment between the two sides over the past few years. On the other hand, it is also because of the strong nationalist sentiment in both countries.

Ikenberry et al. (2015) emphasizes that the United States should give China a certain space in the regional order to accommodate the rise of China and its aspirations, in exchange for Beijing accepting and accommodating the core strategic interests of the United States, including the United States continuing to serve as the leading security guarantor in East Asia. Yan (2019) also believes that there will be no war between China and the United States because, first, both countries have nuclear weapons, and, secondly, the progress of globalization has also prevented the two countries from having a war.

4 US-China Rivalry and Its Implications After the Pandemic

After the outbreak of COVID-19 pandemic, the Trump administration accelerated its actions to force China to delink from U.S. high-tech industrial sectors, and is trying to force its allies to follow this strategy (Niblett and Vinjamuri 2020). Besides, during the pandemic, the economic and technological decoupling between China and the United States has become an irreversible trend, because now there is a lack of mutual trust between these two great powers, and their official relations are almost frozen (Wang 2020).

Additionally, while facing the current pandemic, there's no way any one country can solve the consequent problems by itself. Accordingly, the important thing is that China and the United States should be looking for some common projects. They could do them together to symbolize the fact that they have more to gain from cooperation than from rivalry (Nye 2020). At the same time, in a pandemic situation, if the world's two most powerful countries—the United States and China—cannot put aside a verbal war on who should be held responsible for the crisis and turn to more effective leadership, the credibility of both countries could be seriously damaged (Burns 2020).

5 Historical Resumé of Sino-US Relations: The "Good Old Days"

Before we begin to analyze the current deterioration of Sino-US relations, let us first review the "good old days" since the establishment of Sino-US diplomatic relations.

In 1972, U.S. President Richard Nixon's visit to China marked a thaw in Sino-US diplomatic relations that had been sour since the founding of People's Republic of China. In the late 1970s, China's political leader Deng Xiaoping seized the opportunity to establish ties with the United States and formal diplomatic relations were instated on January 1, 1979. 27 days after the establishment of diplomatic relations, Deng undertook the first head of state visit to the United States in the history of the PRC. After his trip, with the support of the U.S. government, more than 50 Chinese students received full scholarships from the top American universities such as Princeton, MIT and UC Berkeley that year itself. On July 7, the Carter administration also granted MFN status to China which was still under the planned economic system. It can be seen that the United States at that time gave China the greatest encouragement for market opening through preferential policies.

In 1984, U.S. President Ronald Reagan visited China and signed four agreements and protocols to avoid double taxation and prevent tariff evasion, and initialed the Sino-US cooperation agreement on peaceful use of nuclear energy. That is when diplomatic relations between China and the United States were viewed by both sides as having officially entered the "honeymoon period". After Reagan's visit, Sino-US relations developed greatly and became one of the most important bilateral relations in the world.

Since the formal establishment of diplomatic relations between China and the United States, economic and political cooperation between the two sides has been constantly upgraded. With the support of the United States, China successfully joined the WTO in 2001. After the "9/11" incident, Chinese President Jiang Zemin immediately called U.S. President George Bush to express his sympathy, and America's anti-terrorism military actions against the Taliban and Al Qaeda in Afghanistan also received political support from China. After the global subprime mortgage crisis broke out in 2008, the Chinese government purchased a large number of U.S. Treasury bonds, which provided vital economic support to America's rapid economic recovery and the continuous positive growth of GDP from 2010 to 2019.

As the largest and the second largest economy in the world, China and the United States are also each other's largest trading partners. Before the Trump administration imposing tariffs on China, the total trade volume between China and the United States reached an all-time peak in 2018, totaling $659.84 billion, ranking first in global bilateral trade. In addition, China and the United States have also been insisting on expanding access to each other's domestic market. While more American enterprises are entering the Chinese market, more Chinese capital is also entering the American market, which brings employment opportunities to American workers. Both the Foxconn assembly plants throughout Mainland China, and the automobile glass processing plant set up by Chinese Fuyao Glass Industry Group in Ohio, symbolize win–win developments brought about by Sino-US cooperation.

It can be seen that Sino-US bilateral relations imply not only political cooperation and competition between governments, but also the well-being of the people on both sides. In addition, as permanent members of the UN Security Council and sovereign states with the most political influence in the new and old continents, any change in Sino-US relations will inevitably have an important impact on peace in and the development of the whole world. Therefore, many people hope that Sino-US relations can continue to develop smoothly and the two cooperate for a long time.

In the process of long-term competition and cooperation, owing to the differences in political systems, the opposing ideologies, and the competition between geopolitics and global political influence, some contradictions, conflicts and even crises are inevitable. In the past 41 years, although the relations between the two countries have experienced various problems and crises, including America's sanctions against China triggered by the "Yin-he" incident in 1993, the "Accidental Bombing of the Chinese Embassy" in Yugoslavia in 1999, and the "Battleplane Crash in the South China Sea" in 2001, the general direction of Sino-US relations has not been fundamentally shaken.

6 Recent Changes and Conflicts in Sino-US Relations

We now turn to the escalation of the confrontation between China and the United States on economy and trade, geopolitics and military, technology and ideology, since the outbreak of the COVID-19 pandemic. Then we discuss the causes of the deterioration of Sino-US relations, including China's overreach and the US's overreaction. Looking at the changes in Sino-US relations since the outbreak of the COVID-19 pandemic, it is clear that after the pandemic started spreading in the United States in March 2020, tensions between China and the United States have gradually expanded from the dispute over the origin of and accountability for the COVID-19 virus to confrontation and competition that cover five key aspects which we outline below.

6.1 Shrinkage of Financial and Economic Interactions

Trade friction between the two sides has dealt a blow to the investment confidence of both investors, resulted in US-China FDI flows declining from more than $60 billion in 2016 to less than $10 billion in 2019, rapidly falling to the level before 2005. At the micro level, American sanctions against Chinese enterprises have been expanding. In response, China has also begun to impose sanctions on American enterprises including General Motors and Lockheed Martin, to restrict their business and transactions in China. At the international level, the economic confrontation between China and the United States has had a huge, negative impact on global economic development. IMF chief economist Gita Gopinath (2019) said "Under roughly 2 years of US-China economic frictions, economies of 90% of countries and regions in the world have slowed down. If geopolitical and economic risks continue to increase, the world economy will be close to depression."

6.2 Governmental and Social Rivalry Over the Pandemic Accountability Issue

In a speech delivered digitally to the UN General Assembly on September 22, 2020, Trump accused China of controlling the WHO, and demanded that China take full responsibility for the spread of the pandemic. On July 14, 2020 White House Trade Adviser Peter Navarro (2020) had criticized China for "attacking the United States with a deadly, weaponized virus." The United States accused China of being "the manufacturer and original disseminator of COVID-19", and called on the EU and the world to jointly investigate China for the pandemic. At the same time, China has repeatedly criticized the U.S. government for "lack of transparency and concealment of key information" on the issue of pandemic prevention and control, and suggested that the United States may also be the source country of COVID-19. The conspiracy that the outbreak of cowid-19 was caused by the leakage of biochemical virus weapons in Fort De Crete has been widely hyped on Chinese online social media.

From a social perspective, according to survey data from Pew Research Center (2020), as of the second quarter of 2020, 73% of Americans, including 83% of Republican supporters and 68% of Democratic supporters, already held negative views on China. In addition, compared with 2018, in a short period of two years, the American people's concerns about China's continued growth in science and technology and military strength, as well as China's negative impact on the global environment and human rights, have also risen rapidly.

6.3 Conflicts in the Field of Science and Technology

In August 2020, then US Secretary of State, Pompeo announced the launch of the "Clean Network Program". Under this plan, more than 2500 Chinese IT products and services were banned from sale or subscription in America. Products involved in this plan are mostly intelligent terminal technology equipment, software, cloud services, submarine cables, etc. What's more, 7 Chinese ICT enterprises, including Tencent, Huawei and Byte Dance, were specifically targeted in a press conference given by the U.S. government. Pompeo issued a statement saying that software such as Tik-Tok and WeChat would be banned, and data access hitherto granted to various Chinese operators would henceforth be restricted.

Among these restrictions, Tik-Tok is required to implement a property right transfer within a given time limit, and domestic enterprises in the United States would take over all the business and operations management rights. In addition, on May 22, the U.S. Department of Commerce expanded the "entity list" for export control, and a total of 13 Chinese universities involved in domestic military technology were included in the "red-flag 'unverified' list", members of which are restricted from buying specified products containing American technology. As a result, for example, Harbin Institute of Technology (HIT) and Harbin Engineering University (HEU) will not be able to use licensed MATLAB software in an international mathematical modeling competition.

6.4 Military Tensions Over the South China Sea Issue

In the past 10 years, the U.S. Navy's reconnaissance exercises in the South China Sea have doubled, and now it conducts nearly 2000 sorties a year. And the presence of Chinese surface military power in the South China Sea has also increased by 60%, while large-scale military exercises have also increased by about 30%. By the first half of 2020, the United States had dispatched about 3000 fighter planes and 60 warships to the South China Sea, and launched "double carrier operation" in the South China Sea. It can be said that the U.S. Navy has invested far more troops in the South China Sea than in the rest of the world. At the same time, China has also launched several military exercises in the South China Sea which are directed at the Taiwan Army and the U.S. Navy stationed in the Asia Pacific region. Therefore, the South China Sea has become one of the most militarized areas in the world, with maximization of military confrontation between the two powers.

7 Causes of the Mounting Tensions: China's Overreach and US's Overreaction

In the first 10 years of the twenty-first century, there were two major crises in the United States, namely, the crisis triggered by the "9/11" Terrorist Attack in 2001 and the subprime mortgage crisis in 2008, which greatly weakened the economic and political confidence of the United States. In contrast, in the twenty-first century, China has shown a rising trend and gradually shifted its diplomatic approach from keeping a low profile to building up its own leadership in an attempt to change the US-led liberal world order.

Naturally, the result of the collision between the two sides is that the United States has begun to defend its international status by preventing and containing China in an all-round way. Susan Shirk (2019), Assistant Secretary of State for China Affairs during the Clinton administration made a very accurate exposition of the state of play, which can be summed up as "China's overreach and the US's overreaction".

On the one hand, China's overreach is manifest in its expanding nationalistic mentality and its tough stance on international issues. In the promotion of self-confidence at the national level, the assertiveness of many Chinese people and officials has been over inflated, resulting in the "Wolf Warrior Thinking", which has repeatedly resulted in too tough an attitude being presented on the international stage.

After 2010, China's strong actions on issues relating to the South China Sea, Hong Kong, Taiwan and Africa have resulted in a high degree of vigilance from the United States., China's strong economic support for Russia in the blockade following the Crimea Crisis, as well as its commercial relations with Iran (which has violated the Nuclear Non-proliferation Treaty and is also sanctioned by the United States) has been treated as a signal of China's intent to challenge the current US-led world order.

Moreover, China has repeatedly declared that the issues of human rights in Xinjiang and Hong Kong, and sovereignty in the South China Sea and Taiwan, are China's internal affairs, and other countries are not allowed to interfere. However, based on the current world order and the international legal framework, these series of behaviors have shown China to be an economy that has benefited from the US-led global economic system but one that now refuses to acknowledge global concerns about human rights and the pursuit of the freedom on sea voyage.

On the other hand, the United States is obviously overreacting to changes in China's diplomatic posture. At the instigation of the United States, Trump's Hawkish foreign policy making team has turned this misjudgment into a mainstream social consensus. They believe that they have suffered losses in the development of Sino-US relations, that is, China has taken advantage of the open market and open society of the United States, and then turned to its rising power to destroy the whole liberal world order.

At the 18th CPC National Congress in 2012, the need for China to build a "maritime power" was explicitly raised. The strategic policy is that China hopes to further enhance its sea power and realize complete protection and utilization of its surrounding waters. But this is considered by the United States as a major strategic threat to replace the American maritime status in the Pacific region and even across the whole world.

Therefore, the need for taking further containment measures against China to defend the current America's global political leadership has become a strategic consensus between Democratic and Republican parties in the United States. Under this strategic consensus, the political buffer space between China and the United States has been further squeezed, which directly led to the all-round confrontation between the two countries during Trump's presidency. After Joe Biden came to power, although the new U.S. foreign policy team headed by its new Secretary of State Antony Blinken has more professional diplomatic literacy and better understanding of China, whether they can really promote the Sino-US relations back to the "good old days" is still unknown.

8 The Possible Future of Sino-US Relations: A Temporary New Cold War?

In this context, whether China and the United States will move towards escalation of all-round confrontation and finally start a "New Cold War" is a matter of great concern for everyone in all walks of life. It is undeniable that more and more commentators are taking up the new strategic concept that emphasizes the "Sino-US" bipolar global political system. As mentioned above, according to Mearsheimer's analysis of structural contradictions, China and the United States will almost certainly fall into the quagmire of a "New Cold War", and the current trade war represents the opening skirmish. However, even if the "New Cold War" is inevitable, it is still necessary for us to see the difficulties in China and the United States achieving complete decoupling.

8.1 Shaking the Foundations of Sino-US Relations

In essence, any consideration of U.S.-China policy has mainly to be based on 3 aspects: geopolitical considerations, economic interests and political values. The most important factor that prompted the establishment of diplomatic relations between China and the United States in 1979 was geopolitical, because the two countries acknowledged that they had a common adversary, namely the Soviet Union. In other words, the reason why China and the United States came together to begin with was not because they recognized each other's basic values. Moreover, at that time, there were not many common economic interests between the two countries. Later, with the collapse of the Soviet Union, geopolitical considerations no longer played such a decisive role. However, the relationship between China and the United States continued mainly because of the increasing importance of economic interests and, it may seem strange to suggest, political values.

It should be noted here that economic and political factors do not work independently. The United States once hoped to change China by helping it to develop its economy. Its strategic plan was to allow China to enter the post-war international system built and dominated by America, so that China could develop its economy, induce political changes, and establish democracy, finally aligning with American values. This is also the root of the Americans' general adherence to the "engagement" strategy over the past 41 years. From Carter to Obama administration, the United States saw helping China to modernize and integrate into the US-led liberal world order as a strategic intervention in their own interests. The reasoning was that if China promotes modernization with the assistance of the United States, it will gradually form values consistent with its liberal democracy. With these common values, China will have fewer conflicts of interest with the United States, and finally respect America's global leadership. Under the guidance of this assumption and vision, Americans believed they should open up their markets to China, transfer technology, invest capital, and help China modernize itself (by achieving liberal economy and democratic institution).

In fact, China has accepted the so-called modernization on the surface for quite a long period of time, because China does want to change (although subjectively, it does not want to change in the direction of the American policy-makers' aspirations). Therefore, for quite a long period after the establishment of diplomatic relations between the two countries (Deng to Hu), China has abided by its own strategic principle of keeping a low profile, and has not competed with the United States for temporary gains and losses. But now China's pursuit for the status as a great power is manifested.

From an objective perspective, there has been a misplaced consensus between China and the United States, but this misplaced consensus has maintained Sino-US relations for several decades. The reason why this consensus is misplaced is that in essence, there was an unspoken agreement between China and the United States to let only economic factors dominate during this period. Therefore, when America's expectations of change in China's political values failed to materialize, in the view of its strategic decision-makers, the strategic significance of allowing economic factors to play a dominant role is no longer valid. That is to say, at this time, the value factors are no longer important (or have even become negative factors), and the broader strategic goals of the economic factors no longer seem feasible; only the economic interests themselves remain and the foundation of Sino-US relations has thus been shaken.

8.2 *Have China and the US Embarked on a "New Cold War"?*

US-China rivalry has already gone far beyond what may be called trade friction and it is being transformed into a comprehensive confrontation (that is, involving the economy, diplomacy, military, geopolitics, technology and ideology), which is close to the definition of a "Cold War": All hostile actions excepting limited war and total war between two great powers. In terms of all-round confrontation, the United States is exerting comprehensive pressure on China. In summer 2020, US Secretary of State Pompeo proposed "ideological confrontation", which may seem sensational, but it nevertheless serves as an acknowledgment that in the US-China "New Cold War" the ideologies of the two sides are quite different.

However, this new stand-off is not the same as the confrontation between communism and capitalism during the US-Soviet Cold War. Now the competition is to determine the superiority of modes of governance, between the Western democratic system and the "Chinese Model". To further disseminate its national system, China is also trying to promote its own development pattern to third world countries. Moreover, China has established mutually supportive networks with many third world countries, many of which are corrupt, authoritarian and even totalitarian. Among these network relations, the more influential countries are Russia, Iran and DPR Korea, which, like the rest (such as Venezuela and Serbia), are all anti-western powers. Because China is a non-aligned country, the network relationship established by China is relatively loose. The most fundamental foundation of this mutually supportive network relationship is to jointly oppose America's interference in their internal affairs.

In addition, this "New Cold War" represents not only an all-round confrontation, but it also means that contact between the two competing powers is minimized or even cut off. Now the official channels of communication are almost completely suspended. In June 2020, talks between Yang and Pompeo in Hawaii did not produce any groundbreaking results. All levels of official exchanges, non-governmental exchanges, especially the exchange of science and technology are gradually getting eroded. It is clear that we are in the early days of a New Cold War.

For its part, the United States is also building new alliances with countries that share their values and feel threatened by China. Although Trump's isolationist policies have hurt many allies, establishment of an "Anti-China United Front" does not imply leadership by Trump's United States. This rather means that the allies share the common goal of addressing concerns and threats caused by China's rising economic and political power. They all have recognized that China is posing a threat to their way of life and political values. Consequently, these allies have gradually joined a containment Alliance to support America's pressure on China. The United States has tried to dissuade OECD countries from using Huawei's 5G technology and services. Now, the United Kingdom and Australia have closed their market accesses to the installation Huawei's 5G base station facilities.

Besides, the EU's China Strategy Document "EU-China: A Strategic Outlook" released in 2019 pointed out that China is not only the EU's "economic competitor", but also the EU's "systemic rival for implementing a new model of national governance" (European Union 2019). It can be seen that the concept of "institutional competitor" is increasingly emphasized in not only the United States, but also the EU's future China policy agenda. Moreover, Australia, Canada, Japan, and other countries that profess values that are the same as those of the United States are considering joining the containment alliance of the United States to put extreme pressure on China. Therefore, it is obvious that one of the most important factors in the Cold War, a formulation of two camps, is gradually taking shape.

Although the two camps are not as close as they were during the old US-Soviet Cold War, and there are many contradictions within the camps, such as between the United States and the European Union, between China and Russia, and between China and the DPR Korea, the two loose alliances have been formed very clearly. The formation of two mutually exclusive, non-interactive and antagonistic alliances in economic and political spheres is the most distinctive feature of the cold war pattern. Therefore, the trend towards the formation of two camps of allies sharing similar values further confirms that the Sino-US confrontation conforms to the pattern of a "New Cold War".

9 The Infeasibility of the Complete Decoupling of China and the US

In economic matters, China and the United States have a high degree of interdependence and are unlikely to be fully decoupled. This is totally different from the US-Soviet relations. The Soviet Union had greatly deterred the United States militarily, but it was of no importance to the United States economically. The peak value of trade between the two countries was only about $4 billion a year. But at present the annual trade volume between China and the United States is $400–700 billion. Sino-US trade in services has exceeded $125 billion, and bilateral total two-way direct investment amounts to nearly $160 billion. Sino-US economic and trade cooperation has brought tangible benefits to the two countries and their people and contributed to the prosperity and stability of the world economy.

It is not only China that has gained great opportunities and development from its long-term cooperative relationship with the United States. The United States has also obtained capital inflow from China in the course of its economic interactions with China, which include China's various investments in American market, the U.S. Treasury bonds held by China, and the profits from American financial institutions' shares in Chinese financial institutions. According to data from the National Bureau of Statistics of China, in the year 2017, American financial institutions having strategic investments in Chinese financial institutions earned a return of about $32.6 billion.

Moreover, China has a large trade and investment volume not only with the United States, but it has also become one of the top trading partners of almost all of the countries in the world, which means that even if the United States wants to cut off direct trade with China, it cannot ultimately avoid indirect trade with China. Therefore, it is almost impossible for either side to decouple by deterrence or sanctions unilaterally. If Trump or the future presidents insist on "complete decoupling", it will cause great harm to both sides, and undoubtedly American enterprises would be very reluctant to bear the outcome of losing the entire China market.

Additionally, from the perspective of the United States, every time it uses its power based on asymmetric dependence, it also risks the structural basis of its hegemony. When it tries to close the market to Chinese enterprises, it is equivalent to shutting out new technologies, new elements and new business forms representing advanced productive forces, thus suppressing the innovative vitality of the free market economy.

Besides, the pursuit for complete decoupling implies a big problem for the United States since no country or regional alliance can replace China's position in the global industrial chain. Although the WHNTC director Navarro and Finance Minister Mnuchin have been optimistic about the future deployment of American capital withdrawn from China in ASEAN countries such as Vietnam and Malaysia, in terms of global manufacturing capacity, China accounts for 28.22% of global production capacity, while Vietnam and Malaysia only account for less than 0.3%, which is a huge gap in economic scale.

Compared with China, ASEAN countries' biggest problems lie in the supply chain and labor force. Now China not only has a complete industrial chain, but it also has a huge labor and consumer market and complete supporting infrastructure, as well as mature industrial agglomeration, with complete industrial support and high production efficiency. Vietnam, Malaysia and other ASEAN countries may take part in transfer of industrial capacities in the future, but the outcome of this regional competition is unclear. According to Lear's comment, at least in the short run, China's advantages in global supply chain is indispensable.

Finally, the way the COVID-19 pandemic has been controlled by China demonstrates that China has not only a complete domestic industrial system, but also a political leadership with strong organizational power, which is enough to bear internal risks and external threats. China's handling of the pandemic has shown that it has such ability. If the United States wants to promote complete decoupling, it will be a long drawn out, painful process that would consume political capital and require firm strategic determination. Even if a certain degree of decoupling could eventually be achieved, China would have a considerable amount of buffer time to make adjustments.

10 Conclusion: Short Term Cold War, Long Term Peace?

This chapter presents, based on a review of relevant literature, views and arguments proposed by different groups of global scholars on Sino-US relations, including a historical resumé of the "good old days" of relations between China and the United States over the past 41 years. Analysis and exploration of the reasons for the all-round confrontation between China and the United States after the outbreak of the COVID-19 pandemic are presented. Possible directions and patterns of development of Sino-US relations in the future are discussed. We can see that the problems of contemporary Sino-US relations are no longer conflicts around a single point of contention as in the previous "Yin-he" incident or Battleplane Crash incident, but the diverse flashpoints that have flared up in a concentrated way.

According to the argumentation in this chapter, there has been an all-round confrontation between China and the United States in the context of the economy, politics, ideology and technology, etc. At the same time, official and non-governmental channels of communication and interaction between the two countries have tended to stagnate and decelerate. The two major powers are trying to build their own camps to strengthen their respective hands in order to deal with the confrontation.

Our principal finding is that this new normal tendency to engage in conflict is, on the one hand, because of the increase in China's national strength, which has triggered overreaching expectations to change its traditional preference for "keeping a low profile" on a global scale by replacing it with the ability to actively pursue international leadership and provide goods and services to international consumers and clients. On the other hand, the United States has been overreacting to China's overreach, leading an influential group within the Trump administration (represented by Robert O'Brien, Christopher Ford, and Rob Strayer, etc.) to magnify the threat that China may pose to the United States. Eventually a consensus has been formed between Republicans and Democrats to implement a containment policy against China.

Therefore, we can affirm that China and the United States have entered the primary stage of a "New Cold War". However, due to the continuously upgraded and deepened economic and trade cooperation and political interaction in the past 41 years, as well as China's irreplaceable position in the global industrial chain, it is impossible to realize "complete decoupling" between China and the United States, and the "New Cold War" is destined to be a temporary rather than a long-lasting phenomenon.

The issue that begs further discussion is the possibility that the "New Cold War" will grow into a hot war (that is, a limited war or total war). Although leaders of both sides are not willing to engage in direct military combat, the mechanism for preventing a hot war between China and the United States has not yet been established. During the US-Soviet Cold War, various arms control treaties, such as the Strategic Arms Limitation Treaty (SALT) and the Strategic Arms Reduction Treaty (START), had sound international rules and bilateral communication mechanisms to prevent military engagement. In contrast, in the current US-China rivalry, both sides are still in a blank state in terms of establishing a military and arms control mechanism and a platform for conflict resolution. Meanwhile, the two countries have started deploying more and more ships and aircraft in the Western Pacific, the South China Sea and the East China Sea, making it increasingly difficult to avoid gunfire. Therefore, both sides still need to recognize the danger of the absence of a mechanism for preventing military conflict.

Generally speaking, in the post-pandemic era, although actual and potential conflict between China and the United States has risen to an unprecedented peak since the establishment of diplomatic relations, in the long run, the relationship between the two countries must eventually return to peace and cooperation, most urgently because of the need to fight the global epidemic and deal with global governance issues (such as climate change and the global sustainable development goals agenda). It is our view that for the sake of all human beings and global civilization, it is undoubtedly necessary that both China and the United States maintain a rational and developmental relationship, so that an integrated and harmonious global governance mechanism can be guaranteed.

References

Allen, J. (2020) *The History of COVID-19 Will Be Written by the Victors*. Kenya Insights. [online]. Available at: https://kenyainsights.com/how-the-world-will-look-after-the-coronavirus-pandemic/ (Accessed 28 October 2020).

Allison, G. (2017) *Destined for War: Can America and China Escape Thucydides Trap?* London: Mariner Books.

Allison, G. (2015) *The Thucydides Trap: Are the U.S. and China Headed for War?* The Atlantic. [online]. Available at: https://www.hks.harvard.edu/sites/default/files/centers/mrcbg/files/Allison%2C%202015.09.24%20The%20Atlantic%20-%20Thucydides%20Trap.pdf (Accessed 15 November 2020).

Baldacchino, G. (2018) Thucydides or Kissinger? A Critical Review of Smaller State Diplomacy. *International Political Economy Series*, 21–40. London: Palgrave Macmillan. [online]. Available at: https://doi.org/10.1057/9780230246911_2 (Accessed 15 November 2020).

Bartz, D., and Freifeld, K. (2020) *U.S. Puts 37 Chinese Companies and Schools on Red-Flag "Unverified" List.* Reuters. [online]. Available at: https://www.reuters.com/article/us-usa-china-unverified-idUSKCN1RM26T (Accessed 30 October 2020).

Burns, N. (2020) *How to Lead in a Time of Pandemic.* Foreign Affairs. [online]. Available at: https://www.foreignaffairs.com/articles/2020-03-25/how-lead-time-pandemic (Accessed 27 October 2020).

CGTN. (2020) *Chinese FM Responds to MATLAB's Ban on Two Chinese Universities.* CGTN. [online]. Available at: https://news.cgtn.com/news/2020-06-13/Chinese-FM-responds-to-MATLAB-s-ban-on-two-Chinese-universities-Rhx20G3pte/index.html (Accessed 30 October 2020).

Chakraborty, B. (2020) *Pompeo Meets Chinese Counterpart in Hawaii to Talk Trade, Hong Kong, Human Rights.* Fox News. [online]. Available at: https://www.foxnews.com/us/pompeo-chinese-counterpart-hawaii-talks (Accessed 27 November 2020).

Cole, W. (2020) *China Responds to Pompeo: 'South China Sea Is Not U.S. Hawaii'.* Hawaii News. [online]. Available at: https://www.staradvertiser.com/2020/08/03/hawaii-news/china-the-south-china-sea-is-not-hawaii/ (Accessed 31 November 2020).

Coleman, J. (2020) *Navarro: 'It's Incumbent on China to Prove' Lab Played No Role in Coronavirus Outbreak.* The Hill. [online]. Available at: https://thehill.com/homenews/sunday-talk-shows/493570-navarro-its-incumbent-on-china-to-prove-lab-played-no-role-in (Accessed 28 October 2020).

Colombia-Harvard China and the World Program. (2019) *"Overreach and Overreaction: The Crisis in US-China Relations" a Talk by Susan Shirk UCSD.* [online]. Available at: https://cwp.sipa.columbia.edu/events/%E2%80%9Coverreach-and-overreaction%C2%A0-crisis-us-china-relations%E2%80%9D-talk-susan-shirk-ucsd (Accessed 31 November 2020).

European Commission. (2019) *EU-China: A Strategic Outlook.* [online]. Available at: https://ec.europa.eu/commission/news/eu-china-strategic-outlook-2019-mar-12_en (Accessed 14 December 2020).

Fang, J. C., and Zhao, N. W. (2019) *IMF Chief Economist Gita Gopinath Discusses U.S.-China Trade Tensions at JFK Jr. Forum.* The Harvard Crimson. [online]. Available at: https://www.thecrimson.com/article/2019/10/30/IMF-economist/ (Accessed 25 November 2020).

Huntington, S. P. (1997) *The Clash of Civilizations and the Remaking of World Order.* Touchstone: Simon & Schuster.

Ikenberry, G. J., Feng, Z., and Wang, J. S. (2015) *America, China, and the Struggle for World Order: Ideas, Traditions, Historical Legacies, and Global Visions (Asia Today).* London: Palgrave Macmillan.

Lee, J. H. (2019) *Is a China-US cold War Inevitable? Chinese Analysts Say It Can't Be Ruled Out.* South China Morning Post. [online]. Available at: https://www.scmp.com/news/china/diplomacy/article/3022587/china-us-cold-war-inevitable-chinese-analysts-say-it-cant-be (Accessed 16 November 2020).

Mahbubani, K. (2020) *A More China-Centric Globalization.* Kenya Insights. [online]. Available at: https://kenyainsights.com/how-the-world-will-look-after-the-coronavirus-pandemic/ (Accessed 28 October 2020).

Mbe, V. S. S. (2020) *Conversation with Joseph S. Nye, Jr. on Power in the Modern World.* Thought Economics. [online]. Available at: https://thoughteconomics.com/joseph-s-nye-jr/ (Accessed 27 October 2020).

Mearsheimer, J. J. (2018) *The Great Delusion: Liberal Dreams and International Realities*. New Heaven: Yale University Press.
Ministry of Commerce of the PRC. (2019) *Sino-US Trade and Investment in 2018*. [online]. Available at: http://www.mofcom.gov.cn/article/i/dxfw/nbgz/201905/20190502859509.shtml (Accessed 31 November 2020).
Ni, H., and Yan, C. (2019) *Can Vietnam replace China in the Global Industrial Chain?* China Trade News. [online]. Available at: http://www.chinatradenews.com.cn/epaper/content/2019-11/14/content_63920.htm (Accessed 26 November 2020).
Niblett, R., and Vinjamuri, L. (2020) *Op-Ed: Why Democracies Do Better at Surviving Pandemics*. Los Angeles Times. [online]. Available at: https://www.latimes.com/opinion/story/2020-05-26/democracies-autocracies-coronavirus-pandemic-response (Accessed 27 October 2020).
People's Daily. (2013) *'Ocean' Becomes Hot Word in China*. [online]. Available at: http://english.qstheory.cn/politics/201301/t20130115_205805.htm (Accessed 31 November 2020).
Pew Research Center. (2020) *Unfavorable Views of China Reach High in the United States*. [online]. Available at: https://www.pewresearch.org/politics/ (Accessed 30 November 2020).
Pew Research Center. (2020) *Republicans Remain More Unfavorable Toward China, but All Partisans Are Increasingly Negative*. [online]. Available at: https://www.pewresearch.org/politics/ (Accessed 30 October 2020).
Pew Research Center. (2020) *Problems for the US*. [online]. Available at: https://www.pewresearch.org/politics/ (Accessed 30 October 2020).
Project Syndicate. (2019) *An Interview with Joseph S. Nye, Jr*. [online]. Available at: https://www.project-syndicate.org/say-more/ps-say-more-joseph-nye?barrier=accesspaylog (Accessed 16 November 2020).
Rhodium Group, U.S.-China Investment Tracker. (2019) *U.S.-China FDI Flows from 1990 to 2019*. [online]. Available at: https://tradevistas.org/u-s-china-fdi-cold-venture-capital-heats-up/ (Accessed 24 November 2020).
Schake, K. (2020) *America's Built-in Protection Against Bad Leadership*. The Atlantic. [online]. Available at: https://www.theatlantic.com/ideas/archive/2020/05/pandemic-will-make-america-stronger/610912/ (Accessed 27 October 2020).
Statista. (2020) *Total Value of U.S. Trade in Goods (Export and Import) with China from 2009 to 2019*. [online]. Available at: https://www.statista.com/statistics/277679/total-value-of-us-trade-in-goods-with-china-since-2006/ (Accessed 11 October 2020).
U.S. Department of Commerce. (2020) *Commerce Department Prohibits WeChat and TikTok Transactions to Protect the National Security of the United States*. [online]. Available at: https://www.commerce.gov/news/press-releases/2020/09/commerce-department-prohibits-wechat-and-tiktok-transactions-protect (Accessed 30 October 2020).
U.S. Department of State. (2020a) *The Clean Network*. [online]. Available at: https://www.state.gov/the-clean-network/ (Accessed 30 October 2020).
U.S. Department of State. (2020b) *Secretary Michael R. Pompeo Remarks at the Richard Nixon Presidential Library and Museum: "Communist China and the Free World's Future"*. [online]. Available at: https://translations.state.gov/2020/07/23/secretary-michael-r-pompeo-remarks-at-the-richard-nixon-presidential-library-and-museum-communist-china-and-the-free-worlds-future/ (Accessed 24 November 2020).
Wang, J. S. (2020) *China-U.S. Ties Today Worse Than Soviet-U.S. Relations During Cold War*. Caixin. [online]. Available at: https://www.caixinglobal.com/2020-06-18/wang-jisi-china-us-ties-today-worse-than-soviet-us-relations-during-cold-war-101569472.html (Accessed 27 October 2020).
Ziezulewicz, G. (2020) *Two US aircraft Carriers Are Operating in the South China Sea; Air Force B-52 Joins Them*. Navy Times. [online]. Available at: https://www.navytimes.com/news/your-navy/2020/07/06/two-us-aircraft-carriers-are-operating-in-the-south-china-sea-air-force-b-52-joins-them/ (Accessed 31 November 2020).

Global Disorder for the Post-COVID-19 World

Suisheng Zhao and Johnston H.C. Wong

1 Introduction

The COVID-19 pandemic sweeping the globe has cost more than lives and livelihoods. It has rendered a heavy blow to the already shaking America's global leadership established after World War II. Instead of coordinating with its allies and international organizations to fight the common enemy, the Trump administration focused the bulk of its efforts on blaming China and the World Health Organization (WHO). Overwhelmed by the virus and doing a poor job of protecting its citizens, the US set a bad example for the world and offered no leadership to the rest of the world. The world has come to the "post-American" order."

As two prominent American policy analysts Campbell and Doshi (2020) suggested, the Pandemic has reshaped the world order because the Trump administration failed the test of all elements of US leadership. Beijing has moved quickly and adeptly to take advantage of the opening created by U.S. mistakes, filling the vacuum to position itself as the global leader in pandemic response.

Is China ready to step into the breach left by the Trump administration and become a global leader? This chapter argues that while the failure of the US leadership has indeed created a vacuum in global leadership, China is not yet ready to assume

The chapter was based on an article published in the *Journal of Contemporary China*, Vol. 30, No. 128, March 2021, with permission granted by the journal available online at: https://www.tandfonline.com/doi/full/10.1080/10670564.2020.1790900.

S. Zhao (✉)
Director, Center for China-US Cooperation, Josef Korbel School of International Studies, University of Denver, Denver, CO, USA
e-mail: Suisheng.Zhao@du.edu; szhao@du.edu

J. H.C. Wong
Social Work and Social Administration Programme, Division of Humanities and Social Sciences, BNU-HKBU United International College, Zhuhai, Guangdong, China
e-mail: johnstonhuang@uic.edu.cn

S.X.B. Zhao et al. (eds.), *COVID-19 Pandemic, Crisis Responses and the Changing World*, https://doi.org/10.1007/978-981-16-2430-8_3

comprehensive leadership by providing the global public goods, such as coordinating multilateral response to the pandemic, global economic and financial leadership, and enhanced WHO independence. China's success in combating the COVID-19 was grossly undermined by many political leaders who were eager to put the blame of their poor performances on China.

2 The Post-WWII World Order Leadership under Challenge

World order refers to the dominant values, rules, norms, and institutions that define the terms of global governance and give shape and substance to international society at any given time (Zhao 2020). The US-led Post-WWII world order has been embodied primarily in the UN Charter system, appealing to both state-centric principles and globalist aspirations. On the one hand, territorial states are the only legitimate members of the UN and the sole subject of international law, perpetuating the Westphalian principles of state sovereignty, diplomatic equality, and non-intervention in their domestic jurisdictions.

Functional economic institutions under the UN, notably the World Bank, the International Monetary Fund (IMF) and the World Trade Organization (WTO) have looked beyond the territorially bounded nation-state system on a reciprocal and mutually advantageous basis to replace bilateralism and mercantilism, the primary causes of imperial rivalry. With free movement of capital and goods, many states may recognize few reasons to engage in territorial expansion as global enterprises headquartered in the country can acquire resources through open and free markets.

In addition, the relevant UN organizations have been constituted to regulate the behavior of individual states in response to emergence of non-traditional security threats, such as infectious diseases, environmental degradation and transnational crimes. Beyond the UN Charter system, the US and its allies have created and maintained inter-state alliances such as NATO and OECD, to defend their collective security interests and advocate liberal values of democratic states.

China has regarded the existing world order as unfair and unable to reflect the interests and values of developing countries. China is expanding its influence within the present world order which is believed to suppress its rights. Presenting the Chinese vision for the reform of the world order, President Xi put forward the vision of the *Community* of Shared Future for Mankind (CSFM) in 2013. The Chinese government managed to incorporate this phrase into the UN resolution on the UN Commission for Social Development in 2017. It was also endorsed by the UN Security Council, the Human Rights Council and the First Committee of the UN General Assembly. These developments show that the competition for leadership between China and US in some areas of world order and within relevant organizations has been going on for a significant period; however, the Trump presidency has brought the competition into the public glare.

In addition to the increased competition, COVID-19 has further destabilized the world order. An initiating event was that the Trump administration criticized the World Health Organization (WHO) hiding information at China's behest on the initial response to COVID-19. One motive may be Trump's desire to find a scapegoat for his failure to contain the pandemic at home effectively. As a result, he withdrew the US from WHO on the ground that it had been bought by China. Trump obviously exaggerated China's influence.

China contributed only $40 million while the US contributed $450 million to WHO in 2019. China's influence over WHO, which was at the time very much under US's dominance, was not because of money but because of its focused and strategic efforts to cultivate its relationship with this global organization. WHO could not have possibly hidden information at China's behest because the US was well represented in the top ranks of WHO. A week after the US suspension of funding, China pledged $30 million on top of its annual contribution, further advancing its influence in WHO but still far from US's annual contribution. In other words Trump by withdrawal had given up US's leadership of WHO.

3 COVID-19 the Test Case for China

The outbreak was initially predicted as China's Chernobyl moment, a mishandled disaster which could make the Chinese leadership lose political legitimacy. But once the Chinese government realized the scale of the threat, it made the most consequential decision to quarantine the city of Wuhan on January 23, 2020, the epicenter and home to more than 11 million people, and then extended the quarantine to the entire country. Large swathes of the public transportation networks, factories, shops, and schools/universities were shut down. The citizens of Wuhan were demanded to stay home. Two hospitals with a total capacity of 2300 beds were built in Wuhan within 10 days. Requiring people to wear face masks, the government facilitated old and new factories going into overdrive to produce millions of masks every day.

State organs in Wuhan imposed strict controls, assigning community workers and medical staff to set up health and temperature check stations in all residential estates and areas. Big data and monitoring technology were deployed to track individual exposure to the virus. Health rating codes on cellphones were used to identify individuals infected or coming from high-risk places. A green code was set as the entrance requirement for many places to stop the spread of the virus.

The scale and speed of these measures were unseen in history, a testament to the public health governance in times of crisis. China announced zero new domestic cases on March 18 and reported zero coronavirus deaths on April 7. The 76-days lockdown on Wuhan was lifted on April 8, an implicit pushback against some of the criticism about aggressive authoritarian measures. The WHO mission in China in late February reported that "China's bold approach to contain the rapid spread of this new respiratory pathogen has changed the course of a rapidly escalating and deadly epidemic." China's efficient testing, tracking and city lockdown measures gained global attention after China quickly contained the spread of COVID-19.

The stringent social distancing and isolation approach forced a rapid acceleration of the backlash against liberal globalization. America's borders with Canada and Mexico remained open during WWII but were closed this time. Many countries, including liberal democracies of US and European governments, adopted China's approach in exercising authority to fight the borderless virus.

4 Following China's Footprints

South Korea had learned from its bitter experience of fighting SARS in 2003 and MERS in 2015 and used surveillance technologies to enforce quarantines and track people's contacts with the virus during the pandemic. The country has institutionalized the testing and tracking systems by passing legislations in 2015 that authorized the administration to access digital personal data during public health crisis.

Although the adoption of invasive health surveillance systems could have astounding consequences, including a vast increase in state authority, contact-tracing became increasingly attractive as countries struggled to balance concerns about public health and the economy. While China was criticized for its well-disposed contact-tracing systems that facilitate increased surveillance of the citizenry, some democratic countries including UK, France, Finland, Italy, Australia, New Zealand, Ghana, Israel and India are among the diverse liberal democracies that have rushed to develop their own contact-tracing apps. Google and Apple collaborated on refining an anonymized contact-tracing application programming interface.

France passed a decree that people must fill forms every time they leave home. Israel used cellphone location data to track citizens. Greece established the short message service (SMS) system for people to send declaration in advance for approval to leave home. Asian countries, including South Korea, Japan, and Singapore, were more successful than the US in limiting the spread of the COVID-19 virus because they adopted smartphone app-tracking technology for contact tracing among their people. The US refused to use high-tech tracing for the fear of privacy intrusion and became the global epicenter of the pandemic (Oxford University 2020).

5 Trump's Wrestle with COVID-19

Previous to the pandemic, the Trump administration had increased tariffs on some Chinese products and thereby, launched the trade war. Higher prices of imported equipment resulted in depleted inventories, including medical supplies. Parroting the talking points that the virus was under control and predicting a positive ending for the United States, he failed to increase crucial medical supplies or prepare for a surge in demand for medical personnel when the virus casualties surged all over the

US in mid-2020. What more the WHO and China could or should have done is less consequential to the outcome than how the US dealt with the pandemic.

The Trump administration, further, did not coordinate response with allies. Routinely criticizing alliances as burdensome and devaluing them, the Trump administration did not provide a head's up before announcing cancellations of flights to and from European countries.

Tainting the US with his own lonely malice, the Trump's coronavirus response was contradictory, incoherent and in shambles, which resulted in humiliation for the superpower of the world. It is deeply ironic that EU states barred the entry of U.S. citizens when they gradually opened international travel ban in July 2020 due to America's failure to combat the spread.

6 Face Mask Diplomacy and the Pandemic Narratives

After the coronavirus started spreading, China was stung by widespread criticism of its handling of the pandemic. The initial delay in reporting that the coronavirus is capable of transmitting between humans, amplified by the death of a doctor who was reprimanded for speaking about the virus, led to lack of confidence. At the beginning China had probably underestimated the lasting effect of these early incidents which led to the popular mistrust of China.

People around the world suffered greatly from COVID-19 and were looking for those who had made mistakes that worsened their predicament. Some foreign organizations and governments filed lawsuits demanding China compensate them for the damages caused by the pandemic started in China (Fidler 2020). Although it is unlikely that they can hold China legally responsible, the lawsuits were indicative of a negative mood as well as of a tendency to scapegoat China for global ill.

Amid the widespread mistrust around the world towards its success in handling the COVID-19, China began to ship masks, surgical gowns, diagnostic tests, and, in many cases, doctors to pandemic-ravaged countries to position itself as the partner of choice. Medical teams and supplies were sent to more than a hundred countries around the world. Chinese media dutifully reported these events, trying to promote the country's image.

China's face-mask diplomacy amid COVID-19, again due to popular mistrust towards the rising power, has not turned out to be a total success. Recipients in the Netherlands, Spain, the Czech Republic, Canada, and Turkey rejected some early shipments of Chinese medical equipment and supplies, dubbing them substandard. Finland's prime minister fired the head of the country's emergency supply agency for spending millions of Euros on defective Chinese face masks, further feeding distrust of Chinese products' safety standards.

Nevertheless nor did these events make the Chinese approach to fighting the COVID-19 unsuccessful. After the coronavirus was contained, Beijing began to reshape the political narrative. China argued that their efforts, particularly the close down of a big city like Wuhan, had given ample time for the world to take appropriate measures to counteract COVID-19.

The failure of President Trump's efforts in controlling the spread of the virus added credibility to the Chinese propaganda. However, China's narrative appeared too ambitious and overwhelming, seeking to demonstrate in the same message that: (1) The coronavirus did not originated from China, (2) it was not responsible for migration of the virus around the world, (3) China had better managed the epidemic at home thanks to its centralized government; and (4) it was ready to help all other countries facing the pandemic in a disinterested manner.

7 General Mistrust Towards China's Rise

Beijing celebrated the superiority of the Chinese system not only because it quickly contained the virus but also because other countries, including liberal democracies, began to copy China and imposed stringent quarantine and other similar measures, sometimes even more stringent than China, and erect barriers to movement of the people (Oxford University 2020). One article in N*ature* described that "As the new coronavirus marches around the globe, countries with escalating outbreaks are eager to learn whether China's extreme clampdowns were responsible for bringing the crisis there under control." Other nations are now following China's lead and limiting movement within their borders, while dozens of countries have restricted international visitors (Cyranoski 2020).

Very few Americans have, however, expressed any trust in the way China had managed and informed the world about the epidemic, providing additional arguments to push for decoupling with China in sensitive sectors like high-tech and medical supplies. Far from persuading the US to cooperate with China, the crisis brought China to the forefront of the 2020 US presidential campaign when both the Republicans and the Democrats said they would confront China squarely.

The perception that China's aid came with strings attached and targeted at furthering China's strategic objectives and interests, has gained popularity. The Foreign Policy Chief of European Union, Joseph Borrell criticized donation of masks from China as a "battle of narratives" and "politics of generosity" (Stolton 2020). Despite spokesmen from Spain and Italy have rejected Borrell's comments, damage is done (Li 2020).

Interpreting the providing of medical aids as China's eagerness for international recognition, people in the world disregarded the goodwill China has tried to present (Bradsher and Alderman 2020). As Western governments were faulted for mismanaging the pandemic or failing to galvanize an international response, China's standing took a hit. The wave of criticism, sometimes from friendly nations, underscored the challenge facing Beijing's aspirations for global leadership. In this case, while the pandemic hurt US's prestige and compounded global concerns about American competence and reliability, China has thus far been able to match the perhaps overly ambitious rhetoric, asserting a complete leadership for internationally concerted efforts. Facing domestic issues and external barriers resultant from a global pandemic, Chinese leaders have understandably faced challenges in mobilizing resources necessary to rewrite the admirable goals to attain a world order more equable for developing countries.

8 US-Sino Competition for Systemic Supremacy

Liberal globalization that created so much of opportunities for economic growth has also made the world more vulnerable. The growing global connectedness has meant that when things went bad in one place, the trouble could be transmitted farther, faster, deeper and cheaper than ever before. After the outbreak in Wuhan, the COVID-19 moved quickly across borders, forcing national governments to close their borders to contain the virus. Lives and livelihoods were destroyed but governments were often powerless to help their citizens, creating opportunities for a breed of statist governance as an alternative. To US, the success of China in containing COVID-19 represented a systemic challenge, not just in the area of public health but the entire areas of economics and politics.

Behind the US-Sino trade war was the issue of manufacturing supremacy. For this purpose Trump had no problem in emulating China's state capitalism, unleashing a fresh wave of industrial policy measures. Enhancing the state role to rebuild a national instead of a global economy and increasing the levels of redundancy in their manufacturing system regardless of cost and rationality, the Trump administration increasingly stepped in the market place to slap tariffs on foreign products, ban competitive Chinese companies using bogus national security justifications.

It is not only a Trump policy, Hillary Clinton (2020), a quintessential globalist, wrote in October 2020 that "It's time for ambitious industrial policies" to pursue a plan "in innovation and manufacturing" and impose stronger "Buy American" provisions, with the goal of jump-starting domestic production in key sectors, "reshoring sensitive supply chains, and expanding strategic stockpiles of essential goods."

Competition in manufacturing industries has its core in technological supremacy. The U.S. government tightened the restrictions by barring US companies from supplying to Chinese competitors such as Huawei products manufactured with American technology. Wary of China's acquisition of critical technology, countries, such as the United States, Australia, and Japan have tightened the screening of foreign direct investment. National security concerns are increasingly encroaching upon existing webs of economic interdependence. The pandemic has only reinforced the existing trend as Western governments expand their toolkits to restrict trade and investment flows. Using the government to protect US companies against global competition, the Trump administration was as much a proponent of state-led growth as the Chinese.

This was an "all-of-government and enduring strategy built on a coalition of trusted partners" to ban virtually all Chinese information technology products, reflecting elements of China's approach to internet governance, one where cyberspace is tightly controlled by the state. While American lawmakers and tech entrepreneurs have lamented Beijing's refusal to allow Facebook Inc., SGoogle, and other tech giants to operate in China, the US government banned popular Chinese video app TikTok and forced its owner to sell it to a U.S. company.

Although America benefited enormously from having a large open global economy, especially in the technology space, these efforts suggest a reversal of the U.S. liberal policy. Instead of favoring a global open Internet and communications, the US walled off its cyberspace and envisioned a restricted Internet that is cordoned off by governments. Countries around the world, from Britain to India, embraced the idea of Internet sovereignty.

9 China's Internal Issues and External Environment

As the US was caught by the myriad distractions of coronavirus, recession, and racial upheavals, China has moved to a much more active profile to exploit the global leadership vacuum left by the US. But China has not filled the vacuum because it does not yet have sufficient resources to assume the monumental task. China's supplementary contribution of 30 million USD to WHO, was not comparable with US's contribution of 450 million USD in 2019.

It is not clear if China, a recent and rising power, facing immense external and internal huddles to its continued economic growth, could become the first non-western regime to avoid the middle-income trap that had ensnared Latin America and North Africa, which has kept many emerging economies from entering the exclusive club of high-income countries. Internally, suffering environmental destruction, industrial overcapacity and huge debts from local governments, China's one-child policy has hastened the problem of a swiftly aging population. The costs of social security and care for the elderly are increasing (Textor 2021).

Externally, earning rapid achievements by "picking low-hanging fruits during the early decades of catch-up" growth, China enjoyed expanding access to foreign markets and technology. But the fruit of state-driven industrialization has largely exhausted and import-led growth has hit the limits. Decimating its own natural endowments and importing more food and energy than any other nation, China needs unfettered global access to foreign markets, resources and technology to reach the critical break-through achieved by Japan and Korea.

The trade war with the US and COVID-19 further deteriorated China's external environment. Many governments began to re-think China relations and reconsider supply chain strategies to serve national security and public health goals. The Chinese leadership has acted boldly to jump ahead on the technological curve but at the same time has created more conflicts in its external environment.

10 To Lead or not to Lead

COVID-19 is a non-traditional security threat that transcends rivalry and enmity, diluting the concept of zero-sum military-led national security threat. Like an earthquake or climate change, COVID-19 is non-discriminatory and unbiased when affecting people: i.e., it disregards wealth, nationality, democracy or autocracy. Cooperation has brought about benefits while a policy of isolationism has inflicted miseries. The Coronavirus demonstrated that globalization is a double edged sword. The crisis should have galvanized international cooperation within the framework of the UN and other international institutions led by big powers such as China and the U.S. to fight the common enemy even as they competed ferociously in other spheres.

In the 'good old days', the U.S. would have asserted leadership and teamed with its allies and multilateral institutions to coordinate the response to the pandemic. The United Nations Security Council (UNSC) has a track record of responding to pandemics under the US leadership. The U.S. chaired the meeting to pass UNSC Resolution 1308 in July 2000, transforming a public health concern over the HIV/AIDS pandemic in Africa into a matter of international security to coordinate response. The UNSC actions helped galvanize a multilateral response, including the establishment of the Global Fund for AIDS, Tuberculosis, and Malaria in 2002. The U.S. also led the passage of UNSC Resolution 2177 in September 2014, designating the Ebola outbreak in West Africa a threat to international security and created the U.N. Mission for Ebola Emergency Response, the first U.N. emergency mission directed at a public health crisis.

But the U.S. under President Trump displayed virtually no capacity for effective management of the outbreak even within America's borders, let alone for the global leadership. While the Trump administration was slow in reacting to COVID-19 and this led to uncontrollable health risks, China on the other hand was very much occupied with internal issues trying particularly to bring the economy back to recovery.

Despite confronting a public health threat that dwarfs any pandemic since the Great Influenza of 1918, however, the UNSC failed to pass a resolution. China held the rotating presidency of the UNSC in March and insisted that the UNSC involvement in COVID-19 was unwarranted because this public health matter did not fall within the "geopolitical" ambit of the UNSC. Washington also dragged the feet by demanding that any resolution must specify the Chinese origins of the coronavirus. The Chinese blasted Washington for politicizing the outbreak.

While the absence of leadership paralyzed the UN response to the pandemic, the meeting of the G7—the U.S. and its six closest allies—in March 2020 also failed to agree on a joint declaration because US Secretary of State Mike Pompeo insisted on describing COVID-19 as the 'Wuhan virus' and the others gave up in disgust. The G20 meeting on the following day was unable to coordinate a global economic strategy to protect critical global supply chains and avoid deepening the recession. Former Swedish Foreign Minister Carl Bildt tweeted on April 1, 2020 that "This is the first great crisis of the post-American world. The UN Security Council is nowhere to be seen, G20 is in the hands of the Crown Prince of Saudi Arabia and the White House has trumpeted America First and Everyone Alone for years. Only the virus is globalized."

The WHO remains the focal point for COVID-19 response within the U.N. system. It also lacks the authority to cut through the political obstacles ranging from trade barriers to border closures, travel restrictions, supply chain interruptions and impediments to sharing vaccines. Turning the tide on the global crisis requires international cooperation, including prompt collective decisions on matters that are fundamentally political, rather than purely technical.

11 Conclusion: Is Shared Leadership Possible?

A trustful global leadership is needed urgently to harness the multilateral institutions to smash through on pandemic response and global macroeconomic management. Unfortunately, the global leadership was absent when it was required most urgently.

The U.S. global leadership has been seriously damaged by President Trump's America First and ultimately America alone policy and the US is not willing to defend and pay for the Post-WWII order. The world is moving toward the jungle of disorder where it's everyone for themselves and the strong do what they can and the weak suffer what they must. The lack of cooperation in initiating a global policy for a global pandemic has an obvious disastrous consequence. Yet China is not ready to assert itself as the global leader in reconstructing the new world order. The world has not rushed for a China-led order, and China too appears to have no intention to rush into a leadership role.

COVID-19 could be a moment for China and the US to tackle the shared challenge and mitigate their growing tensions. It has, however, added fuel to the simmering U.S.-China rivalry and turned global public health crisis into yet another battleground for power rivalry. As the coronavirus spread, mistrust between the two countries eviscerated the global coordination that such a crisis required. COVID-19 worsened the US-China geopolitical tensions and brought in a gloomy global disorder in which every country is for itself and major powers such as the US and China failed to provide the leadership that their size and power warrant. Both the US and China were insecure, distracted by internal tensions and threats, and fought a zero-sum game. The two major powers were so hesitant and inward-looking that they were not just absent but actually had a chilling effect on global relations.

Since the writing of the article, Trump's Presidency is taken over by Biden, not smoothly but eventually, and the U.S. has rejoined the WHO under the new administration. Biden administration is eager to reassume its leadership of the World Order, but there are many obstacles. In the first place the COVID-19 continues to spread in the United States with accumulative deaths of over 500,000. The curve of new cases in America has fortunately peaked off in early January (WHO 2021). I addition, recovery of local economy and providing assistance to the most needy will be high on Biden's agenda to prevent social unrests.

Shaun Breslin (2017) discussed about the power struggles in the world order, suggested that power shifts were occurring with more actors able and willing to provide leadership roles, it is not likely to see the clear transfer of leadership roles from one country to another, as in the traditional unipolar order. Rather, we are in transition to a multipolar order in which there are multiple sites of authority but no longer with fixed and stable forms of alliances. The new forms of global governance including different and multiple sites of authority, and different forms of leadership will be welcomed by European Union, South East Asian countries and China. Competition for global leaderships will continue and shared leaderships will perhaps take shape in 2021. As mask diplomacy is replaced by vaccine diplomacy, the struggle for technological supremacy need not be interpreted negatively. Properly monitored, technological competition could benefit the whole mankind.

References

Bradsher, K., & Alderman, L. (2020) The World Needs Masks. China Makes Them, but Has Been Hoarding Them. *New York Times*, March 13. Available at: https://www.nytimes.com/2020/03/13/business/masks-china-coronavirus.html.

Breslin, S. (2017). Leadership and Followership in Post-Unipolar World: Towards Selective Global Leadership and a New Functionalism? *Chinese Political Science Review* 2, 494–511. Available at: https://doi.org/https://doi.org/10.1007/s41111-017-0082-y.

Campbell, K. M., & Doshi, R. (2020) The Coronavirus Could Reshape Global Order. China Is Maneuvering for International Leadership as the United States Falters. *Foreign Affairs*, March 18. Available at: https://www.foreignaffairs.com/articles/china/2020-03-18/coronavirus-could-reshape-global-order?utm_campaign=Foreign%20Policy&utm_content=85046008&utm_medium=email&utm_source=hs_email.

Clinton, H. (2020) A National Security Reckoning: How Washington Should Think About Power. *Foreign Affairs*, November–December. Available at: https://www.foreignaffairs.com/articles/united-states/2020-10-09/hillary-clinton-national-security-reckoning?utm_medium=newsletters&utm_source=pre_release&utm_campaign=&utm_content=20201009&utm_term=PressCFR%2C%20Members%2C%20and%20Staff.

Cyranoski, D. (2020) What China's Coronavirus Response Can Teach the Rest of the World. *Nature*, March 7. Accessed June 2 2020. Available at: https://www.nature.com/articles/d41586-020-00741-x.

Fidler, D. (2020) COVID-19 and International Law: Must China Compensate Countries for the Damage. *Just Security*, March 27. Available at: https://www.justsecurity.org/69394/covid-19-and-international-law-must-china-compensate-countries-for-the-damage-international-health-regulations/.

Li, W. (2020) Mask Diplomacy Is a Tool to Bash China. CGTN.COM, 2020–04–05 16:04. Available at: http://www.81.cn/jwywpd/2020-04/05/content_9785263.htm.

Oxford University. (2020) *Oxford COVID-19 Government Response Tracker*. Available at: https://www.bsg.ox.ac.uk/research/research-projects/coronavirus-government-response-tracker.

Stolton, S. (2020) What Is a Mask. *Brussels Times*, March 27. Available at: https://www.brusselstimes.com/brussels-behind-the-scenes/103103/what-is-a-mask/.

Textor, C. (2021). China Population Growth from 2000 to 2019. *Statista*. Available at: https://www.statista.com/statistics/270129/population-growth-in-china/.

World Health Organization. (2021). Weekly Operational Updates on COVID-19, Feb 1, 2021. Available at: https://www.who.int/publications/m/item/weekly-operational-update-on-covid-19---1-february-2021.

Zhao, S. (2020) A Revisionist Stakeholder: China and the Post-World War II World Order. *Journal of Contemporary China*, 27, 113, 2018. Accessed June 2, 2020. Available at: https://www.tandfonline.com/doi/full/https://doi.org/10.1080/10670564.2018.1458029.

Post-pandemic De-globalization? Analysis of Likely Changes in Global Supply Chains

Simon X.B. Zhao and Zekai Gong

1 Introduction

Since the end of the cold war in the 1990s, globalization has rapidly swept the world, with one result being the development of global supply chains. Globalization of supply chains is mainly affected by two factors. One is tradability—the rapid increase in the number of goods and services due to dramatic reduction in the cost of transportation and the opening up of service sectors around the world. The continued decline in costs attendant on this opening up has prompted many companies to switch to global sourcing models, enabling them to take advantage of lower labor, material, land and other expenses. The other factor is the increasing application of subcontracting. Subcontracting is becoming more common for many reasons, including the increased complexity of components, the need for expert manufacturing processes, and the desire of manufacturers to have more flexible production schedules because of the rising volatility in demand. All this leads to deeper tiering of supply chains, whereby suppliers draw upon their own suppliers who in turn draw on further suppliers in multistage production networks (Shih 2020). In a well-developed subcontracting network, it is difficult for companies to know the true identities of all suppliers, a situation which paves the way for hidden dangers that are nowadays coming to light. In addition, there have been many incidents in the past decade that go against the inherent logic of supply chain globalization. The internal logic is that "the transformation of supply chains to global multistage production networks took place in a benign environment of falling trade barriers and an implicit willingness to accept increasing interdependence and the associated risks" (2020). At the same

S. X.B. Zhao (✉) · Z. Gong
Division of Humanities and Social Sciences, Beijing Normal University-Hong Kong Baptist University United International College, Zhuhai, Guangdong, China
e-mail: sxzhao@uic.edu.cn

Z. Gong
e-mail: 1730007001@alumni.uic.edu.cn

S.X.B. Zhao et al. (eds.), *COVID-19 Pandemic, Crisis Responses and the Changing World*, https://doi.org/10.1007/978-981-16-2430-8_4

time, there have been several events that have gone against that internal logic, such as the East Japan earthquake and the flooding in Thailand in 2011, Sino-US trade disputes since 2018, and, the focus of this chapter, the COVID-19 pandemic in 2020.

Since the first novel coronavirus pneumonia was diagnosed in December 2019, the pandemic has spread rapidly to most countries in the world. As of August 31, 2020, the total number of confirmed cases in the world has exceeded 25 million. The impact of the pandemic and the emergency policy measures taken in response to it have led to unprecedented losses in the global supply chain. In particular, as the world's manufacturing center, China's role in the global supply chain post pandemic is highly controversial. This chapter aims to explore the changing trends in the global supply chain since the pandemic. We begin with a summary of the different views of American and Chinese scholars on the likely impact of the pandemic. After briefly describing the trend towards deglobalization of global supply chains between the world financial crisis in 2008 and the pandemic in 2020, the chapter focuses on the arguments for no change and for changes in the supply chains in the post-pandemic era. Particular attention is paid to the reasons for and effects of foreign-funded corporations' accelerated withdrawal from China in the post-pandemic period, from a diversity of perspectives.

The views of scholars on the impact of the COVID-19 pandemic on the global supply chain and even on the global economy vary. The first viewpoint emphasizes the negative impact of the pandemic on globalization, spotlighting the closure of the economies of several countries, the decoupling of the hitherto integrated economies of different countries and the daunting risks that have come to the fore during the pandemic. The pandemic, from this perspective, will boost a preference for autonomy and nationalism, which may lead to "a less open, prosperous and free world" (Walt 2020). Because of the epidemic situation, all kinds of governments are unveiling emergency measures in an attempt to control the crisis. When the crisis is over, many of them will be reluctant to relinquish these newly acquired powers. In the view of Niblett, the pandemic will accelerate the decoupling of the economies of China and the United States: "Once countries are no longer willing to protect the common interests brought about by global economic integration, the global economic governance structure established in the twentieth century will shrink rapidly" (2020). Wang agrees with the idea that the economic and technological decoupling of China and the United States is irreversible: "Official relations are almost frozen, the lack of strategic mutual trust is becoming increasingly serious, and people's feelings of mutual antipathy are unprecedented" (2020). Haass is also negative, predicting that the pandemic will prompt most countries to pay more attention to domestic affairs for at least a few years: "The country will take greater steps towards selective self-sufficiency (and the subsequent decoupling) because of the fragility of the supply chain" (2020).

In contrast, some other scholars hold a more optimistic view. O'Neil supports the idea that the new post-pandemic supply chain will reduce profitability but increase supply chain stability (2020). On the one hand, an increasing number of enterprises are opting for a more detailed understanding of the supply source even at the cost of efficiency, in exchange for a stable and sufficient inventory. On the other hand, governments will also intervene to force industries that they consider to be of strategic value to develop domestic back-up plans and reserves. As Menon observes, "the new outbreak does not represent the end of interconnectedness among countries in the world, because the epidemics themselves are proof of human interdependence" (2020). Of course, this is not to deny that governments are emphasizing internal economic development and autonomy. In response, Garrett proposes "a dramatic new stage in global capitalism," proceeding to predict that "The supply chains will be closer to home and full of surpluses in order to avoid future damage, which may reduce short-term profits of enterprises but will make the whole system more flexible" (2020).

Finally, some scholars believe that the pandemic will create great opportunities for China's manufacturing industry. Huang envisions two main opportunities for China. First, China's outstanding control of the epidemic will promote further transfer of world manufacturing to China. China's cluster production mode reduces the risk of purchasing parts from different sources in the world, and shows its competitiveness during the epidemic. Second, fiscal and monetary policies implemented by various countries to fight the epidemic and resume production will objectively inject large-scale liquidity into the Chinese market (Huang 2020).

Also, there are some strategic suggestions from macro and micro perspectives proposed by several scholars. From macro perspective, former US Secretary of State, Henry A. Kissinger, calls for "safeguarding the principles of the liberal world order" (2020). He believes that "a global retreat from balancing power and legitimacy will cause the social contract to disintegrate both domestically and internationally." Hence, "Restraint is necessary on all sides in both domestic politics and international diplomacy" (2020). From micro perspective, Shih provides a series of specific suggestions for transnational enterprises in global supply chains. First, he urges, "consider regionalization". The Sino-US trade dispute makes the regionalization of the manufacturing industry once again the focus of enterprise strategy. Second, he recommends that we "develop second sources or additional safety stocks." Although setting up more alternative sources of supply and safety stocks means an increase in costs, the long-term benefits of the supply chain will also be greater. Third, Shih suggests expanding the diversity of suppliers. Shih takes the Taiwan Semiconductor Manufacturing Company (TSMC) as an example. So far, the production process of TSMC still relies upon advanced lithography systems provided by a single Dutch supplier. In addition, the production process of the Dutch supplier requires optical engines supplied by a single German factory. Finally, Shih wants us to "rethink size and product mix". He points out that production processes benefit from minimum effective scale, such as automobile assembly. That's why many companies rely on factories that focus on producing similar products on a single platform and transport finished products to different countries (2020).

From a political and social perspective, the latest study by the Nobel laureate and (de)globalization theorist, Joseph Stiglitz, suggests that there is a close relationship between the pandemic and inequality—the pandemic has not only exposed the existence of inequality within and among countries, but also deepened that inequality (Stiglitz 2020). Firstly, the pandemic is exacerbating inequalities among different classes of society, particularly among low skilled labor. Enterprises will have to consider the potential epidemic risk and replace low-skilled laborers with robots in manufacturing and service industries, which will further increase unemployment and reduce the average income of the poor. Second, the pandemic has also exposed inequalities between countries. Poor health conditions in the least developed economies have led to inadequate preparedness of local health systems for the pandemic. From this political and social consideration, it is necessary for manufacturing industries to reposition their global supply chains.

2 A Brief Overview of the De-globalization of Global Supply Chains

2.1 From 2008 to 2017: "Manufacturing Back to America" Proposed by the Barack Obama Administration

From 2007 to 2008, the global financial crisis caused by the subprime mortgage crisis forced the U.S. government to rethink the loss of manufacturing businesses. The lack of a "real" economy has caused a series of problems in American society, such as the steady shrinkage of domestic industry, serious structural unemployment problems and a deterioration in the foreign trade balance. In December 2009, then Vice President Joe Biden convened a meeting of cabinet members and manufacturing executives to discuss the future of US manufacturing. Subsequently, the Obama administration issued *A Framework for Revitalizing American Manufacturing*, aimed at factors that were driving costs at each step in the manufacturing process. It put forward a comprehensive policy and framework of measures for the US government to support the development of the American manufacturing industry. In July 2010, the US House of Representatives followed this initiative by launching the "Made in America" Agenda. The agenda aimed to encourage businesses to create products and boost innovation in the United States by strengthening infrastructure and increasing investment in key areas such as education and energy, thereby creating more job opportunities for Americans. In August 2010, President Obama signed The U.S. Manufacturing Promotion Act. This Act planned to invest about $17 billion in manufacturing. The federal government hoped to ease the burden on U.S. manufacturers by temporarily eliminating or reducing tariffs on raw materials imported by the U.S. manufacturing industry. In fact, even without the policy influence, the global manufacturing industry should have returned to the United States. From 2004 to 2014, the average annual wage growth rate in mainland China was maintained at 10 to 20%. At the same time, the labor productivity of American equipment manufacturing industry was about six times higher than that of China. Therefore, the comparative cost advantage of China's equipment manufacturing industry was not very large. In addition, there are a number of factors conducive to the return of manufacturing to the United States, among them automation without labor and better responses to changes in the North American market. Among the American technology giants, Apple is the representative enterprise that uses Chinese factories to produce assembly parts. Let's take Apple's top 200 suppliers in 2016 as an example.

Apple's Chinese suppliers, which include parts suppliers and other suppliers, accounted for more than 97% of Apple's global raw material, manufacturing and assembly procurement expenditure in 2016. Table 1 shows that, based on the actual suppliers, only 23 of the 200 suppliers own Chinese enterprises, accounting for only 11.6% of the total. On the other hand, based on the actual locations of the manufacturing plants, only 346 of the 759 manufacturing plants of the 200 suppliers are located on the Chinese mainland, less than half of the total. If we only look at the suppliers of iPhone (Apple's most famous and most profitable series of products) in 2015, this phenomenon is more obvious: among the 759 iPhone supplier subsidiaries, three main sources accounted for a large proportion (80.2%): 32.7% (Japan), 28.5% (the United States) and 19.0% (Taiwan). The remaining suppliers include 6.5% European suppliers and 7.5% Asian suppliers, of which only 3.95% are mainland Chinese enterprises.

Finally, there is a more intuitive and clearer set of data, as shown in Table 2, which reflects the proportion of foreign-funded enterprises in China's imports and exports of electronic products from 2005 to 2015. In value terms, the share of exports dropped sharply from 87% in 2005 to 69% in 2015, and the proportion of imports decreased rapidly from 84% in 2005 to 69% in 2015. This clearly shows that the trend of foreign-funded enterprises withdrawing from China had begun to appear before the 2020 pandemic.

2.2 *From 2018 to 2020: Sino-US Trade Disputes Initiated by Donald Trump Administration*

The reasons for the U.S. manufacturing enterprises to return to the United States include not only the tax cuts granted by the US government to American enterprises but also the tariff increase in imports from China, which caused the comparative advantage of China's supply chain almost to disappear. On March 22, 2018, US President Trump signed a presidential memorandum at the White House. Based on 301 trade investigations launched against China, the U.S. government imposed tariffs on about $60 billion of imports from China, mainly steel and aluminum products. On April 4, 2018, the U.S. Trade Representative's Office released a list of Chinese products on which the increased tariffs would apply. Worth about $50 billion, the proposed list covered about 1300 items, including the top 10 areas of "Made in China 2025", which include aerospace, information technology, robotics, machinery manufacturing and pharmaceuticals. Later, the Chinese government countered this measure. Since then, trade friction between the two countries has intensified. According to a report issued by Kearny on April 7, 2020, entitled "Trade

Table 1 Subsidiaries in China by country of origin for Apple products

Country of origin	Core components	Percentage in China (%)	Non-core components	Percentage in China (%)	Assembly	Percentage in China (%)	Total subsidiaries	Percentage in China (%)
United States	141	22.7	51	52.9	24	50	216	32.8
Europe	33	12.1	14	42.9	4	75	51	25.5
Japan	98	23.5	133	27.8	18	33.3	249	26.5
Taiwan	39	69.2	52	82.7	54	83.3	145	79.3
Korea	32	40.6	11	27.3	N/A	N/A	43	37.2
Hong Kong	4	100.0	6	100.0	4	100.0	14	100.0
Singapore	1	N/A	9	100.0	2	100.0	12	91.6
China	8	100.0	16	100.0	2	100.0	29	100.0
Total	356		292		111		759	44.2

Source Grimes and Sun (2016)

Table 2 The share of China's import and export of electronic products by foreign invested enterprises in 2005 and 2015

	2005 (%)	2015 (%)
Share of exports by (by values)	87	69
Share of imports by (by values)	84	69

Source https://www.bnext.com.tw/article/46271/iphone-x--supplier-apple-success-fail

War Spurs Sharp Reversal in 2019 Reshoring Index, Foreshadowing COVID-19 Test of Supply Chain Resilience", the Manufacturing Import Ratio (MIR) of US manufacturing industry in 2019 was 12.1%. This marked the first obvious decline in MIR since 2011, ending five consecutive years of growth. From 2018 to 2019, U.S. manufacturing imports from China fell by 17%, or about $90 billion. In 2019, U.S. manufacturing imports from other low-cost countries or regions in Asia increased by $31 billion. In addition, U.S. manufacturing imports from Mexico increased by $13 billion. Another Kearney index report, called the China Diversification Index (CDI), tracks the shift of US manufacturing imports from China to other low-cost countries or regions in Asia. Although China remains the major importer of U.S. manufactured goods, the share of manufactured goods in China's total imports from the U.S. declined for six consecutive years. In 2013, manufactures accounted for 67% of China's total imports from US. By the fourth quarter of 2019, this had dropped to 56%. Nearly one half (46%) of the $31 billion worth of goods earlier imported by the United States from China were shifted to other low-cost countries or regions in Asia like Vietnam. In 2019, Vietnam's exports of manufactured goods to the United States increased by $14 billion compared with 2018. Prior to the Sino-US trade dispute, the trend towards reducing imports from China and increasing imports from other low-cost countries or regions in Asia had lasted for several years because of cost considerations. Even if China and the United States can finally resolve their trade disputes, the manufacturing industry shift driven by cost considerations that was evident before 2018 will no doubt continue.

It is worth noting that Mexico may be the biggest beneficiary of Sino-US trade disputes. Sino US trade friction and USMCA accelerated the growth of the manufacturing industry in Mexico. Between 2017 and 2018, due to the 301 tariffs imposed by the United States on China, imports of goods defined by NAICS 33 (87% of Mexico's exports to the United States) from Mexico increased by 11%, which was the largest annual increase since 2011. In 2019, with the expansion of the scope of 301 tariff to China, US imports of related goods from Mexico increased by 4% ($11 billion). These figures indicate that some U.S. manufacturers have begun to replace China with Mexico as a source of imports of manufactured goods (Bossche 2020).

3 In 2020: The Pandemic that Interferes Global Supply Chains

In various types of global supply chains, the degree of globalization of electronic products supply chain is particularly significant. This section takes Apple and Samsung as examples to describe the direct impact of the epidemic on the global supply chain. One of the most important industrial cities in South Korea, Daegu has also been one of the centers of the epidemic. To curb the epidemic, health authorities forced all local smartphone factories to shut down. As a result, in April 2020, Samsung closed its manufacturing plant in Gumi, another Korean city near Daegu. The plant is responsible for the production of what is currently Samsung's latest flagship smartphone, Galaxy S20, and the foldable Galaxy Z flip for Korean consumers. These models are crucial for Samsung. In response to the epidemic, Samsung decided to urgently transfer part of its mobile phone production to Vietnam, in order to ensure stable production of its high-end smart phones. In total, production of about 200,000 high-quality smart phones a month will be transferred to Vietnam. However, in order to prevent the spread of infection, the Vietnamese government has also imposed restrictions on land transportation between China and Vietnam, which has made it difficult for those of Samsung's parts sourced in China to reach Vietnamese factories.

Apple, too, was able to ship less than 500,000 iPhones in February, down about 60% from the same period last year, according to a report from the China Institute of Information and Communications Technology. In addition, the demand side has been hit hard. Apple's 42 retail outlets in Mainland China all closed during the outbreak. By the end of February, only 29 Apple stores were back in business. The Chinese market accounts for nearly 15% of Apple's total sales. That Apple will not be able to meet its revenue target for the second quarter is due to the impact of the coronavirus outbreak on China's production. A special survey conducted by the U.S. Institute for Supply Management shows that the outbreak has led to supply chain disruptions for nearly three consecutive quarters. The survey received responses from 628 manufacturing companies in the United States. Of the companies surveyed, 80% affirmed that the supply chain would be affected. As a large proportion of parts manufactured by the affected Chinese factories are micro accessories, such as resistors, thermistors and sheet metal parts, most American downstream suppliers did not recognize the seriousness of the problem in time. Peter Quarraia, the head of Bain Inc, estimates that up to 60% of executives know nothing about parts of the supply chains except direct suppliers. The lag effect of parts and raw materials shortages has been much more severe than was expected.

In addition, the pandemic has triggered plans for the return or relocation of manufacturing units proposed by the governments of developed countries. On April 9, 2020, the Japanese government announced a 220-billion yen subsidy to encourage Japanese enterprises to move from China to Southeast Asian countries or Japan, the subsidy from the supplementary budget for fiscal year 2020. Of this amount, 23.5 billion yen was dedicated to promoting the geographical diversification of production bases from China to Southeast Asia. On July 17, 2020, Japan's Ministry of Economy,

Trade and Industry announced the list of the first batch of 87 Japanese manufacturing enterprises (with a total subsidy of 70 billion yen), including Sharp, Shionogi, Terumo and Kaneka. The products of these Japanese enterprises cover many fields, such as aviation parts, automobile parts, fertilizers, medicines and paper products. Fifty-seven Japanese enterprises will move back from China to Japan. For example, Iris Ohyama, Inc., a manufacturer of household products, currently produces masks at factories in Dalian and Suzhou, purchasing non-woven fabrics and other major materials from Chinese companies. With the help of subsidies, the company will start making masks at its Kakuda factory in Miyagi Prefecture, Japan. All materials will be prepared locally, independent of overseas suppliers. Saraya, another manufacturer of hygiene products, which includes alcohol based disinfectants, will also receive subsidies. The other 30 companies will shift production to Southeast Asia. For example, Hoya, which makes hard disk components, will move to Vietnam and Laos, Sumitomo Rubber will produce nitrile rubber gloves in Malaysia, while Shinyue Chemical will transfer production of rare earth magnets to Vietnam (Cheng 2020).

4 Argument for No Post-pandemic Change in the Global Supply Chains

First of all, it must be understood that China is still the center of the world's manufacturing industry and will continue to trade with the outside world for a long time to come. According to Q. F. Huang, the former Chongqing mayor and currently a high-profile theorist who is active in think tanks on the Chinese economy and reform, one of the effects of the pandemic is the clustering of supply chains. As a country with one of the most complete manufacturing sectors in all the world, China will obviously be a beneficiary of supply chain adjustment in the post-pandemic era, which suggests that, despite a degree of readjustment, there may be no really substantial change in supply chains after the COVID-19. This view is rather prevalent among Chinese scholars and policy-makers and supported by such recent trading figures as are shown in Table 3.

As Table 3 shows, from January to August 2020, although the total value of imports and exports decreased by 0.6% year-on-year, export

Table 3 China's trade volume with major economies from January to August 2020 (Trillion yuan)

	Trade value	Export volume	Import volume	Trade surplus
ASEAN	2.93(+7.0%)	1.64(+6.9%)	1.29(+7.1%)	0.34(+6.2%)
EU	2.81(+1.4%)	1.72(+5.3%)	1.09(−4.1%)	0.63(+26.9%)
USA	2.42(−0.4%)	1.87(−0.5%)	5.49(+0.2%)	1.32(−0.8%)
Japan	1.40(+1.0%)	0.64(+0.3%)	0.77(+1.6%)	0.13(+8.7%)

Source The General Administration of Customs of China (2020)

Table 4 China's export volume of mechanical and electrical products (Trillion yuan)

	Export volume	Growth rate (%)
Automatic data processing equipment and its components	0.90148	8.4
Mobile phone	0.48873	8.9
Total mechanical and electrical products	6.47	2.1

Source The General Administration of Customs of China (2020)

volume increased by 0.8%, which resulted in an increase in China 's trade surplus. In addition to the unexpected decline in the total trade volume between China and the United States (by 0.4%), the trade volume between China and ASEAN, the EU and Japan has increased to a certain extent. As the new largest trading partners, ASEAN and China had a total trade of 2.93 trillion yuan (a year-on-year increase of 7%), accounting for 14.6% of China's total foreign trade. This overall growth of trade between China and ASEAN includes imports from and exports to ASEAN countries. China's total trade with the EU, its second largest trading partner, was 2.81 trillion yuan (up 1.4% year-on-year), accounting for 14% of China's total foreign trade. It is worth noting that China's imports from the EU have declined significantly (4.1% year-on-year), which has further increased China's trade surplus with the EU. Accordingly, in the first seven months of 2020, China surpassed the United States as the largest trading partner of the EU for the first time. From January to July, EU imports from China increased by 4.9% year-on-year, while imports from the United States decreased by 11.7%. EU exports to the United States and China declined, but the decline in exports from the EU to the United States was much greater than in the case of China (Table 4).

China's exports of mechanical and electrical products, textiles and plastic products in the first eight months of 2020 indicate there will be some growth in exports of these products in 2020. From January to August, exports of mechanical and electrical products reached 6.47 trillion yuan (up 2.1% year-on-year), accounting for 58.5% of the total export value. Among them, exports of mobile phones reached 488.73 billion yuan, an increase of 8.9% points year-on-year.

5 Changes in Post-pandemic Supply Chains

As the "world's factory", China is the center of the global manufacturing industry. It has the largest number of OEM [Original Equipment Manufacturer] factories and the largest labor force in the world. Accordingly, this section describes China's decoupling from the outside world to demonstrate the fact that the global supply chain *is* in the process of deglobalization. As described in the foregoing section, in the late 2010s, supply chains of many multinational companies tended to withdraw from China. Indeed, the 2020 pandemic has just accelerated a process that was already ongoing; the pandemic has only strengthened the determination of multinational companies to shift supply chains from China to other locations.

1. **Analysis of Foreign-Funded Corporations' Withdrawal**

As Q. F. Huang has said, the cluster production mode of China's supply chains, the scale of its manufacturing capacity and its diverse range of products has reduced the risk of the epidemic to a certain extent. However, it is still unable to stop the trend of foreign companies leaving China. This section of the chapter turns not to an examination, from economic and political perspectives, of the key issues of the process and reasons for the withdrawal of foreign companies from China.

(a) **The Actual Capacity of China's Manufacturing Industry and Rising Challenges from New Asian Economies**

The root cause of the withdrawal of foreign-funded enterprises from China is economic in nature and can be explained from two aspects. On the one hand, China's manufacturing industry has not been able to transform and upgrade in the global industrial chain, particularly in the upstream. Despite the promotion of some policies by the Chinese government, such as the "Innovation driven Development" and "Made in China 2025" strategies, while Chinese enterprises have achieved a certain degree of independent innovation in some manufacturing sectors, on the whole, China's manufacturing industry remains at the level of OEM, the lowest stream. As part of the "Made in China 2025" strategy, an assessment report on China's manufacturing industry is issued by the Chinese Academy of Engineering every year. In the 2019 annual report, shown as Table 5, China ranked fourth in the world (the first in the third matrix) in the composite index after the United States, Germany and Japan. Not surprisingly, based on scale development, the fourth column, China ranked first in the world, far more than the United States, in second place. However, in terms of the quality benefit, the fifth column, China only surpassed India among the nine countries assessed.

Table 5 Report on the development index of China's manufacturing power in 2019

Rank	Country	Comprehensive index	Scale development	Quality benefit	Structural optimization	Sustained development
1	U.S	170.99	35.81	55.60	48.49	31.09
2	Germany	124.96	28.47	26.22	45.93	24.34
3	Japan	111.84	19.99	30.01	32.65	29.20
4	China	108.94	54.97	14.52	23.56	15.88
5	S.Korea	78.11	17.16	24.37	15.98	20.60
6	France	67.82	10.58	23.98	16.27	16.99
7	Britain	63.46	9.26	23.34	13.65	17.21
8	India	43.80	5.79	13.25	11.91	12.86
9	Brazil	32.96	3.62	15.09	3.30	10.96

Source Chinese Academy of Engineering (2019)

Table 6 Apple's suppliers location and ownership (2016)

	Within China	Outside China	Total	Percentage in China (%)
Ownership (Based on the actual suppliers)	23	176	199	11.6
Location (Based on the actual location of manufacturing plants)	346	413	759	45.6

Source Grimes and Sun (2016)

A further, specific example is shown in Table 6, the data on suppliers of core components, non-core components and the assembly for Apple Inc, including the countries of origin of these subsidiaries, and the proportion of subsidiaries of specific countries (or regions) established in the Chinese mainland. As Table 6 indicates, the top four sources of suppliers' subsidiaries that provide core parts production (upstream of supply chain) are the United States, Japan, Taiwan and Europe. Only 22.7% and 23.5% of the suppliers of the US and Japan are located in mainland China. In addition, only 12.1% of the subsidiaries from Europe are located in the Chinese mainland. Although 69.2% of Taiwan's subsidiaries are located in mainland China, Taiwan-funded enterprises that provide manufacturing services to Apple have also begun to leave the mainland, for example, the Wistron Group and Kecheng Technology. The top three sources of supplier subsidiaries that provide assembly business (downstream of the supply chain) are Taiwan, the United States and Japan. The proportion of suppliers from Taiwan, the US and Japan to mainland China is 83.3%, 50% and 33.3%, which is generally higher than that of the first-class subsidiaries in mainland China. It shows that the overall level of China's manufacturing industry has not yet fully reached the upstream of the global supply chain.

Furthermore, China's so-called "world factory" is in fact substantially contributed to by foreign-funded & owned firms, particularly in the electronics industry. As indicated by official data shown in Table 7, the total foreign trade volume by foreign funded enterprises occupied near 43% in 2018 and 40% in 2019 in China's total foreign trade. As far as we know, in the electronics sector, the most hi-tech and advanced industry, the proportion of foreign-funded firms, largely Taiwanese, S. Korean, Japanese and American firms, is much higher, up to nearly 70% in 2015 as shown in Table 2 above. These foreign funded and owned firms, the so-called FDI

Table 7 Total foreign trade volume of foreign funded enterprises and proportion of foreign funded enterprises in China

	2018	2019
Total foreign trade of foreign funded enterprises in China (Yuan Trillion)	19.68	12.57
Proportion of foreign funded enterprises in China in China's total foreign trade (%)	42.57	39.9

Sources Observer Network (2020) and Department of Foreign Investment, Ministry of Commerce (2020)

multinational corporations (MNCs), are very fleet of foot, by nature prone to moving easily away from host countries since they are particularly sensitive and vulnerable to cost & tariff rises. These MNCs are inherently transient, always seeking low-cost production bases, and in fact they have started moving away from China, gradually since 2010, and the incentive to leave China has only been increased by the Sino-US trade war and the COVID-19 pandemic (Zhao et al. 2020).

Another factor in the flight of the MNCs from China is the general rise in labor costs and China's rapidly aging population. A comparison of the population structure of China and India is illuminating in this respect. From 2011 to 2018, China's working age population (18–59 years old) maintained a downward trend for seven consecutive years, with a total decrease of more than 26 million people. By comparison, India's working age population (18–64 years old) has been increasing for seven consecutive years, from 806 million in 2011 to 916 million in 2019. The proportion of the working age population in India has continued to rise from 64.43% in 2011 to 67.0% in 2019 (Kuaiyi Financial Management Network 2020). This means that India's population structure is becoming younger and the "demographic dividend" is growing. As a result, compared with Southeast Asia and South Asia, where there are more low-income people, China's rising labor cost and aging population are making China less attractive to the OEM part of the global supply chain.

Thus, the important factors that made China the "world factory" after the period of reform and opening up, such as abundant cheap labor and low land prices, have rapidly been changing and may be overridden by new factors like the rise of labor cost and aging population (due to Chinese living improvement), Tax & Tariff-rises imposed by Sino-US trade war and, of course, the fallout from the COVID-19 pandemic.

(b) **Analysis on Diplomatic Disputes, Security Considerations and Ideological Conflicts**

The reasons for foreign enterprises withdrawing from China involve not only economic factors such as declining profits but also some political considerations. As mentioned above, the high tariff caused by Sino-US trade frictions since 2018 has already prompted some US-funded enterprises to leave China. Although the first phase of the Sino-US economic and trade agreement was signed on January 15, 2020, the sudden outbreak of the epidemic made this agreement irrelevant. Before 2010, among all foreign-invested manufacturing enterprises in China, the investment scale of Japanese enterprises had long ranked in first place. However, the Diaoyu Islands issue, the negative feelings generated by the Yasukuni Shrine incident and the East China Sea oil and gas field dispute continue to simmer and have resulted in the deterioration of Sino-Japanese relations. During the 2010s, with the escalation of the Chinese people's boycott of Japanese goods, Japanese enterprises began to leave China one after another. During the decade when Japanese enterprises withdrew from China, Korean enterprises at one point ranked first among foreign-invested manufacturing enterprises, including automobiles and spare parts, consumer electronics and fine chemicals. However, in 2016, China-South Korea relations deteriorated rapidly owing to the Sade missile incident, and Korean enterprises (such as Samsung Electronics and Lotte Group) suffered a devastating blow in the Chinese market.

At the beginning of 2020, the Japanese government announced a supplementary budget to support the subsidy program because of political and public security considerations. First, trade frictions and conflicts between the United States and China had intensified, which has increased the risk of unexpected disruption of the supply chain of Japanese enterprises. Japan thus needs to maintain localized production of key components. Secondly, in the early stage of the pandemic, Japan encountered serious challenges in procurement of masks, medical protective clothing, etc. At that time, most of the supply chain for emergency medical supplies was located in China. But China has been unable to meet demand from Japan in the face of rapidly increasing global demand.

The economic and technological decoupling promoted by the US government is based more on information security considerations. After a series of security reviews of Chinese companies, on August 5, 2020, then U.S. Secretary of State Pompeo announced the "Clean Networks" program, including clean operators, clean stores, clean applications, clean clouds and clean cables.

In short, due to the structural defects of China's manufacturing industry and the rising comparative advantage of emerging Asian economies, the trend of foreign-funded enterprises leaving China had already become visible by 2018. After 2018, the trade war and political friction between China and the United States greatly accelerated this trend. Finally, the pandemic in 2020 was the last straw for foreign-funded enterprises to either reduce their presence in China or leave it altogether.

(2) **Impacts of Foreign-funded Corporations' Withdrawal from China: National Strategy, Economic Order and International Relations**

(a) **Adjustment of National Strategies: American and Japanese Strategies of Digital Economy and Chinese Internal Circulation Policy**

The pandemic has certainly had an impact on the economic strategies of all countries in the short or long term. This chapter has taken the American and Japanese strategies for the digital economy and the internal circulation policy proposed by China to illustrate some of the impacts. The U.S. government recognizes the positive value and effectiveness of its digital economy strategy in response to the epidemic. From the perspectives of epidemic prevention and health care, the U.S. Department of Health and Human Services believes that the relevant practices launched by American technology enterprises have been beneficial to public early warning, crowd tracking and material allocation during the epidemic period. The Digital Economy Advisory Committee of the U.S. Department of Commerce has determined that from the perspective of an industrial economy, the digital economy has been able to help alleviate the impact of the epidemic on the tertiary industry. However, its effect on primary and secondary industries has been relatively limited. The main reason is that the global supply chain system has been deeply impacted by the epidemic, which to a large extent has hindered the value of the U.S. digital economy to strengthen the traditional industries. From the perspective of epidemic prevention and medical security, Japan's Ministry of Health, Labor and Welfare believes that the existing digital economic foundation has played a positive role in restricting personnel flow, security of material supplies and social welfare distribution. In terms of industrial economy, the Japanese government is most concerned about how to use digital economy to alleviate the impact of the epidemic on catering, food, publishing, wholesale and manufacturing sectors (especially small and micro enterprises). At the same time, three major priorities of the Japanese government's digital economy work include innovation in digital infrastructure, stabilization of the global industrial chain and the expansion of export channels. In addition, other representative measures including relaxing the issuance of e-payment licenses for domestic enterprises, laying out manufacturing and warehousing logistics bases in ASEAN countries, and accelerating the implementation of the US-Japan and EU-Japan trade agreements.

The Chinese government has emphasized the need to address the impact of counter globalization on China's economic growth by forming a strong internal circulation in the domestic economy. At the meeting of the Political Bureau of the CPC Central Committee held on July 30, 2020, an earlier statement regarding "expanding domestic demand" has been upgraded from a simple "strategy" in previous years to a "strategic base point" in 2020. On the one hand, the Chinese government will further promote consumption through a variety of measures, including a more equitable income distribution to include low-income groups, the reform of basic public services (education, health care and pension) and housing price restriction policies. Furthermore, the Chinese government will promote more productive investment in manufacturing. Of course, manufacturing investment is led by private enterprises. The supporting measures that the government needs to provide include improving the business environment and reducing taxes and fees.

(b) **Reconstruction of New Economic Order: Decentralization of Global Manufacturing Center**

Based on the above analysis, it can be predicted that the pandemic will accelerate the reshaping of the global economic order. Instead of relying too much on China, manufacturing supply chains will move back to their home countries (North America, Europe and Japan) or more suitable regions for accumulation (Southeast Asia and South Asia). This will further promote the wider geographical dispersion of global manufacturing hubs, from one center of gravity to multiple centers of gravity.

Compared with India, Vietnam is particularly attractive to supply chains in the short term. Vietnam not only has an almost perfect infrastructure but also has a more open economic policy. On June 30, 2019, Vietnam and the EU signed a free trade agreement and an investment protection agreement, which means that the two sides will gradually reduce the tariff of 99% in bilateral goods trade. This has made Vietnam more attractive to labor-intensive industries, which have difficulty moving back home because of cost problems. After closing its Dongguan plant in 2016, Samsung announced the closure of its foundry in Huizhou, a city in Guangdong Province in October 2, 2019, which is also its last foundry unit in mainland China. The global manufacturing base of Samsung mobile phones will henceforth be located at two factories in Vietnam, in Beining province and Taiyuan Province. In fact, during 2008–2019, Samsung's total investment in Vietnam has risen from a relatively modest $630 million to an impressive $17.3 billion, with eight additional plants (Qian 2020).

In addition, the rapid rise of Vietnam's color TV manufacturing industry also poses a threat to China's industry in the world market. For example, between 2019 and 2020, India imported $781 million worth of color TV products of which $293 million of products were from China but the value of products from Vietnam was as high as $428 million (Sina Technology 2020).

(c) **Continuing Deterioration of International Relations: Absence of Economic Cooperation as the Foundation**

Diplomatic relations between countries largely depends on the interdependence of their economies. With the economic decoupling of some countries and progress in the process of deglobalization, relations among some countries are deteriorating at an unprecedented pace. Taking Sino-US relations as an example: since the normalization of Sino-US relations in 1972, bilateral relations reached their lowest point in 2020. Both sides have not only accused each other of being responsible for the epidemic (in March 2020) but have also begun to consider qualitative and strategic risks of bilateral relations. On July 24, 2020, then U.S. Secretary of State Pompeo delivered a speech at the Nixon Library, marking the Trump administration's recognition of the failure of the US government's policy of engagement with China since the Nixon era. On August 6, 2020, President Trump signed an executive order that prohibits US companies from trading with Tik Tok and WeChat. Tik Tok is by far one of the most globally successful Internet products by a Chinese company and the ban will require ByteDance to sell its U.S. business to Microsoft. Thus, as a non-traditional security threat, the pandemic not only does not promote public health cooperation between China and the United States but also raises issues and provides platforms for escalation of conflicts between the two countries. At the same time, the pandemic has promoted the rise of nationalism in various countries, which has led to further acceleration of inward looking attitudes of economies that, to some degree, have already been experiencing deglobalization.

6 Conclusion: Summary and Prospects for the Future

To sum up, based on the analysis above, we tend to acknowledge that the pandemic will further deepen the de-globalization trend of global supply chains. This process in fact significantly predates the eruption of the COVID-19 pandemic in 2020, but now it seems even more predictable, even inevitable, given the upcoming restructuring of the global economy in the post-pandemic era. The argument that there will actually be no substantial change in the structure of the global supply chain, which is supported by a recent strong performance in China's trade figures, neglects the fact that the robustness in the Chinese economy will be short-lived and its current buoyancy could be largely because of the ongoing closedown and lockdown situations across most of the world. As the momentum for restructuring the global supply chain gathers force and accelerates, we can reasonably foresee that multinational manufacturing firms will migrate to two main directions. Those supply chain firms with a higher degree of automation will move back to their country of origin or a nearby area, although the process of doing so will necessarily be tough. This deglobalization could lead to a grand, new phenomenon, that might be designated a trend towards the regionalization or 'continentalization' of the global supply chain, in which many multinational supply chain firms reposition themselves in their home or neighboring regions in order to avoid catastrophic events and minimize risks.

Those supply chains firms that rely on low production costs will accelerate migration to developing countries with large-scale cheap labor, reasonable transportation infrastructure and open market policies. Among such potentially favorable destinations, Vietnam, India and Mexico appear to be high on the agenda. Currently these countries appear to be relative winners in repositioning themselves globally to attract FDI and supply chains firms. However, this rise in new competitors doesn't mean China's role will decline significantly. As long as China is well prepared for this new trend, adjusts its role according to the changing global situation, and keeps opening up and integrating with the outside world, China will definitely have an obvious positive contribution to make in the future to this new process of global regionalization of supply chains. As demonstrated by the newly-born RCEP in November 2020, which consists of ASEAN + 5 countries (S. Korean, Japan, Australia, New Zealand, and China), China will certainly continue to play an important role in this largest trade block as well as in global supply chains.

References

Bossche, P. (2020). U.S. manufacturing trends are reversing, but will not return to prosperity. Available at: https://www.sohu.com/a/392419470_611421?_f=index_businessnews_1_8&spm=smpc.home.business-news22.3.1588308757462yJ59sMO (Accessed 8 August 2020).

Cheng, M. (2020) The Japanese government announced the first batch of 87 funded enterprises to leave China. Available at: https://mp.weixin.qq.com/s/wzl_ZPmHg91fSQAXWYj-0g (Accessed 18 August 2020).

Chinese Academy of Engineering. (2019) Report on the development index of China's manufacturing power in 2019. Available at: http://www.cae.cn (Accessed 22 August 2020).

Department of Foreign Investment, Ministry of Commerce. (2020) Import and export profile of foreign invested enterprises from January to December 2018. Available at: http://www.fdi.gov.cn/1800000121_33_11808_0_7.html (Accessed 24 October 2020).

Garret, L. (2020) A dramatic new stage in global capitalism. *Foreign Policy*. Available at: https://foreignpolicy.com/2020/03/20/world-order-after-coroanvirus-pandemic/ (Accessed 6 August 2020).

Grimes, S., & Sun, Y. (2016) China's evolving role in Apple's global value chain. *Area Development and Policy*, 1(1), 94–112.

Haass, R. (2020) More failed states. *Foreign Policy*. Available at: https://foreignpolicy.com/2020/03/20/world-order-after-coroanvirus-pandemic/ (Accessed 6 August 2020).

Huang, Q. (2020) Three thoughts on the restructuring of global industrial chain under the spread of COVID-19. Available at: https://baijiahao.baidu.com/s?id=1662487825914770798&wfr=spider&for=pc (Accessed 21 August 2020).

Kissinger, H. (2020) The coronavirus pandemic will forever alter the world order. Available at: https://www.henryakissinger.com/articles/the-coronavirus-pandemic-will-forever-alter-the-world-order/ (Accessed 13 August 2020).

Kuaiyi Financial Management Network. (2020) India's total population of young and middle-aged and the gradually entering the working age group (15–64 years old) over the years. Available at: https://www.kylc.com/stats/global/yearly_per_country/g_population_15to64/ind.html (Accessed 3 August 2020).

Menon, S. (2020) This pandemic can serve a useful purpose. *Foreign Policy*. Available at: https://foreignpolicy.com/2020/03/20/world-order-after-coroanvirus-pandemic/ (Accessed 6 August 2020).

Niblett, R. (2020) The end of globalization as we know it. *Foreign Policy*. Available at: https://foreignpolicy.com/2020/03/20/world-order-after-coroanvirus-pandemic/ (Accessed 6 August 2020).

Observer Network. (2020) General Administration of Customs: Private enterprises surpassed foreign-funded enterprises for the first time and became the largest foreign trade subject in China in 2019. Available at: https://www.sohu.com/a/366755874_115479 (Accessed 24 October 2020).

O'Neil, S. (2020) Lower profits, but more stability. *Foreign Policy*. Available at: https://foreignpolicy.com/2020/03/20/world-order-after-coroanvirus-pandemic/ (Accessed 6 August 2020).

Qian, Z. (2020) Samsung and Apple are facing a crisis as the epidemic affects the global mobile phone manufacturing supply chain. Available at: https://baijiahao.baidu.com/s?id=1664756138058886197&wfr=spider&for=pc (Accessed 15 August 2020).

Shih, W. (2020) Is it time to rethink globalized supply chains? The COVID-19 pandemic should be a wake-up call for managers and prompt them to consider actions that will improve their resilience to future shocks. *MIT Sloan Management Review*, 61, 16–18.

Sina Technology. (2020) Development of Vietnam's color TV manufacturing industry. Available at: https://tech.sina.com.cn/roll/2020-08-18/doc-iivhuipn9307582.shtml (Accessed 27 August 2020).

Stiglitz, J. (2020) Conquering the great divide. Available at: https://www.imf.org/external/pubs/ft/fandd/2020/09/covid19-and-global-inequality-joseph-stiglitz.htm/ (Accessed 8 October 2020).

The General Administration of Customs of China. (2020) China's foreign trade import and export increased by 3.6% in the first eight months of this year. Available at: http://www.customs.gov.cn/customs/xwfb34/302425/2586202/index.html (Accessed 5 September 2020).

Walt, S. (2020) A world less open, prosperous, and free. *Foreign Policy*. Available at: https://foreignpolicy.com/2020/03/20/world-order-after-coroanvirus-pandemic/ (Accessed 6 August 2020).

Wang, J. (2020) *China-US relations in the context of COVID-19*. [Lecture] Peking University, 26 March.

Zhao, X.B., Wong, D.W.H., Wong, D.W.S., & Jiang, Y.P. (2020) Ever-transient FDI and ever-polarizing regional development: revisiting conventional theories of regional development in the context of China, Southeast, and South Asia. *Growth and Change*, 51(1), 338–361.

Actions Across Government and COVID-19: The Experience of Mainland China, Macao and Hong Kong

Edoardo Monaco, Kwok Cho Tang, Wah Kwan Cheng, Huixin Liu, and Bijun Pan

Abstract This chapter begins with a general overview of how actions have traditionally been taken across government agencies to prevent and control major causes of mortality and morbidity, with particular regard to infectious diseases. Three case studies then follow, detailing how the Whole-of-Government (WoG) and Health in All Policies (HiAP) approaches have been used to combat COVID-19 in Mainland China as well as in the Macao and Hong Kong Special Administrative Regions respectively, primarily in the period between the end of December 2019 and September 2020. A concluding synthesis of the case studies' inferences and implications is then provided, setting out what has worked in these contexts, as well as the few key issues that may warrant further attention and research.

1 Introduction

It is evident that there are many determinants of health, and the great majority of them lie outside the mandate of health authorities alone. To prevent and control major causes of both noncommunicable and communicable diseases, actions must,

E. Monaco (✉) · K. C. Tang
Globalisation and Development (GAD) Programme, Beijing Normal University-Hong Kong Baptist University United International College (BNU-HKBU UIC), Zhuhai, China
e-mail: emonaco@uic.edu.cn

K. C. Tang
e-mail: kwokchotang@uic.edu.cn

W. K. Cheng
Department of History and Heritage Studies, University of Saint Joseph, Macao SAR, China
e-mail: wkcheng@usj.edu.mo

H. Liu
Hong Kong Institute of Asia-Pacific Studies, The Chinese University of Hong Kong, Shatin, Hong Kong

B. Pan
Graduate School of Public and International Affairs, University of Pittsburgh, Pittsburgh, PA, USA

S.X.B. Zhao et al. (eds.), *COVID-19 Pandemic, Crisis Responses and the Changing World*, https://doi.org/10.1007/978-981-16-2430-8_5

therefore, be undertaken by authorities beyond those in the health sector, at the international level by the United Nations (UN) and World Health Organization (WHO), at the national level by central and provincial governments and at the local levels by city and district governments. Examples of how major causes of noncommunicable diseases can be affected by actions beyond the health sector include: lowering occupational deaths and injuries through work related measures mandated by labour authorities; lowering road deaths and injuries through improving road and motor vehicle designs as well as traffic flow, led by road and traffic authorities; preventing cardiovascular diseases and strokes through reducing consumption of salty, sugary and fatty foods overseen by food administrations; increasing life expectancy through improving access to higher education through the action of education authorities; reducing cancers, heart and respiratory diseases through effective implementation of tobacco control measures—such as tax increases and bans on tobacco advertising and sponsorship—by the combined efforts of various government authorities (Tang et al. 2014; WHO 2015).

Actions across sectors are also essential to combatting communicable diseases. Measures including quarantining of sick people, provision of piped water and sanitary sewers, reduction of overcrowding and improvement of air ventilation, proper disposal of garbage, avoidance of contact with body fluids of infected people, and improvement of personal hygiene such as handwashing have been proven over centuries to be keys to the preventing and controlling of pandemics such as the black death, tuberculosis, cholera, SARS, Swine flu and Ebola. These measures built on the foresight of public health pioneers, more notably in Sweden in the seventeenth century (Asp 2007; Räsänen 2007), in the UK in the mid-nineteenth century (Chadwick 1842; Snow 1855) and in the US in the early twentieth century (Winslow 1920). They all agreed on the need to address issues beyond personal hygiene and quality health care and to look particularly at basic living and working conditions (Winslow 1920). Quarantine as a public health practice to combat communicable diseases was also established in China as early as the seventh century when it was used to detain sailors and foreign travelers suffering from plague (WHO 2007). To provide people with a decent work and living environment, particularly in countries or local areas where root causes of poor health such as weak infrastructure, lack of essential services and social protection are prevalent, it is essential that public and water works, urban services, social welfare, civil affairs as well as finance and planning authorities take charge. To enforce effective quarantine measures, actions by the custom and police authorities are also required (Tang et al. 2014).

Action across sectors has also been adopted by governments since the 1990s and subsequently was recognized by the UN in 2001 for the effective action against HIV AIDS, as it was deemed simultaneously a health, a development and a humanitarian crisis (UN 2001).

2 Action Across Sectors: "Health in All Policies" and "Whole-of-Government" Approaches

"Action across sectors" broadly refers to work undertaken together by two or more government ministries or agencies to develop and/or implement policies, programmes or projects that work towards achieving a set of goals and targets. In essence, they are vertical actions across national, provincial and local governments and horizontal actions between ministries or public agencies within one government level. Traditionally, the health sector has facilitated action across sectors for health and health equity mainly through the "Health in All Policies" approach and the "Whole-of-Government" approach (WHO 2015).

''Health in All Policies" (HiAP) is an approach to public policies across sectors that systematically takes into account the health implications of decisions, seeks synergy and avoids harmful health impacts. It aims to improve population health and health equity (WHO 2014). The "Whole-of-Government" (WoG) approach is one in which public service agencies work across portfolio boundaries, formally and informally, to achieve a shared goal and an integrated government response to particular issues. It aims to achieve policy coherence in order to improve effectiveness and efficiency. This approach is a response to departmentalism and focuses not only on policies but also on programme and project management (APSC 2004).

Both the HiAP and WoG approaches are commonly used to address major causes of morbidities and mortalities. The HiAP approach focuses on health and health equity, is led by the health minister and implemented only on a ministry level, not by the whole by government. Whereas the WoG approach focuses on effectiveness and efficiency in achieving policy coherence of the entire government and is led by the head of government. Obviously, the WoG approach is the most powerful and comprehensive single approach to achieving health and health equity as it is led by the head of government and requires alignment from all government agencies. There are, however, invariably competing priorities in a government and cutting health spending is therefore not uncommon when economic development is at the top of the public agenda. Moreover, it is also important to note that sustained whole of government action on a given health issue is usually not employed unless the problem is both a health and development issue like HIV/AIDs or a pandemic like COVID-19.

3 The 2020 COVID-19 Pandemic

The COVID-19 pandemic is, indeed, more than a health crisis: it is, at the very same time, an economic crisis, a humanitarian crisis, a security crisis, and a human rights crisis, within and across countries. As a consequence, emerging from such crises requires leadership and actions not only by health authorities but also by the "whole-of-government" at every level (UN 2020; WHO 2020a).

At the global level, in fact, the UN has urged its member states to take immediate measures to strengthen the capacity of health systems to respond to COVID-19; help people who face adversities in life through social protection and basic services; protect jobs through economic recovery programmes; provide and implement fiscal and financial stimulus for the most vulnerable; invest in community-led resilience and response systems, and strengthen multilateral and regional responses (UN 2020). In order to ultimately contain the spread of the virus, stem the deterioration of human rights, social cohesion and livelihoods, and protect disadvantaged groups particularly vulnerable to the pandemic, the WHO, as the lead UN health agency, has provided global guidance on COVID-19. It has worked with member states to maintain access to essential health services, providing essential supplies, training health workers and supporting the development of a multi-sectoral response to COVID-19 via mainstream public health measures (WHO 2020a).

Along with the WHO, some 30 UN entities including agencies, funds and programmes[1] have developed policies and plans to respond to the pandemic. A UN inter-agency fund mechanism has also been set up to support low- and middle-income countries to deal with the pandemic, particularly its socio-economic impact upon the most disadvantaged populations.

Similarly, the WoG and HiAP approaches have also been used at the national, provincial and local levels worldwide. In this chapter, the extent to which they have been effectively used in the combat of COVID-19 in Mainland China, the Hong Kong Special Administrative Region (HKSAR) and the Macao Special Administrative Region (MSAR) will be detailed and synthesized. The key issues in their effective application for achieving better health and sustainable development will also be highlighted and discussed.

4 The Case of Mainland China

In late December 2019, several pneumonia cases with unknown aetiology were detected in Wuhan, Hubei Province, China. Upon learning of the emerging situation, between 27 and 29 December 2019, local hospitals promptly reported to the Centre for Disease Control (CDC) in the Jianghan district of Wuhan, as well as to the municipal and provincial Health Commissions (Li et al. 2020).

The Chinese government paid close attention to the development of the disease and informed the WHO on 31 December 2019 (WHO 2020b). However, by 3 January 2020, the Wuhan Municipal Health Commission announced that there were already 44 cases diagnosed as "unknown pneumonia". The situation quickly worsened, culminating in a much larger outbreak of COVID-19: the epidemic rapidly spread throughout other regions in China during the following two weeks and, ultimately,

[1] UNICEF; UNDP; UNESCO; WFP; FAO; WHO; UNEP; UNODC; UNFPA; UNHABITAT; UN Women; ILO; UNHCR; IOM; IMO; ITU; IFAD; UNIDO; UNWTO; UPU; WIPO; UNAIDS; UNITAR; UNRWA; IAEA; ICAO; WB; IMF.

globally, determining the onset of what the WHO eventually defined, on 11 March 2020, a "pandemic" (BBC 2020).

Although Mainland China was the first to experience the severe impact of COVID-19, within only one month, it went from the peak of a single-day increase in domestic cases of 15,152 on 12 February, to the double digit (+46) daily increase reported on 8 March (China Daily 2020a): since then, and up until the end of August 2020, China has consistently recorded, at the most, double-digit daily increases, except for a few occasional spikes—the highest of which on 17 April (+352) and second highest on 31 July (+276)—reaching an overall total of just over 90,000 confirmed cases (USNews 2020; WHO 2020c). The economic impact was also significant, with a GDP reduction of 6.8% in the first quarter of 2020 and the closure of about 460,000 Chinese businesses, but not as prolonged and severe as elsewhere around the globe (Time 2020). Overall, China was, therefore, able to contain the first wave of the outbreak and recover relatively swiftly due to a well-coordinated range of prevention and response measures adopted by various government agencies across different domains—well beyond the mere health sector, as surveyed below.

In doing so, China ultimately established a paradigm to combat the virus that would represent a key benchmark for other countries to follow and that highlights the effectiveness of WoG and HiAP approaches to curb the spreading of infectious diseases like COVID-19.

4.1 Health

Local authorities in Hubei provided a quick response once they received early reports from hospitals: three institutions were assigned to conduct epidemiological research on 29 December 2019 including Wuhan and Jianghan CDC and Jinyintan Hospital, a designated hospital for infectious diseases (Sohu 2020). One day later, the Wuhan Municipal Health Commission sent out an emergency notice to all medical institutions asking for reports of any pneumonia patients with unknown causes in a timely manner (China Daily 2020a). The National Health Commission (NHC) started to investigate the cause of unexplained pneumonia on 30 December 2019. On the morning of the next day, a working team and expert group organized by the NHC were sent to Wuhan to guide relevant work and help with any ongoing investigations. On 17 January 2020, similar groups were dispatched to various provinces to supervise and help provincial governments with implementing preventative measures (Huanqiu 2020).

At the same time, other institutions actively joined and supported the epidemic control work. By 13 February 2020, for instance, the People's Liberation Army (PLA) had already dispatched more than 4,000 medical staff to Wuhan (Dong 2020). The central government and local governments from other provinces sent 346 medical teams with 42,600 personnel to support Hubei province by 8 March 2020 (Peng 2020). The Central Steering Group—a central government team led by Chinese Vice

Premier Sun Chunlan—arrived in Wuhan on 3 February 2020. After on-site investigations, this unit proposed to convert gyms and exhibition centres into temporary hospitals in an effort to address the bedding shortage (CGTN 2020a). These so-called "Fangcang" shelter hospitals were used for isolating patients with mild symptoms from the communities, while medical treatment and basic life care were provided (Chen et al. 2020). To expand capacity for patients with severe conditions, in early February, two temporary hospitals with 2,600 beds were set up within 10 days in Wuhan—"Huoshenshan" and "Leishenshan" (Wang et al. 2020).

A collaborative effort was also made to efficiently collect and publish relevant data and discoveries regarding the transmission, clinical manifestations, management and treatment of the coronavirus. In order to foster national research activities on the disease, the NHC ordered the Chinese Centre for Disease Control and Prevention, the Chinese Academy of Medical Sciences, the Chinese Academy of Sciences, and the Chinese Academy of Military Medical Sciences to jointly conduct tests on received patients' samples. The NHC itself published daily updates on nationwide transmission trends and guidelines on disease prevention (Huanqiu 2020).

4.2 Transportation

Following the outbreak, tight traffic controls for non-emergency vehicles were imposed around the country. The Ministry of Transport (MOT) suspended public transportation in many cities: on 27 January 2020, Tianjin, Zhejiang, Anhui, Shanghai, and Qinghai provinces suspended inter-provincial highway bus services (Xia 2020). Additionally, airports, railway stations, bus stations, and port passenger terminals enforced strict body temperature screening on passengers especially people from Wuhan (Ministry of Transport of the PRC 2020a). On 19 January 2020, the MOT issued a notice that transportation of emergency materials, patients, and doctors would have priority to pass on highways and be exempt from any toll charges (Ministry of Transport of the PRC 2020b). This policy ensured efficient and unobstructed emergency transportation of critical resources. Furthermore, all available transportation was leveraged to mobilize resources nationwide. Between 24 January to 10 March 2020, twenty-nine domestic airlines were organized by the Civil Aviation Administration of China to carry out 411 missions to transport medical supplies and teams from various Chinese provinces to Hubei (Civil Aviation Administration of China 2020a).

The Civil Aviation Administration (2020b) also limited international routes of both domestic and foreign airlines to, at the most, one flight per week. At the same time, once the domestic crisis was brought under control and thus imported cases became a major focus, the National Immigration Administration and the Ministry of Foreign Affairs introduced a uniquely stringent temporary ban on all foreign nationals—even those holding valid visas and residence permit—from 28 March (Xinhua 2020a) up until 28 September 2020 (Ministry of Foreign Affairs 2020).

4.3 Education

To help control the movement of students and reduce student densities that might further exacerbate the outbreak, the Ministry of Education (2020a) issued a notice on 27 February 2020 requiring schools at all levels to appropriately delay the start of the upcoming semester. However, postponing the opening of campuses would not mean the termination of learning activities altogether: schools were in fact asked to provide on-line teaching to ensure the normal fulfilment of their educational mission. No mandatory reopening date was given in this document. Yet, schools were required to follow unified deployment of the local education department, under the supervision of the national Ministry of Education (Minister of Education 2020a).

In late March and April 2020, several provinces and areas including Shanghai, Jiangsu, Guangdong, Hebei announced the reopening of school activities (CGTN 2020b). Daily health inspections were made compulsory for students and staff. Any individuals who experienced symptoms such as a fever or coughing, had been in high-risk areas, or had close contact with confirmed patients were sent to designated quarantine sites. In the education sector, the transition back to school was made successful through local coordination and a controlled approach. According to the Ministry of Education (2020b), by 14 July 2020, 200 million students at all education levels across China went back to class—making for a resumption rate of about 75%.

4.4 Finance

On 28 January 2020, in order to make sure that patients would seek and receive timely medical treatment regardless of socio-economic status, as well as to ease financial pressure on hospitals, the Ministry of Finance (MOF) and National Healthcare Security Administration decided that individual expenses arising from COVID-19 medical treatments would be fully covered by the government. Both confirmed and suspected patients could therefore get completely free medical care (Liu et al. 2020).

The steady reopening of the country resulted in an increased demand for personal protective equipment—such as face masks, face shields, and body suits. Therefore, to meet this need, the National Development and Reform Commission and the MOF officially included relevant protective materials in the national resource reserve list on 11 February 2020. The government declared its readiness to purchase any surplus of medical grade protective equipment, also encouraging manufacturers to produce more masks and other protective necessities by means of fiscal incentives and credit facilitation (Beijing Youth Daily 2020).

On a more macro-economic level, Premier Li Keqiang in May 2020 unveiled a massive stimulus package of about 4 trillion yuan, which was similar in size to the one devised after the 2008 financial crisis and aimed primarily at "preserving employment, people's livelihoods and helping market entities" by reducing costs for struggling businesses through tax cuts, lower bank interest rates and prices for utilities, as well as by allocating 2 trillion yuan of additional fiscal spending and government bond issuance (SCMP 2020).

4.5 Provincial and Local Governments

As per tradition within the strictly hierarchical Chinese administrative system, provincial and municipal government agencies continued to strictly execute orders emanating from the higher national authorities, and provided regular reports on their implementation, as well as, in general, on local trends and challenges. Yet, during the COVID-19 crisis, provincial and municipal governments were also empowered with special autonomy to adjust policies and directives from the central government in accordance with the local circumstances. Usually, such "adjusted" deliberations were made collectively by leading groups formed by officials spanning across all sectors of the local government (China Daily 2020b).

Horizontal communication and cooperation across government entities helped to share successful experiences among governments. Once an initiative achieved success, that would be swiftly replicated elsewhere. For instance, Zhejiang was the first province to utilize health QR codes when reopening workplaces. Residents were required to input their personal information, travel history and health condition into the apps supported by Alipay and Tencent. A coloured QR code was then generated automatically identifying different levels of health risk. Without this code, residents were not allowed to enter public and residential areas. This tool, which leveraged big data and technological advances in surveillance systems, helped government easily monitor residents' movements and undertake contact tracing. Consequently, this practice was quickly adopted by Jiangsu, Guangxi, Shanghai and Yunnan and then by the whole country (Tan 2020).

4.6 Neighborhood Committees

Neighborhood committees—the most "grassroots" level of government in charge of civil affairs—played a significant role in containing the spread of coronavirus in China. During quarantine time, residents' movement outside their homes was restricted. This was most severe in Wuhan, when lockdown measures were enacted between 23 January to 8 April 2020. Every three days, only one family member per household would be allowed to leave their residence to purchase daily necessities. If residents wished to leave for any other reason, permission from the competent neighbourhood committee was needed. While this was without doubt a challenging constraint for all ordinary citizens, the hard work of four million neighbourhood committee workers across the country contributed to the successful management of the problem. Apart from providing food, medical supplies and other daily necessities for residents—especially vulnerable groups—neighbourhood committee workers also gathered information about residents' movements through door-to-door visits, assisted residents to measure body temperature, sterilized the entrance of each residential block and offered help for people in self-quarantine (Lu 2020).

4.7 Cooperation Platforms

Due to its institutional strength, China could easily facilitate cooperative efforts across sectors. At the central government level, the Joint Prevention and Control Mechanism of the State Council was set up. It consisted of thirty-two government departments ranging from health care, disease prevention and control, science and publicity to foreign affairs and others, and aimed at better allocating resources countrywide (Xinhua 2020b). Within this coordinated system, leading administrators of multiple ministries could collaboratively resolve urgent problems in a timely manner. At the provincial level, the Ministry of Commerce organized to establish a joint supply guarantee mechanism through coordinating with provincial departments of commerce in Hubei, Shandong, Anhui, Jiangxi, Henan, Hunan, Chongqing, Guangxi and Yunnan province. These provinces transported rice, flour, meat, eggs, fruit, vegetables, and masks to Wuhan and Hubei to ensure adequate supply of daily necessities and medical resources support for Hubei (Ministry of Commerce 2020).

In conclusion, China managed to turn itself from the most severe epicentre to a successful response model in the time span of merely three months—from January to March 2020. This appears to be due to a series of factors, including but not limited to a solid government infrastructure of top-down, strict supervision of socio-economic activities; sound epidemiological monitoring and science-based decision-making processes; a unique capacity for swift mobilisation of resources and effective implementation of emergency response measures on a vast scale and at short notice; strengthening and optimisation of coordination between central and local administrations. The successful paradigm—in essence, a major example of an effective "whole of government" approach in response to a multifaceted public health emergency—was de facto established, and could be replicated in response to similar future emergencies, just like the SARS response "model" was partially re-utilized and significantly revised during the COVID-19 crisis: for instance, the National Infectious Disease Information System (IDIS) set up in 2004 after the SARS outbreak was also crucial in gathering relevant statistics during the COVID epidemic. Similarly, the strategy of constructing temporary hospitals to relieve the overstressed medical system in Wuhan is also a replication of the practice developed during the SARS epidemic (AlTakarli 2020).

5 COVID-19 Impact and Response in Macao Special Administrative Region (MSAR)

Macao saw its first case of novel coronavirus infection on 22 January 2020. Within a week, six more cases were reported, bringing the number of infections to seven. All seven patients were visitors from Wuhan, the epicentre of the coronavirus outbreak. Then three more cases were confirmed in the first week of February. This time, all infected were residents of Macao (Special Webpage against Epidemics: Statistics, n.d.). In addition, while patient number 8 was diagnosed on 2 February, the 64-year-old woman was first admitted to hospital as early as 27 January (Macao News 2020b). The 9th case involved a 29-year-old woman who apparently got infected when she visited patient number 8 on 24 January (Macao News 2020c). The 10th confirmed coronavirus patient was a 57-year-old man residing in Macao who traveled frequently to Guangzhou (Macao News 2020d). This turn of events, ten confirmed cases in rapid succession, looked ominous, as it suggested that a community outbreak may have taken hold.

We now know that these ten cases constituted the entirety of the first wave of the coronavirus outbreak in Macao. For nearly a month and a half, no new infections were reported. All ten patients would eventually recover (Leung 2020a).

As residents started to return to the city from overseas, the second wave of coronavirus infection began to mount in force. From 15 March to 8 April, a slew of thirty-five cases were confirmed (Special Webpage against Epidemics: Statistics, n.d.). These were all imported cases. By then, a mandatory quarantine programme for arrivals to Macao was already in place, effectively intercepting the infections at the points of entry to the city or in quarantine. It would not be another two-and-a-half months before the 46th coronavirus patient—and the last reported case to date—was identified (Macao Post Daily 2020a).

As summer gave way to fall, there had been no new domestic infection cases for nearly six months and no imported cases for nearly three. There had been no community outbreak, no coronavirus fatality, and no healthcare or medical personnel infected (Leung 2020a). Except for one short episode of face mask panic buying (The Star 2020) daily life in Macao remained calm and orderly. All forty-six confirmed coronavirus patients recovered, with the last discharged from the hospital on 6 March 2020 (Government Information Bureau 2020c).

5.1 Multi-dimensional Challenges

This is not to say that Macao has not been severely impacted by the coronavirus outbreak. We have remarked earlier that the coronavirus pandemic is by its very nature a multi-dimensional crisis. Indeed, the onset of the pandemic immediately presented the Macao authorities with two grave and interrelated challenges beyond public health. First, Macao's economy relies disproportionally on the gaming and tourism industry. The severe tightening of border movements brought about an immediate economic fallout unprecedented in both depth and scale (Sullivan 2020; Macao News 2020h). Second, the normal functioning of Macao society depends immensely on a fluid and sustained flow of goods and labor across the border from China and, to a lesser but not insignificant extent, overseas. The extraordinary measures needed to combat the coronavirus pandemic could stress the social and economic fabrics into a state of disarray and even unrest, as witnessed in other countries.

Even allowing that health and infectious disease control measures take the front line in the fight against the coronavirus pandemic, the Macao authorities could not but confront a complex of diverse and compelling demands affecting every aspect of society's wellbeing.

5.2 *WoG Central Command and Coordination*

One of the first critically important actions on the part of the authorities at the onset of COVID-19 in Macao was the creation of a central, top-down WoG command centre to coordinate government-led measures in a whole-city anti-pandemic effort that fully recognized the multi-dimensionality of the undertaking.

When knowledge of an infectious outbreak in Wuhan first became known, the city reacted quickly by setting up, on 5 January, an "Interdepartmental Working Group Against Pneumonia of Unknown Cause" under the Health Bureau. On 21 January, one day before the first coronavirus infection was reported, Chief Executive Ho Iat Seng ordered the formation of the "Novel Coronavirus Response and Coordination Centre" directly under his office to replace the Working Group (Macao Printing Bureau 2020). Significantly, Ho appointed the Secretary for Social Affairs and Culture as co-chair of the Coordination Centre, clearly establishing the government's intention to take a broad, holistic approach to the task at hand. The Centre's membership comprised the heads and representatives from all the topline government agencies (Au 2020; Macao Printing Bureau 2020). This WoG message was clearly and consistently impressed on the public in the Coordination Centre's regular press conferences in which a panel of top government representatives answered questions from the press in live broadcasts.

5.3 *Isolation, Containment, and Prevention*

When the first coronavirus cases began to appear in Macao, the immediate urgency was to identify the infected individuals and those who could be at risk by contact, as well as to put in place measures to prevent escalation of the threat. This was to be done by a well-coordinated system of screening, tracing, quarantine, and medical care. Body temperature screenings and health declarations were implemented at all points of entry into Macao by mid-January, whereas compulsory medical observation was imposed on people entering Macao from mid-February 2020 (Au 2020). Within a week of the first reported case, opening hours were drastically reduced at the Border Gate (rthk.hk 2020). And before the month was over, the government had identified 1,113 travelers from Hubei who were still in Macao for quarantine (Bian et al. 2020). Then on 28 January, Beijing agreed to suspend the issuance of visitor's permits to mainlanders to enter Macao, effectively if not completely locking down the city (National Immigration Administration 2020).

On 23 January when Macao confirmed its second case of infection, the Tourism Office immediately canceled all Chinese New Year celebrations, including the New Year Parade (Marques 2020a). This was followed by an announcement from the Education and Youth Affairs Bureau that the Chinese New Year holidays were to be extended until at least 10 February (Macao News 2020a). It would not be until early May when senior secondary schools began to resume classes (Macao News 2020f). The next day, the Sports Bureau announced the closing of all sporting facilities (Health Bureau 2020). Government workers, except for those in emergency and critical services, were asked not to report to work from 8 February to 16 February, resulting in an effective shutdown of public services (Government Information Bureau 2020d). Beginning in mid-February, testing would be administered for groups: e.g., tour bus drivers, at high risk of infection (Government Information Bureau 2020b). In an unprecedented move, all casinos were ordered to shut down on 4 February for 15 days (Lahiri 2020; McAlinden 2020). Other public spaces such as cinemas, theatres, internet cafés, beauty salons, gyms, health clubs, etc., were to be closed until further notice (Office of the Chief Executive 2020).

5.4 Economic Relief

Given that in recent years, gaming alone contributed over 80% of Macao's total tax revenues, over 70% of visitor entries to Macao were from China, and nearly 40% of Macao's labor force were employed in the gaming, hospitality, and restaurant industries (DSEC 2019), the pandemic's impact was immediately felt throughout the economy. This can be attested in the reported figures of a 99.7% year-on-year decline in visitors in April (Blaschke 2020) and a 90% year-on-year drop in casino gross gaming revenue (GGR) in September (Newsdesk 2020).

As early as 31 January, the Secretary for Economy and Finance, Mr. Lei Wai Nong, announced the early distribution of the Wealth Partaking Scheme to Macao residents. He also reported that meetings were held with the Macao Chamber of Commerce, representatives of local SMEs, and property developers' associations to discuss support measures for local enterprises, and that the Economic Bureau was ready to assist eligible local businesses regarding financial subsidies (Government Information Bureau 2020a).

Then on 13 February, a comprehensive, multi-faceted economic relief plan was announced by the government that includes reduction of taxes and fees for local businesses and residents; financial subsidies to SMEs to support the continued existence of enterprises; measures to assist families and individuals at risk of penury;

and measures to protect work and wages (Scher 2020). A major focus of the government's economic subsidies is to incentivize job retention. In addition to direct aid to the city's workers, government subsidies for businesses are pegged to the retention of employees (Sénécaut 2020).

One measure of note in the government's economic relief effort was the support given to the local SMEs by putting money directly in the hands of the consumers. To date, there had been two rounds of electronic consumption card distribution totaling MOP 8,000 for each resident (Macao News 2020e). These cash cards have a daily consumption limit of MOP 300, ensuring that the SMEs are the main beneficiaries (Sénécaut 2020). In the same vein, the Macao Government Tourism Office spearheaded a subsidized domestic tourism scheme for local residents in support of tourism businesses (TTG Asia 2020; Siu 2020).

5.5 *Social Order and Livelihood*

With memory of the SARS outbreak in 2003 still fresh, there was an early consensus about the importance of face masks in the fight against the coronavirus pandemic among Macao's residents and the authorities. Even before the first local coronavirus infection case was reported and despite the Health Bureau's assurance of sufficient supply, there was a run on face masks on 10 January, leading to reports of shortages in a number of pharmacies (Macao Daily 2020). Following the report of Macao's first confirmed case, the Health Bureau immediately imposed a system of mask rationing in the city whereby residents and non-resident workers could purchase up to 10 masks per person every 10 days (Macao News 2020g; Marques 2020b). On the same day, the Guaranteed Mask Supply for Macao Residents Scheme was introduced together with the announcement that the government had ordered 20 million masks to sell to the public at cost (Novel Coronavirus Response and Coordination Centre 2020).

As part of the coordinated effort to maintain a sense of normalcy in the city's daily life in the middle of a developing pandemic, the Economic Affairs Bureau and Consumer Committee dispatched inspectors to monitor grocery prices and inventory on a regular basis (Au 2020). When a local grocery chain was found in May to have jacked up the prices of a number of grocery items, taking advantage of the knowledge that residents were in possession of government-issued electronic coupons, the authorities promptly revoked the company's eligibility to partake in the scheme (Macao Post Daily 2020b).

6 COVID-19 Action in Hong Kong Special Administrative Region (HKSAR)

6.1 The COVID-19 Outbreak and Its Impact

As of 15 December 2020, over 7722 confirmed cases (6345 of whom already discharged) and 122 deaths were registered in Hong Kong (HKSAR Government 2020a).

The first wave of COVID-19 began with the first confirmed case of COVID-19 found in late January 2020. Many Hong Kong citizens proceeded to purchase various personal protective equipment, mindful of the lessons learnt during the difficult SARS outbreak in 2003. To this date, it remains unclear whether the epidemic was initially sparked in the city by visitors or returning Hong Kong citizens and residents—a conundrum that may highlight initial Immigration Clearance shortcomings. In response to the crisis, public transportation organisations, such as the Hong Kong Railway and the Hong Kong Airport Authority, enforced enhanced cleaning and disinfection measures on the Guangzhou-Shenzhen-Hong Kong High Speed Rail and planes. Infrared thermometers were placed in all Immigration Clearance stations and additional manpower was assigned to boundary control stations. The HKSAR Government also mandated that incomers who had visited Wuhan (where the virus was first detected in Mainland China) within the last 14 days showing fever and respiratory symptoms would be instantly transferred to hospitals for treatment and isolation. Moreover, the Compulsory Quarantine of Certain Persons Arriving at Hong Kong Regulation and the Prevention and Control of Disease Regulation were set up to further control the COVID-19 outbreak.

The second wave of COVID-19 started at the end of March 2020 when a large number of Hong Kong residents and students studying abroad started to return from overseas. The HKSAR Government then started implementing mandatory quarantine for those who had been to foreign countries in the previous 14 days. The wave was well controlled, and no new confirmed cases of COVID-19 were recorded for 23 consecutive days from April to May. This possibly contributed to complacency and negligence among some sections of the population: following reports of breaches of quarantine measures, in fact, the HKSAR Government was forced to deploy more resources to random-check inbound travelers, including citizens and residents. In addition, foreign domestic helpers' employers were required to make home quarantine arrangements for their helpers upon their arrival in Hong Kong.

The third wave of COVID-19 started at the beginning of July 2020, largely due to an existing exemption—justified by economic reasons—from strict quarantine requirements of some 200,000 people, including mostly aircrew members and seafarers (Cheung 2020). More than 100 confirmed cases per day were detected from mid-July to the end of July. To effectively deal with the third wave of COVID-19, the HKSAR Government started to impose more stringent quarantine measures among aircrew members and seafarers and social distancing regulations, in particular prohibiting group gatherings. The Prevention and Control of Disease (Prohibition on

Group Gathering) Regulation was enforced to tighten the number of people allowed in a group gathering from 4 to 2, and on-the-spot fines were also issued for breaches of the two-person rule (HKSAR Government 2020b). Flexible work arrangements for government employees were also implemented (HKSAR Government 2020c).

A fourth wave of COVID-19 started in November 2020, mainly due to two big clusters—a dancing group and a team of construction workers—who failed to properly use masks and social-distance during close contact activities and manual work. The HKSAR Government reacted quickly and closed specific venues, in addition to further tightening social distancing measures, and requiring particular groups to undergo mandatory COVID-19 testing. The HKSAR Government also launched the "LeaveHomeSafe" mobile app on 11 November 2020 and encouraged the public to record their whereabouts and set up more specimen collection points in various districts across the territory and MTR Stations.

In Hong Kong too, the pandemic has had persisting and wide-ranging effects that transcended the public health dimension, severely affecting also the local economy and citizens' overall wellbeing.

The economy of Hong Kong performed poorly in the second quarter of 2020, with a drastic drop of 9% in real GDP, and forecasts of further contractions between—6% to—8% (HKSAR Government 2020d). Tourism in Hong Kong was severely affected due to the mandatory 14-day quarantine regulation: total visitor arrivals from January to June 2020 fell by 89.9% compared to the same period in 2019 (Hong Kong Tourism Board 2020). This significant drop in the number of visitors also hit the aviation and accommodation industry: the Hong Kong Airport Authority reported a year-on-year drop of 98.6% in the number of passengers arriving at Hong Kong Airport and 73.2% in the number of flights (Hong Kong International Airport 2020). The accommodation industry also suffered significantly, with various hotels—especially high-end ones—facing the concrete threat of permanent closure. In addition, the retail industry saw a 33.3% drop in consumer sales from January to June 2020 (Leung 2020b). The Hong Kong Retail Management Association reported that 96% of companies had suffered losses in their business due to the outbreak and that around 5,200 retail stores were closed by the end of May because of the unprofitable business environment in Hong Kong (Leung 2020c). Under the prohibition on gathering regulation, many restaurants suffered significant losses, reported in the range of 5 billion Hong Kong Dollars in July and 6.5 billion in August (Yau et al. 2020). With many businesses forced to close temporarily or permanently, the unemployment rate in the July-September quarter of 2020 stood 6.4%—more than double the rate of 2.9% in the same period of 2019 and dangerously close to the all-time high of 8.5 recorded in 2003, during the SARS pandemic (HKSAR Government 2020e).

The economic downturn and the rising unemployment rates negatively impacted citizen's quality of life. According to a study from the University of Hong Kong, for instance, three fourths of Hong Kong citizens showed moderate-to-high symptoms of depression during the COVID-19 outbreak (Choy 2020). Faced with repeated COVID-19 waves and the traditionally high costs of living in Hong Kong, socio-economically vulnerable groups were particularly hard hit. Already in March 2020 a research conducted by the Hong Kong Council of Social Service pointed out that the majority of its beneficiaries had difficulty in paying household expenses, with more than half of the respondents stating that their household income had decreased by at least 50%, and more than 30% stating that the decrease reached 70% or above (HKCSS 2020).

6.2 Actions Undertaken by the HKSAR Government to Combat the Outbreak

The COVID-19 outbreak in Hong Kong proved itself to be as much about "life" as it was about "livelihood": related actions, therefore, had to be undertaken across the whole government. Notable examples of these actions are:

The Department of Health set up thematic hotlines and a website for public enquiry; held daily press conferences to provide updates on the latest new cases; implemented special measures in public hospitals to cope with outbreak events (e.g. suspension of visiting arrangements); informed all private hospitals, doctors and Chinese medicine practitioners to refer suspected cases; amended the Prevention and Control of Disease Ordinance (Cap. 599) and made COVID-19 a statutorily notifiable infectious disease; handled compulsory quarantine of all incomers; kept enhancing virus testing capabilities and provided more COVID-19 testing services; investigated the infection sources and conducted a series of infection control actions with various governmental departments; launched funding to support the two medical schools of Hong Kong University & Chinese University of Hong Kong to conduct COVID-19 research.

The Financial Committee launched three rounds of measures totaling 287.5 billion Hong Kong Dollars to help both the public and various industries by "supporting enterprises, safeguarding jobs and relieving financial burdens" (HKSAR Government 2020f); the "supporting enterprises" component of the scheme would provide financial support to affected enterprises in sectors such as tourism, retail, and catering, temporarily waive some governmental fees, introduce low-interest loans, and reduce electricity, water and properties hire charges; jobs would be "safeguarded" by providing wage subsidies to employers for retaining employees, by providing a one-time subsidy to self-employed persons, by creating 30000 jobs in the public and private sectors in the coming two years (with the HKSAR Government hiring 10,000 civil servants and creating 5000 short-term internships for young people) as well as by encouraging employees to learn new skills and assisting enterprises to use technology; the "financial burden relief" would consist of 10,000 Hong Kong Dollars paid to Hong Kong permanent residents aged 18 or above, the provision of transport subsidies to all citizens, the reduction of salary taxes, the temporary waiving of domestic property taxes, as well as the provision of electricity charge subsidies to each residential electricity account and more allowance to citizens at the grassroots level.

The Education Bureau disseminated related information to schools; made appropriate arrangements for different examinations; suspended classes for the first time in February and then constantly adjusted the school resumption arrangements; kept improving the development of e-learning and provided necessary help to students in need.

The Transport Department broadcasted related information to transport sectors; required management companies to intensity disinfection on public transport; checked whether members of the public wore masks when taking public transport.

The Housing Department reminded personal households and shops to keep good hygiene; strengthened the cleaning and disinfection measures in the common areas of all Housing Authority public housing estates and provided adequate personal protective equipment to frontline cleaning staff.

The Food and Environmental Hygiene Department inspected restaurants to determine whether social distancing and body temperature checking regulations were followed, as well as hawker stalls to ascertain whether the appropriate hygiene was maintained; kept arranging free COVID-19 testing services for high-risk groups.

The Leisure and Cultural Services Department devised arrangements on body temperature checking and access to venues according to the relevant trends in COVID-19 outbreak; set up an online resource centre for the public to access cultural entertainment.

The Social Welfare Department supplied protective gear to vulnerable groups; kept providing relief materials and psychological services to people in quarantine; kept arranging free COVID-19 testing services for high-risk groups; gave anti-virus coating spray to care homes for the elderly and for people with disabilities.

The Labour Department distributed information material to key working stations to share health advice; appealed to foreign domestic helpers to stay at home on their rest days; appealed to employers to make flexible work arrangements.

To ensure effective action across government, accurate information must be shared and competing interdepartmental priorities must be holistically managed. To these ends, inter-departmental mechanisms are required. To combat COVID-19, even as early as 2 January 2020 when no cases were confirmed in Hong Kong, the local government had already organized an inter-departmental meeting to share information and discuss possible response prevention measures (HKSAR Government 2020d). To manage competing priorities among departments, the Chief Executive of the HKSAR Government, with the assistance from the Executive Council, reviewed anti-pandemic measures submitted by various bureaus and department across the government, and decided how and when to devise social distancing measures. The HKSAR Government constantly kept adjusting these actions during the outbreak so as to strike a constructive and sustainable balance between public health emergency and socio-economic needs, a policy of moderation boding well for the future of the city in its fight against COVID-19.

7 Synthesis and Conclusions

7.1 *Strong and Effective Government Leadership*

Our three case studies of China, Hong Kong, and Macao clearly show why the WoG and HiAP approaches are necessary in combating a pandemic such as COVID-19.

There are two aspects of a pandemic crisis that accentuate the importance of strong and effective government leadership. First, when confronting a pandemic outbreak, time is of the essence. Decisive and bold government actions are critical, particularly at the onset of the crisis, in helping to frame and condition the ultimate parameters of the anti-pandemic undertaking. Second, pandemics are systemic threats that require a multi-dimensional response. Only the government has the necessary institutional tools and resources at its disposal to quickly implement a comprehensive master plan to control and manage the outbreak.

All three government authorities in our case studies acted quickly at the outset of the pandemic with a multi-front, multi-agencies campaign to isolate and contain the coronavirus outbreak. A comprehensive system of screening, testing, contact tracing, medical care and treatment, and quarantine was immediately put in place, together with strong and decisive actions to reduce the movements of people to a necessary minimum, including strict border control, reduction of public transportation and government services, temporary work and school stoppage, shelter-in-place measures, social distancing and group congregation restrictions, and, when the prospect of full-blown escalation appeared imminent, even city-wide lockdowns.

Needless to say, the effectiveness of the WoG and HiAP approaches in a pandemic crisis correlates closely to how well and consistently the government authorities are able to coordinate the multitude of moving parts, in both the public and the private sectors, of the total endeavor. If the three cases under study reveal variations in the degree of success in different facets of the anti-pandemic efforts, these divergences can be explained in terms of this correlation. It is more than plausible, therefore, that the urgent, diverse and intertwined needs of governance in a time of pandemic may be more effectively addressed with a master action plan formulated by the head of government and executed through a set of coordinated action plans by various ministries and departments, similar to those devised by the UN and its specialized agencies, funds and programmes to achieve a common goal. Ideally, the continuity and sustainability of such concerted efforts should also become a concern beyond the most acute phases of the public health emergency: the sound, permanent incorporation of the WoG and HiAP approaches into broader national (and international) sustainable development governance frameworks, in fact, would likely yield benefits that would transcend the solution of a single given ongoing crisis and significantly help mitigate, if not prevent altogether, the next.

7.2 Civil Commitment and Inclusion

As evidenced in our three case studies, among the most delicate and vital anti-pandemic tasks undertaken by the government authorities was the management of its relationship with the public. In principle, it can be argued that one way to put the pandemic quickly under control is to strong-arm an immediate, up-and-down shut down of civil society—a sort of induced temporary stasis, so to speak—for the duration of the virus's infectious period, which in COVID-19's case is about two weeks. However, a total lockdown of this magnitude and thoroughness, even for a short period, requires an inordinate amount of mobilization and resources, lest we run into the classic paradox of the cure being more deleterious than the illness. Of the three cases we studied, only China was able to pull off an operation successfully with such strong and forceful measures. But as we have noted when discussing China's anti-pandemic experience, not only does China benefit from a strong and strictly hierarchical administrative system and a tradition of social regimentation, it had the advantage of having the capacity to bring in massive amount of aid and assistance to Wuhan from other parts of the country, including fielding over forty thousand medical personnel from other provinces, construction of two temporary field hospitals in less than two weeks, not to mention the deployment of the People's Liberation Army for enforcement and security needs. This is a luxury unavailable to Hong Kong or Macao.

For Hong Kong and Macao, therefore, the authorities must strike a careful balance between taking strong and decisive anti-pandemic measures and mitigating the resulting systemic disruptions to the daily life of the residents, hence the wide array of extraordinary social and economic relief programmes put in place by the respective governments, all of which demand an incredible degree of WoG leadership to orchestrate multi- and inter-agencies actions.

In all the three contexts surveyed, in fact, the contraction in economic output has been substantial. To lessen the enormous impact on livelihood, the respective governments have indeed come up with a wide range of stimulus packages like lump sum payments to households, wage subsidies, reductions and deferments of rent payments, loans and subsidies to businesses, and more. Without these relief packages, government mandated social distancing restrictions could not have been enforced, and the different waves of the pandemic could not have been controlled. Nevertheless, equality implications have emerged, with people from the lower socio-economic strata faring worse for various reasons, including loss of income due to social distancing and increased exposure to COVID-19 infections. This suggests the need to accompany the macro-economically essential financial support to big firms with relief measures targeting directly and specifically those disadvantaged population groups.

As our case studies show in particular regard to Hong Kong and Macao, strong and effective government leadership is critical and necessary, but it may not be sufficient. Precisely because of the relative autonomy of Hong Kong's and Macao's civil society, in order for the anti-pandemic endeavor to have better than a fighting chance, the public must, first, have sufficient confidence in government leadership and, second, hold a shared perception that they as individuals and groups have ownership in the collective effort. It is for the fostering of this government-civil society partnership that we emphasized above the importance of the government in managing its relationship with the public.

Take, for example, the issue with face masks. It is true that, as our three case studies have shown, there was an early and universal recognition among the public in China, Hong Kong, and Macao of the importance of wearing face masks as a preventive anti-pandemic measure, most likely due to their memory of the SARS epidemic in 2003. In Macao, following the panic run on face masks on 10 January, the government immediately put in place the Guaranteed Mask Supply for Macao Residents Scheme and a city-wide rationing programme for face mask distribution. The latter is carried out in a public clinics-private pharmacies partnership that ensures not only sufficient but also easy access to face mask supply for the city's residents. As if that was not enough, Chief Executive Ho Iat Seng reassured the public in early February that his team would seek to procure masks and other medical supplies in the global market at all cost (Hong Kong Economic Journal 2020).

In this respect, the Macao government's performance compares favorably with its counterpart's in Hong Kong, where images of the city's residents in long lines scrambling to buy face masks became a point of discontent about the government's shortcomings (Pao 2020; Crawford 2020). This is by no means to downplay Hong Kong's remarkable achievements in the fight against COVID-19. There should be no denying that the Hong Kong government's swift actions on multiple fronts in the anti-pandemic fight have played a critical role in stabilizing what could easily have been a much more volatile state of affairs (Saiidi 2020).

However, to the extent that in some respects Hong Kong civil society's own anti-pandemic initiative may have taken perhaps half a step ahead of its confidence in the government, it does highlight that the civil society's proactive commitment to combating the pandemic is an indispensable weapon no WoG or HiAP approach should or can afford to ignore.

References

Al Takarli, N. (2020) China's response to the COVID-19 outbreak: A model for epidemic preparedness and management. *Dubai Medical Journal*. Available at: https://www.karger.com/Article/Pdf/508448 (Accessed 7 September 2020).

Asp, N. (2007) Health claims for foods in focus. *Scandinavian Journal Food Nutrition*, Volume 51, 90.

Au, A. (2020) Communicating prevention in the COVID-19 epidemic: Case study on Macao SAR. *Research Square*. Preprint. Available at: https://doi.org/10.21203/rs.3.rs-16832/v1 (Accessed 20 September 2020).

Australian Public Service Commission. (2004) Connecting government: Whole of government responses to Australia's priority challenges. Available at: http://www.apsc.gov.au/publications-and-media/archive/publications-archive/connecting-government (Accessed 4 May 2015).

BBC. (2020) Coronavirus confirmed as pandemic by World Health Organization. Available at: https://www.bbc.com/news/world-51839944 (Accessed 7 September 2020).

Beijing Youth Daily. (2020) Keep mask producing machine working! national development and reform commission: Please do not hesitate to increase production. Available at: https://www.sohu.com/a/372114402_148781 (Accessed 17 June 2020).

Bian, X., Yao, L. & Bian, Y. (2020) Effective COVID-19 prevention and control in areas of ultra-dense population: Lessons from Macao SAR. *Journal of Clinical Intensive Care and Medicine* [Online], Volume 5 (1): 22–25. Available at: https://doi.org/10.29328/journal.jcicm.1001031 (Accessed 20 September 2020).

Blaschke, B. (2020) Macao GGR down 90.0% to MOP$2.21 billion in September [Online]. Available at: https://www.instapaper.com/read/1347868645 (Accessed 1 October 2020).

CGTN. (2020a) 40 Days in Hubei: The central government team's role in coronavirus epidemic control. Available at: https://news.cgtn.com/news/2020-03-06/Central-government-s-40-days-in-coronavirus-hit-Hubei-ODwhH9ahUc/index.html (Accessed 17 June 2020).

CGTN. (2020b) Shanghai, most of China to reopen schools by end of April, Beijing and Hubei yet to decide. Available at: https://news.cgtn.com/news/2020-04-09/Shanghai-most-of-China-reopen-schools-by-end-of-April-Pyp87FuTpm/index.html (Accessed 7 September 2020).

Chadwick, E. (1842) Report on the sanitary condition of the labouring population and on the means of its improvement. i6 Editorial. Downloaded from http://heapro.oxfordjournals.org/ by guest on September 14, 2014 http://www.deltaomega.org/documents/ChadwickClassic.pdf (Last accessed 30 April 2014).

Chen, S., et al. (2020) Fangcang shelter hospitals: A novel concept for responding to public health emergencies. *The Lancet*. Available at: https://www.thelancet.com/journals/lancet/article/PIIS0140-6736(20)30744-3/fulltext (Accessed 17 June 2020).

Cheung, H. (2020) COVID-19: Why Hong Kong's 'Third Wave' is a warning. Available at: https://www.bbc.com/news/world-asia-china-53596299 (Accessed 2 October 2020).

China Daily. (2020a) White paper – Fighting COVID-19: China in action. Available at: https://covid19.chinadaily.com.cn/a/202006/08/WS5edd8bd6a3108348172515ec.html (Accessed 5 September 2020).

China Daily. (2020b) China's fight against COVID-19. Available at: https://covid-19.chinadaily.com.cn/a/202004/21/WS5e9e2c62a3105d50a3d17880_1.html (Accessed 7 September 2020).

Choy, G. (2020) One-two punch of protests, coronavirus playing havoc with mental health in Hong Kong, study finds. *South China Morning Post*. Available at: https://www.scmp.com/news/hong-kong/health-environment/article/3096326/one-two-punch-protests-coronavirus-playing-havoc (Accessed 2 October 2020).

Civil Aviation Administration of China. (2020a) *Airplane information released on 'fight against epidemic and quickly support Wuhan*. Available at: http://www.caac.gov.cn/XXGK/XXGK/TZTG/202003/t20200319_201530.html (Accessed 17 June 2020).

Civil Aviation Administration of China. (2020b) *Notice on continue reducing international flights during epidemic*. Available at: http://www.caac.gov.cn/XXGK/XXGK/TZTG/202003/t20200326_201746.html (Accessed 17 June 2020).

Crawford, A. (2020) Panic buying in Hong Kong amid 'alarming' spread of coronavirus. Available at: https://news.sky.com/story/panic-buying-in-hong-kong-amid-alarming-spread-of-coronavirus-11924399 (Accessed 2 October 2020).

Dong, Z. (2020) Chinese military sends additional 2,600 medical personnel to Wuhan. Available at: http://eng.mod.gov.cn/news/2020-02/13/content_4860355.htm (Accessed 17 June 2020).

DSEC. (2019) Macao Statistics 2019. Macao: Macao SAR Bureau of Statistics and Survey.

Government Information Bureau. (2020a) *Fresh government measures support Macao residents, SMES amid coronavirus control work*. Available at: https://www.gov.mo/en/news/122454/ (Accessed 20 September 2020).

Government Information Bureau. (2020b) *Updates for the press–Expand the testing, testing of tour bus drivers*. Available at: https://www.gov.mo/zh-hant/news/317900/ (Accessed 20 September 2020).

Government Information Bureau. (2020c) L*ast COVID-19 patient in Macao discharged after successful treatment.* Available at: https://www.gov.mo/en/news/125402/ (Accessed 20 September 2020).

Government Information Bureau. (2020d) *To combat the epidemic: Government employees do not report to work from 8 to 16 February.* Available at: https://news.gov.mo/detail/zh-hant/N20BGROZbm (Accessed 23 September 2020).

Health Bureau. (2020) *Temporary suspension of services at sports bureau sporting facilities starting from 4 pm this afternoon.* Available at: https://www.gov.mo/zh-hant/news/315058/ (Accessed 20 September 2020).

HKSAR Government. (2020a) *Latest developments.* Available at: https://www.hkeconomy.gov.hk/en/situation/development/index.htm (Accessed 2 October 2020).

HKSAR Government. (2020b) *Frequently asked questions on new requirements to reduce gatherings.* Available at: https://www.coronavirus.gov.hk/eng/social_distancing-faq.html (Accessed 2 October 2020).

HKSAR Government. (2020c) *Public services to resume in a safe and orderly manner* [Press release]. Available at: https://www.info.gov.hk/gia/general/202008/20/P2020082000520.htm?fontSize=1 (Accessed 2 October 2020).

HKSAR Government. (2020d) *Government holds inter-departmental meeting on cluster of pneumonia cases in Wuhan* (with photo) [Press release]. Available at: https://www.info.gov.hk/gia/general/202001/02/P2020010200831.htm (Accessed 2 October 2020).

HKSAR Government. (2020e). *Unemployment and underemployment statistics for July - September 2019.* [Press release]. Available at: https://www.info.gov.hk/gia/general/201910/18/P2019101800410.htm (Accessed 2 October 2020).

HKSAR Government. (2020f). *Budget speech by the financial secretary* (1) (with photos/video). [Press release]. Available at: https://www.info.gov.hk/gia/general/202002/26/P2020022600169.htm?fontSize=1 (Accessed 2 October 2020).

Hong Kong Council of Social Service. (2020) *Survey on the living conditions of disadvantaged groups under the epidemic.* Available at: https://www.hkcss.org.hk/%e3%80%8c%e7%96%ab%e6%83%85%e4%b8%8b%e5%bc%b1%e5%8b%a2%e7%a4%be%e7%be%a4%e7%9a%84%e7%94%9f%e6%b4%bb%e7%8b%80%e6%b3%81%e8%aa%bf%e6%9f%a5%e3%80%8d/?lang=en (Accessed 2 October 2020).

Hong Kong Economic Journal. (2020) What our CE can learn from her Macao counterpart. Available at: https://www.ejinsight.com/eji/article/id/2371826/20200206-What-our-CE-can-learn-from-her-Macau-counterpart (Accessed 2 October 2020).

Hong Kong International Airport. (2020) COVID-19 pandemic continues to impact air traffic in July AA receives two awards in recognition of its excellence in nurturing young talent. Available at: https://www.hongkongairport.com/en/media-centre/press-release/2020/pr_1470 (Accessed 2 October 2020).

Hong Kong Tourism Board. (2020) *Monthly report-visitor arrivals statistics: Jun 2020.* Available at: https://partnernet.hktb.com/filemanager/intranet/pm/VisitorArrivalStatistics/ViS_Stat_E/VisE_2020/Tourism%20Statistics%2006%202020.pdf (Accessed 2 October 2020).

Huanqiu. (2020) The National Heath Commission: The current situation of COVID-19 is still under control. Available at: https://china.huanqiu.com/article/9CaKrnKoYBB (Accessed 17 June 2020).

Lahiri, T. (2020) The world's gambling capital is taking no chances with coronavirus. Available at: https://qz.com/1796500/macau-shuts-casinos-over-coronavirus-fears/ (Accessed 20 September 2020).

Leung, K. (2020a) Macao's last COVID-19 patient recovers, with no new cases for a month. *South China Morning Post.* Available at: https://www.scmp.com/news/hong-kong/health-environment/article/3074025/macau-discharges-last-recovered-coronavirus (Accessed 20 September 2020).

Leung, K. (2020c) Estimated 10,400 retail workers axed, 5,200 shops to close in Hong Kong by end of May as coronavirus hammers sector, trade body warns. *South China Morning Post.* Available at: https://www.scmp.com/news/hong-kong/health-environment/article/3080271/estimated-10400-retail-workers-axed-5200-shops (Accessed 2 October 2020).

Leung. K. (2020b) Coronavirus: Hong Kong retail shrinks by a third for first half of 2020 as COVID-19 crisis pummels sector. *South China Morning Post.* Available at: https://www.scmp.com/news/hong-kong/hong-kong-economy/article/3095334/coronavirus-hong-kong-retail-shrinks-third-first (Accessed 2 October 2020).

Li, X., Cui, W., & Zhang, F. (2020) Who was the first doctor to report the COVID-19 outbreak in Wuhan, China? *The Journal of Nuclear Medicine.* Available at: http://jnm.snmjournals.org/content/61/6/782.full (Accessed 7 September 2020).

Liu, C., Xu, K., & Du, Q. (2020) China's flexible fiscal arrangements offer adequate medical expenses for treating COVID-19 patients. Available at: https://www.globaltimes.cn/content/1182599.shtml (Accessed 7 September 2020).

Lu, H. (2020) Nearly 4 million community workers fighting on front line of epidemic control: Official. Available at: http://www.xinhuanet.com/english/2020-02/10/c_138771330.htm (Accessed 7 September 2020).

Macao Daily. (2020) News flash. Available at: http://www.macaodaily.com/html/2020-01/10/content_1408320.htm (Accessed 20 September 2020).

Macao News. (2020a) Schools are closed until February 10 due to coronavirus cases. Available at: https://macaunews.mo/schools-are-closed-until-february-10-due-to-coronavirus-cases/ (Accessed 20 September 2020).

Macao News. (2020b) 8th coronavirus case confirmed in a Macau resident. Available at: https://macaunews.mo/8th-coronavirus-case-confirmed-in-a-macau-resident/ (Accessed 20 September 2020).

Macao News. (2020c) 9th case of coronavirus infection in Macau. Available at: https://macaunews.mo/ninth-case-of-coronavirus-infection-in-macau/ (Accessed 20 September 2020).

Macao News. (2020d) 10th coronavirus case confirmed. Available at: https://macaunews.mo/10th-coronavirus-case-confirmed/ (Accessed 20 September 2020).

Macao News. (2020e) Consumption subsidy smartcard spending starts today. Available at: https://macaunews.mo/consumption-subsidy-smartcard-spending-starts-today/ (Accessed 20 September 2020).

Macao News. (2020f) Senior secondary school pupils return to their classrooms. Available at: https://macaunews.mo/senior-secondary-school-pupils-return-to-their-classrooms/ (Accessed 20 September 2020).

Macao News. (2020g) SSM stands at forefront of COVID-19 fight. Available at: https://macaunews.mo/ssm-stands-at-forefront-of-covid-19-fight/ (Accessed 20 September 2020).

Macao News. (2020h) Macao to recover in 2021, reliant on Chinese tourism. Available at: https://macaunews.mo/macao-to-recover-in-2021-reliant-on-chinese-tourism/ (Accessed 20 September 2020).

Macao Post Daily. (2020) Macau confirms 46th COVID-19 case, 1st in 78 days. Available at: https://macaupostdaily.com/article8623.html (Accessed 20 September 2020).

Macao Post Daily. (2020) Royal supermarket apologises for 'price confusion'. Available at: https://www.macaupostdaily.com/article8241.html (Accessed 20 September 2020).

Macao Printing Bureau. (2020) *Establishment of the novel coronavirus infection contingency coordination centre.* Available at: https://bo.io.gov.mo/bo/i/2020/03/despce_cn.asp#23 (Accessed 20 September 2020).

Marques, R. (2020a) Tourism board cancels all CNY events and activities. Available at: https://macaudailytimes.com.mo/tourism-board-cancels-all-cny-events-and-activities.html (Accessed 20 September 2020).

Marques, R. (2020b) 2019-NCoV | face mask stocks sufficient, more arriving on February 2. Available at: https://macaudailytimes.com.mo/2019-ncov-face-mask-stocks-sufficient-more-arriving-on-february-2.html (Accessed 20 September 2020).

McAlinden, T. (2020) Macau tells casinos to close over Wuhan Virus - RTHK. Available at: https://news.rthk.hk/rthk/en/component/k2/1506543-20200204.htm?spTabChangeable=0 (Accessed 20 September 2020).

Ministry of Commerce. (2020) *Ministry of Commerce spokesperson talked about the work of nine-province joint supply guarantee mechanism.* Available at: http://scyxs.mofcom.gov.cn/article/baogong/202003/20200302941257.shtml (Accessed 17 June 2020).

Ministry of Education. (2020a) *Notice for schools at all levels to delay the start of the Spring Term.* Available at: http://www.moe.gov.cn/jyb_xwfb/gzdt_gzdt/s5987/202001/t20200127_416672.html (Accessed 17 June 2020).

Ministry of Education. (2020b) *Ministry of Education: Over 200 million students went back to class, resumption rate reached 75%.* Available at: http://www.bjnews.com.cn/edu/2020/07/14/748597.html (Accessed 7 September 2020).

Ministry of Foreign Affairs. (2020) *Ministry of Foreign Affairs of The People's Republic of China National Immigration Administration announcement on entry by foreign nationals holding valid Chinese residence permits of three categories.* Available at: https://www.fmprc.gov.cn/mfa_eng/wjbxw/t1817370.shtml (Accessed 23 September 2020).

Ministry of Transport of the PRC. (2020a) *Urgent notice of the Ministry of Transport on the prevention and control of the epidemic and transportation coordination.* Available at: http://xxgk.mot.gov.cn/jigou/ysfws/202001/t20200130_3328400.html (Accessed 17 June 2020).

Ministry of Transport of the PRC. (2020b) *Notice of the Ministry of Transport on the guarantee of the emergency transportation of materials and personnel for the prevention and control of the novel coronavirus pneumonia epidemic.* Available at: http://xxgk.mot.gov.cn/jigou/ysfws/202001/t20200130_3328387.html (Accessed 17 June 2020).

National Immigration Administration. (2020) *The bureau of immigration management suspends issuance of visitor permits to Hong Kong and Macau.* Available at: https://www.nia.gov.cn/n741440/n741542/c1214127/content.html (Accessed 20 September 2020).

Newsdesk. (2020) Macau casino GGR up 66pct m-o-m in Sept: Govt. GGRASIA. Available at: https://www.GGRAsia.com/macau-casino-ggr-up-66pct-m-o-m-in-sept-govt/ (Accessed 1 October 2020).

Nielsen. (2020) Nielsen: Eating at home will remain the new reality for Asian consumers, especially Hong Kong, post COVID-19. Available at: https://en.prnasia.com/releases/apac/nielsen-eating-at-home-will-remain-the-new-reality-for-asian-consumers-especially-hong-kong-post-covid-19-278643.shtml (Accessed 2 October 2020).

Novel Coronavirus Response and Coordination Centre. (2020) *Local mask supply is sufficient, masks delivered to Macao totals 9.8 million at present and are up to quality standards.* Available at: https://www.gov.mo/en/news/122281/ (Accessed 20 September 2020).

Office of the Chief Executive. (2020) *Printing bureau - Executive order of the chief executive.* Available at: https://bo.io.gov.mo/bo/i/2020/05/despce_cn.asp (Accessed 20 September 2020).

Pao, J. (2020) Virus-panic buying hits Hong Kong supermarkets. *Asia Times.* Available at: https://asiatimes.com/2020/01/virus-panic-buying-hits-hong-kong-supermarkets/ (Accessed 2 October 2020).

Peng,Y. (2020) The national health commissions: 346 medical teams and 42,600 personnel were sent to support Wuhan and Hubei. women contribute to 2/3 of the population. Available at: http://news.china.com.cn/txt/2020-03/08/content_75788717.htm (Accessed 17 June 2020).

Porter, R. (1997) *The greatest benefit to mankind: A medical history of humanity.* London: HarperCollins.

Räsänen, L. (2007) Of all foods bread is the most noble: Carl von Linne´ (Carl Linnaeus) on bread. *Food and Nutrition Research,* Volume 51, 91–99.

Rosen, G. (1993) *A history of public health.* Baltimore: JHU Press.

Rthk.hk. (2020) Macau announced reduction of opening hours to 3 hours per day at the border gate crossing. Available at: https://news.rthk.hk/rthk/ch/component/k2/1504833-20200125.htm?archive_date=2020-01-25 (Accessed 20 September 2020).

Saiidi, U. (2020) How Hong Kong beat coronavirus and avoided lockdown. *CNBC.* Available at: https://www.cnbc.com/2020/07/03/how-hong-kong-beat-coronavirus-and-avoided-lockdown.html (Accessed 2 October 2020).

Scher, I. (2020) Macau to give residents cash to boost local economy - Insider. Available at: https://www.insider.com/macau-to-give-residents-cash-to-boost-local-economy-2020-2 (Accessed 20 September 2020).
Sénécaut, B. (2020) Tourism and COVID-19: The case of Macau. Available at: https://www.eias.org/news/tourism-and-covid-19-the-case-of-macau/ (Accessed 20 September 2020).
Siu, R. (2020) Policy pragmatism key to Macau's COVID-19 success. *East Asia Forum*. Available at: https://www.eastasiaforum.org/2020/09/30/policy-pragmatism-key-to-macaus-covid-19-success/ (Accessed 1 October 2020).
Snow, J. (1855) *On the mode of communication of cholera*. London: John Churchill.
Sohu. (2020) The doctor and hospital that firstly discovered and reported epidemic were exposed. Available at: https://www.sohu.com/a/370109572_99988005 (Accessed 7 September 2020).
South China Morning Post. (2020) China pledges largest-ever economic rescue package to save jobs and livelihoods amid coronaviruses. Available at: https://www.scmp.com/economy/china-economy/article/3086569/china-pledges-largest-ever-economic-rescue-package-save-jobs (Accessed 30 August 2020).
Special Webpage against Epidemics: Statistics. n.d. Available at: https://www.ssm.gov.mo/apps1/PreventCOVID-19/en.aspx#clg17458 (Accessed 4 August 2020).
Sullivan, L. (2020) Macau's gaming revenue fell 88 percent in February. *Casino Review* (blog). Available at: https://www.casino-review.co/macau-gaming-revenue/ (Accessed 20 September 2020).
Tan, S. (2020) China's novel health tracker: Green on public health, red on data surveillance. Available at: https://www.csis.org/blogs/trustee-china-hand/chinas-novel-health-tracker-green-public-health-red-data-surveillance (Accessed 7 September 2020).
Tang, K. C., Ståhl, T., Bettcher, D., & De Leeuw, E. (2014) (Ed.) Rhetoric to action, health in all policies. *Health Promotion International*, Volume 29 (1), 1–8.
The Star. (2020) Face mask supplies run out across in Asia due to virus panic. Available at: https://www.thestar.com.my/business/business-news/2020/01/24/face-mask-supplies-run-out-across-in-asia-due-to-virus-panic (Accessed 20 September 2020).
Time. (2020) 'How can I get through this?' The impact of coronavirus on China's economy is only just beginning. Available at: https://time.com/5824599/china-coronavirus-covid19-economy/ (Accessed 14 September 2020).
TTG Asia. (2020) Macau rolls out subsidised tours for locals. Available at: https://www.ttgasia.com/2020/06/18/macau-rolls-out-subsidised-tours-for-locals/ (Accessed 20 September 2020).
UN. (2001) *Summary of the declaration of commitment on HIV/AIDs*. Available at: https://www.unaids.org/sites/default/files/sub_landing/files/jc668-keepingpromise_en.pdf. (Accessed 30 August 2020).
UN. (2020) *United nations comprehensive response to COVID-19: Saving lives, protecting societies, recovering better.* United Nations.
USNews. (2020) China reports 61 new COVID-19 cases for Sunday, highest daily domestic infections since March 6. Available at: https://www.usnews.com/news/world/articles/2020-07-26/china-reports-61-new-covid-19-cases-for-sunday-highest-daily-domestic-infections-since-march-6 (Accessed 7 September 2020).
Wang, J., Zhu, E., & Umlauf, T. (2020) How China built two coronavirus hospitals in just over a week. *The Wall Street Journal*. Available at: https://www.wsj.com/articles/how-china-can-build-a-coronavirus-hospital-in-10-days-11580397751 (Accessed 17 June 2020).
WHO. (2007) *Quarantine as a public health practice in China in 7th century*. Available at: http://www.who.int/whr/2007/07_chap1_en.pdf (Accessed 30 August 2020).
WHO. (2014) *Health in all policies: Helsinki Statement. Framework for country action*. Available at: https://www.who.int/publications/i/item/9789241506908 (Accessed 4 May 2015).
WHO. (2015) *Framework for country action across sectors for health and health equity*. Available at: https://www.who.int/nmh/events/2015/action-across-sectors-framework/en/ (Accessed 3 August 2020).

WHO. (2020a) *COVID-19 response*. Available at: https://www.who.int/health-cluster/news-and-events/news/COVID19/en/ (Accessed on 19 August 2020).

WHO. (2020b) *Novel coronavirus (2019-nCoV) situation report -21 January 2020*. Available at: https://www.who.int/docs/default-source/coronaviruse/situation-reports/20200121-sitrep-1-2019-ncov.pdf?sfvrsn=20a99c10_4 (Accessed 7 September 2020).

WHO. (2020c). Available at: https://covid19.who.int/region/wpro/country/cn (Accessed 14 September 2020).

Winslow, C. (1920) The untilled fields of public health. *Science*, Volume 51, 23–33.

Xia, H. (2020) China extends holidays, strengthens control of coronavirus epidemic. *Xinhua*. Available at: http://www.xinhuanet.com/english/2020-01/27/c_138736690.htm (Accessed 17 June 2020).

Xinhua. (2020a) China suspends entry by foreign nationals holding Chinese visas, residence permits. Available at: http://english.www.gov.cn/statecouncil/ministries/202003/27/content_WS5e7d3587c6d0c201c2cbf8c8.html (Accessed 17 June 2020).

Xinhua. (2020b) The National Health Commission and relevant departments jointly cope with novel coronavirus. Available at: https://baike.baidu.com/reference/24316908/cf43Cc9yjlVyvev8N61C3AiuiRTTxx8dzeiSqMZm1O9eYyvZB0KpUua9QeGiaDYJ9UEvQuYZC85D0Pg8qZZOF1tWjhDj4NaoOBnp2ARZYzjw2eDo (Accessed 17 June 2020).

Yau, C., Tsang, D., & Ngai, M. (2020) Further ease Hong Kong social-distancing rules to prevent catering sector from collapsing, say industry leaders. *South China Morning Post*. Available at: https://www.scmp.com/news/hong-kong/hong-kong-economy/article/3098835/hong-kongs-industry-leaders-call-further-easing (Accessed 2 October 2020).

COVID-19 and the Political Economy of the European Union: New Crisis, Old Concerns

Michal Vavrik and Edoardo Monaco

Abstract The COVID-19 crisis has clearly hit the European Union (EU) hard, and at its very heart: member states' governments have struggled to prepare and respond, while the whole regional block has lacked the coordinated action that would be expected of a cohesive, established and ambitious supra-governmental organisation. The present article investigates the impact of the pandemic on the political economy of the EU, reviewing some estimates of both the scope and depth of an economic downturn that bears a close resemblance the aftermath of the 2008 financial crisis. This timely analysis focuses, in particular, on Italy and Spain: flailing economies already registering stuttering growth and mounting public debt when the Coronavirus entered their borders in early 2020. Concerted solutions are available but require a convergence of intentions which are traditionally hard to come by, in a regional context marked by increasing diversity of economic performances. Further, the public health crisis posed by COVID-19 has brought out fissures in the integration process of Europe between low and high-performing economies.

Keywords Coronavirus · Pandemic · Economic impact · The European Union · Recovery

1 Introduction: The Diffusion of Covid-19 Across the European Union (EU)

In early spring 2020, Europe became the second world region where citizens' lives were altered by the global spread of COVID-19 virus. Besides the devastating impact on health, the pandemic adversely affected the way people worked, spent free time and conducted everyday activities. While the social, economic and political effects

M. Vavrik (✉) · E. Monaco
Globalisation and Development (GAD) Programme, Beijing Normal University-Hong Kong Baptist University United International College (BNU-HKBU UIC), Zhuhai, China
e-mail: michalvavrik@uic.edu.cn

E. Monaco
e-mail: emonaco@uic.edu.cn

S.X.B. Zhao et al. (eds.), *COVID-19 Pandemic, Crisis Responses and the Changing World*, https://doi.org/10.1007/978-981-16-2430-8_6

Table 1 COVID-19 in the EU countries (only countries with over 200 cases/100,000 are listed), June 2020

Country	Sum of cases	Cases per 100,000 population
Spain	246,752	528.1
Italy	238,833	395.2
Germany	191,449	230.9
France	161,267	240.7
Sweden	60,837	597.4
Belgium	60,810	532.4
Netherlands	49,722	288.6
Portugal	39,737	386.5
Ireland	25,391	523.1
Denmark	12,561	216.7
Luxembourg	4,133	680

Source European Center for Disease Prevention and Control (2020)

of the disruption are yet to fully manifest themselves, currently available statistics already indicate the expected scope.

Italy became the first to experience the spread on a massive scale, but the virus soon directly affected all other countries in the EU. However, the impact in Spain, Germany, and France was particularly severe in terms of absolute numbers, but, relative to their size, some smaller countries were affected just as gravely. For example, already by late June, the number of cases per 100,000 inhabitants reached almost 600 in Sweden and well over 500 in Belgium (European Center for Disease Prevention and Control; ECDC 2020).

Table 1 shows the most affected EU countries as of June 2020. They are spatially widely distributed across the continent: particularly within the southern (Spain, Portugal, Italy), western (Germany, France, Belgium, the Netherlands, Luxembourg, Ireland) and northern (Sweden, Denmark) regions. A notable exception in the south has been Greece, where the spread of the virus remained limited, despite the risks posed by vulnerable immigrants living in refugee camps. On the other hand, Central and Eastern Europe have been affected relatively less; the exception in Poland which showed 85.6/100,000 cases in June (European Center for Disease Prevention and Control; ECDC 2020). The crisis even led the government to postpone presidential elections (Wanat 2020).

2 Early Reaction and Measures to Support European Economies

During the months of January and February 2020, as the coronavirus epidemic was spreading in East Asia, the EU-level reaction mainly concerned the repatriation of EU citizens, delivery of solidarity aid to China and efforts to coordinate the joint procurement of medical supplies (European Commission 2020a). It was in March, when the virus did eventually spread to Italy, countries within the union began, by and large, to introduce more or less stringent containment measures. Further, the European Commission made, in response, its first coordinated attempt to mitigate the immediate impact of the pandemic. For example, it issued updated guidance regarding free movements of critical workers, and recommendations to preserve essential freight by air (European Commission 2020a). However, a complex response came only on May 27, when the European Commission presented a recovery package integrated with a long-term common EU budget (European Commission 2020a). This section briefly reviews such early measures, while the recovery plan will be discussed at the conclusion of this paper.

We follow Bénassy-Quéré and Weder di Mauro (2020), who divide the measures to protect and support European economies into three policy areas ("axes"): (1) monetary and banking policies, (2) state aid and fiscal rules, and (3) funding. The distinction is practical, because even though the EU-level institutions can be said to have acted in all three areas, the degree to which the actions have been unevenly integrated.

1. Monetary and banking policy

As of 2020, altogether nineteen member countries of the European Union use the single currency, the Euro. Collectively known as the "Eurozone", they comprise most of Europe's major economies, including Germany and France. The institution responsible for the monetary policy of the Eurozone is the European Central Bank (ECB). National central banks of the Eurozone countries act as mere branches of the ECB, and due to the Eurozone's combined economic weight, their unified monetary policy inevitably influences economies well beyond the single-currency block.

The ECB reaction to the emerging economic consequences of the pandemic is generally seen in expert circles as swift (Bénassy-Quéré and Weder di Mauro 2020). Its first steps included measures aimed at making it easier for financial institutions to provide credit to firms and households at reasonable costs. Namely, they included relaxation of the ECB's supervision over the banking systems, lowering interest rates, increasing short-term loans available to the banking system, loosening collateral requirements in its long-term lending, and expansion of existing asset-purchasing policies (European Central Bank 2020a; Lane 2020).

Regarding the last category of measures, the most visible was "*Pandemic Emergency Purchase Programme*" (PEPP) set up in March 2020. The Programme involved the purchase of assets and was intended to combat the threat of general tightening of financing conditions, including lack of liquidity and availability of credit. As ECB President Christine Lagarde argued with a clear reference to the ECB's central aim, "when private spending is heavily constrained, worsening financing conditions for the public sector – which in the euro area amounts to broadly half of the economy – can be a threat to price stability" (Lagarde 2020).

After successive decisions of the ECB Governing Council, the PEPP can make use of up to 1, 350 billion euro for the purchase of public and private securities. To deal with potentially controversial issues concerning the allocation of the resources across different countries, a benchmark will be applied based on the ECB's capital key but with a degree of flexibility allowing for fluctuations over time (European Central Bank 2020b). The PEPP essentially preserves eligibility criteria previously used in existing purchasing instruments, and it is temporary, intended for the duration of the crisis only (European Central Bank 2020b). As Lagarde emphasized, the PEPP is an instrument fitted for dealing with exogenous shocks and detached from economic fundamentals (Lagarde 2020). In other words, it should not be interpreted as a shift to more generous asset-purchasing policies.

2. State aid and fiscal rules

State aid and fiscal rules are two areas in which national governments, with a view of building single market and economic and monetary union, accept the constraints on the scope of policy action (Article 107(1) and Title IV, esp. Art. 121 and 126 *Treaty on the Functioning of the European Union*). Constraints on aid and fiscal guidelines have often become embroiled in controversy but, in the context of the crisis, it is difficult to imagine an alternative.

The state aid rules regulate the degree to which governments can directly intervene in domestic markets by providing support to enterprises. It is defined as "direct aid granted by the state or derived from state resources, which either distorts or may distort competition, by favoring certain undertakings resulting in an impact on trade between Member States" (Fairhurst 2016). It concerns not only obvious measures, such as subsidies but also, for example, government guarantees for loans, or government purchases of shares in a company that are in financial difficulty (ibid.).

The pandemic created a dilemma: in the absence of government aid many firms would not be able to survive, and the sharp rise in the bankruptcy rate would have serious negative impact on employment, tax revenues and prospects of quick recovery. However, if permitted, state aid could create potential inequalities between firms who did receive aid and those who did not. This may reflect different overall economic performance across countries, among which some can afford generous aid packages and some cannot (Motta and Peitz 2020a). It was exactly this consideration of possible competition distortions or escalation of support for domestic industries that justified the calls for an EU-level aid fund (Motta and Peitz 2020b).

However, as an early recovery measure, the European Commission as the institution charged with monitoring the state aid mechanisms (Fairhurst 2016) had to accept the idea that the main fiscal response would consist of massive help from national governments' budgets. On March 19, the Commission updated the rules to allow for more flexibility, in order "to enable Member States to use the full flexibility foreseen under State aid rules to support the economy in the context of the COVID-19 outbreak" (European Commission 2020a). In a wave of successive decisions, national aid measures such as loan guarantees and funds directed towards production and supply of medical material were ultimately approved (European Commission 2020b). The support was not limited to emergency-related activity, and some governments extended support to their domestic firms, including some important airlines. The French government, for instance, injected 7 billion euro into Air France,

Italy provided 3 billion to Alitalia and Germany 9-billion euro to Lufthansa (Amaro 2020).[1]

The European Commission sought further to adjust guidelines on fiscal discipline. Originally, the rules based on *Stability and Growth Pact* were intended "to prevent fiscal policies from heading in potentially problematic directions, [or] to correct excessive budget deficits or excessive public debt burdens" (European Commission 2020c). In such cases, governments have been required to introduce austerity measures. In 2020, however, as early as March 20 the Commission activated the so-called "*general escape clause*" of the *Stability and Growth Pact* "to allow Member States to undertake measures to deal adequately with the crisis" (European Commission 2020a). The escape clause allowed member states temporary permission to increase budgetary and public debt deficits (European Commission 2020b).

3. Funding

Early reaction in the form of direct assignment of financial funds or opening credit lines took place via several institutions, namely the European Commission, the European Investment Bank and the European Stability Mechanism. A prominent role was played by the Commission's "*Temporary Support to mitigate Unemployment Risks in an Emergency*" scheme (SURE), created to cover "part of the costs related to the creation or extension of national short-time work schemes", and would consist of loans for countries to support employers who would otherwise find it necessary to lay off employees (European Commission 2020b). The scheme was developed to address concerns that the original supply-side shocks caused by the immediate impact of the pandemic will translate into a sustained period of unemployment as well as a long-term recession.

European Investment Bank (EIB) set up the "*Pan-European Guarantee Fund*" as an additional source of funding. The Fund was meant to function as a safety net for small and medium-sized enterprises. It made use of 26 billion euro to back up loans channeled to recipients via participating banks and financial intermediaries in member countries.

Finally, an emergency funding facility was made available via the European Stability Mechanism (ESM). Established as an independent international organization in 2012 with the aim to safeguard financial stability of the euro area countries, the ESM has notably been described as the Eurozone's IMF. The main instrument the ESM used was the *Pandemic Crisis Support* credit line set up in May 2020 to help fund emergency measures taken to protect public health and to tackle the immediate impact of the pandemic. The loans could reach up to 2% of a country's GDP,

---

[1] And they were challenged in a manner parallel to above-mentioned criticism. The granting of state aid to Lufthansa by the German government, and its approval by EU competition authorities was criticized by Ryanair's CEO Michael O'Leary. He argued that rather than being necessary for Lufthansa's survival, the government support would be used to increase its market share: "How can airlines like Ryanair, EasyJet and Laudamotion be expected to compete with Lufthansa in the short haul market to and from Germany, now that it has €9bn worth of German Govt subsidies to allow it to engage in below cost selling or buy up even more competition for the next number of years" (Ryanair 2020).

and, theoretically, up to 240 billion euro for the whole Eurozone (European Stability Mechanism 2020).

Despite the EU's determination to play an active part in dealing with the pandemic and its consequences manifested in such early response measures, as the pandemic progressed it became apparent that grave macroeconomic consequences were to follow in the medium/long-term. The overall debate over emergency measures, therefore, soon evolved into one on broader solutions that could support sustainable economic recovery over time. It was increasingly clear that existing institutional mechanisms, from ECB's asset purchasing, to EU budget allocations or loans from the ESM, would not be sufficient and/or would not be supported by a solid political consensus in the long term. New measures required would be broader in scope and more fundamental in nature than those previously described. Due to the global character, such measures would necessarily be the product of extensive coordination that, nevertheless, demonstrated sensitivity to the diversity of the stakeholders. In order to evaluate the challenges of this endeavor, we first review the economic consequences of the pandemic, before proceeding to assess existing vulnerabilities, and the overall potential consequences for further European integration.

3 Symmetric and Asymmetric Consequences

There is no doubt that the COVID-19 pandemic will have serious economic consequences, which have the potential to significantly influence the future patterns of European integration as a whole. Besides, in fact, an "emotional" impulse for unity and convergence brought about by shared hardships, the economic impact itself threatens to further exacerbate the existing cleavages among competing ideas on European integration.

The clash of different, at times competing, "visions" for the future of the EU is certainly not a novelty. Obviously, if such divisions descend into heated disputes over resources that member governments (and their electorates) perceive as vital for their most basic economic recovery, they have the potential to undermine the "common ground" which the policies and the very identity of the EU have become centered upon. Most importantly, the coronavirus crisis has come at a time when European economies had only just begun to recover from the lingering effects of the 2008 financial crisis. To this crisis it already appears closely related, given the similar asymmetric effects it seems to produce across member countries.

The socio-economic impact of COVID-19 resembles, in fact, the massive exogenous shock that typically triggers economic recessions (McKibbin and Fernando 2020; Financial Times 2020; Horowitz 2020; Jonung and Roeger 2006).

In the first weeks, the epidemic increased health-related expenditure of governments, firms as well as individual citizens, who have had to cope with, at times, severe short-term losses of income and purchasing power.

Soon after the onset of the pandemic, European businesses began to feel the effects of a reduced consumer demand and of the disruption of supply chains caused by lockdowns and border closures (OECD 2020c). “Social distancing” rules and travel restrictions affected service sectors and non-essential construction. Even though the manufacturing sector was in general less affected, specific sub-sectors like transport equipment were primarily shut down because of impediments in obtaining supplies from other countries (OECD 2020c). Large numbers of shipping containers have been held in ports because of logistical restrictions, thereby contributing to supply shortages and rising transport prices elsewhere; costs and time of unloading ships increased as a by-product of the implementation of public health protection measures, and cargo flights’ availability and capacity was significantly reduced (OECD 2020d).

A similar strain was inevitably reflected in firms’ financial performance: even generally healthy businesses encountered “existential” challenges, as “when they [ran] out of cash and [were] unable to cover operating expenses, taxes due and costs of existing debt” resulting in severe liquidity issues. According to a recent OECD report, “the risk of liquidity shortages is high for a large portion of firms”, especially in case of limited government intervention (OECD 2020a).

In the long run, economies worldwide will have to aim to achieve a limited recovery in a context of reduced investment and trade, and of disruptions in capital flows between countries. Capital outflow, especially from emerging economies such as Brazil, is already more significant than after 2008: in Europe, the situation may be regarded as less dramatic, but a divide does exist between inflows in the North and outflows in the South (OECD 2020e).

It is, therefore, hardly surprising that predictions are, indeed, gloomy: the *World Economic Outlook Update* published by the International Monetary Fund in June 2020 projects a global contraction in economic output of 4.9% in 2020; the corresponding figure being 8% among advanced economies, and 10% for the Eurozone (IMF 2020). Job losses and quality deterioration would be obvious: the International Labour Organisation (ILO), has estimated that 5.4% of global working hours were lost, equivalent to 155 million full-time jobs during the first quarter of the year alone (ILO 2020).

Focusing on the European Union, Table 2 measures four macroeconomic indicators to estimate the estimated impact of COVID-19. The figures emerging from the economic forecast of the European Commission in May 2020 were even more alarming than the IMF’s as they estimated an EU-wide 7.5% GDP contraction accompanied by the unemployment rate reaching 9%. Similar negative trends are expected for the government deficit and public debt. According to the same forecast, the

Table 2 The EU-27 post-pandemic economic forecast (spring 2020)

	2019 (%)	2020 (%)	2021 (%)
GDP growth	+1.9	−7.5	+6
Unemployment rate	6.7	9	8
Government deficit (% GDP)	0.6	8.5	3.5
Public debt (% GDP)	79.4	95	92

Source European Commission (2020d)

recovery should occur from 2021 onwards, but, at present, its speed depends on a number of little-known variables (European Commission 2020d).

When confronting an economic downturn of such unprecedented proportions, national governments have felt compelled to support their ailing economies by fiscal and other measures, including but not limited to tax deferrals or moratoria, guarantees for corporate loans, partial funding of firms' wage bills, direct injections of liquidity into firms or even their partial take-over etc. However, already high levels of debt significantly constrain the scope of action and can have further generated additional medium-term challenges (IMF 2020). One such critical development might be the potential for a new wave of sovereign debt crises in Europe involving two major yet traditionally troubled economies: Italy and Spain.

4 Italy and Spain: Too Big to Fail, Too Big to Bail

From a longer perspective, the most serious challenge for the EU is not the temporary decline in economic performance per se, but an uneven pattern of future recovery across and within member countries. This trend has been already discerned in the aftermath of the 2008 crisis (Jespersen 2016; Flassbeck and Lapavitsas 2015; Parker and Tsouharas 2018; Stiglitz 2016): in that respect, while most EU regions recovered their pre-2008-crisis per capita GDP within five years, many regions of Spain and Portugal recovered only between 2015 and 2017, while in some areas in Italy and, particularly, Greece, output appeared still below the pre-2008-crisis levels when the COVID-19 pandemic started (Eurostat 2019).

Similar patterns have been apparent in the degree to which EU governments achieved financial stability. Even prior to 2008 many of them struggled with large government debt, despite the limits set by the Stability and Growth Pact of 1997. In fact, even Germany, a strong promoter of the Pact, failed to curb its own excessive deficit (Pinder 2008). In the aftermath of the financial crisis, public debt increased even more and amounted to a "sovereign debt crisis" when Greece (2010), Ireland (2010), Portugal (2011), Spain (2012) and Cyprus (2012) required assistance from European institutions and the IMF to avoid sovereign defaults. Throughout the 2010s, the trend of rising government debt was reversed in notably Germany, Sweden, the Netherlands, and Slovakia. However, in others, including Spain, Italy and Greece, the debt problem persisted, or even grew (Table 3).

Such divergencies can be problematic for regional integration as they hint at the potential for the rise in conflicts over the optimal shape of common policies in the short and long term. What the data above confirm, for example, is a lasting divergence between countries of the European "North" and the "South". Northern countries are also sometimes referred to as "neo-mercantilist" as they are characterized by a high degree of international competitiveness and export orientation, reflected in current account surpluses (Becker et al. 2015; Flessbeck and Lapavitsas, 2015) or, "ordoliberal" for their rule-based strict economic governance emphasizing wage restraint,

Table 3 General government gross debt in selected countries, % GDP (2008–2014; 2018)

	2008	2009	2010	2011	2012	2013	2014	2018
Germany	65.5	73.0	82.3	79.7	81.1	78.7	75.6	61.8
Italy	106.2	116.6	119.2	119.7	126.5	132.5	135.4	134.4
Spain	39.7	53.3	60.5	69.9	86.3	95.8	100.7	97.4
Greece	109.4	126.7	147.5	175.2	161.9	178.4	180.2	186.2
Euro-19	69.6	80.2	85.8	87.7	90.7	92.6	92.8	85.8

Note General government gross debt, including loans and debt securities
Source Eurostat

stable prices and balanced government budgets (Young 2014). The periphery is characterized by mixed market economies with a weak capacity for wage coordination and important segments of unskilled work. They rely on a demand-led growth strategy based on stimulating consumption at the expense of private or public debt (Parker and Tsouharas 2018). Some argue that the monetary union imposed the single currency on what were previously "distinct varieties of capitalism" (Parker and Tsouharas 2018; Hall and Soskice 2001). It is significant because the European economic and monetary union and its key institutions were inspired by the northern European model of capitalism, the genesis suggesting a challenge for southern Europe to adapt to a different history and intellectual construct (see Soskice and Iversen 2012).

In reality, the two models have been interconnected, and the relationship between them has been more dialectical than antithetical. The citizens and firms of all countries interacted in the single market and monetary union, but instead of creating convergence, the divergence became even more pronounced. This paradoxical, and decidedly negative, outcome has been labelled "*Mezzogiornofication*" (Daianu and Kumar 2014) or "dependent financialization" in Southern Eurozone countries (Becker et al. 2015).

The establishment of the Eurozone as a single monetary area without federal-type fiscal policy was a key development. Once the single currency had removed devaluation risk, capital accumulated in the export-driven economies flowing to the South. In fact, German industrial exports provided external capital that was crucial for the import capacity of European peripheral countries (Becker et al. 2015). Lending to Italy, Spain, Greece, Portugal and Ireland increased from 14% of total bank foreign lending of German banks in 1999 to 20% in 2009 (Mitchell 2015).

Meanwhile in Spain, Greece, Italy and Portugal relatively easily available credit helped fuel both private and public borrowing and contributed to a creation of bubbles in certain attractive sectors. Partly as a consequence of the common market regulations which preclude use of protectionism for the sake of domestic industrialization, Southern European economies continued to focus on tourism, services and the construction industry (Becker et al. 2015).

This model nearly collapsed when the credit necessary to roll-over maturing public debt became more expensive as a result of financial crisis, tax collection during recession decreased, and the situation was further aggravated by government bailouts of collapsing banking sectors (Parker and Tsarouhas 2018).

Since then, the political economy of the Eurozone has been focused on managing conflicts over how to share the burden of structural adjustments (Frieden and Walter 2017; Nölke 2016). The development leading up to the previous crisis was clearly unsustainable, but the period of austerity did not restore a balance either. At the moment they were hit by the pandemic, the economies of the South displayed multiple fragilities making them particularly vulnerable to exactly this kind of shock. Greene (2020) discusses three risk factors that can be seen as specific embodiments of these vulnerabilities.

First, the pre-pandemic level of government debt should be considered as a major impediment, limiting the resources that national governments can deploy to support and stimulate their economies. High levels of debt in Italy and Spain, not to mention Greece, make their governments reluctant to risk further borrowing on a relevant scale (Greene 2020).

Second, in contrast to the 2008 crisis, the COVID-19 crisis will have a disproportionate impact on micro, small and medium enterprises or MSMEs (OECD 2020d; Greene 2020). The MSMEs have less means at their disposal than large enterprises to fight off short-term consequences of any economic downturn. They are typically more vulnerable to "social distancing" rules, find it more difficult to rebuild disrupted supply chains and encounter relatively higher costs when shifting to teleworking (OECD 2020f). In general, therefore, they register higher levels of risk and lower resilience related to their size (OECD 2020f). Moreover, empirical data show that "there is an above average representation of SMEs particularly affected by the crisis", in sectors such as construction, transport manufacturing, accommodation and food services, and personal services (OECD 2020f).

Finally, the recovery may be hindered if the economy is heavily reliant on sectors strongly affected by the pandemic, such as the tourist industry (Greene 2020). Globally, the decline of international tourism is estimated to range between 60 and 80%. In Europe, approximately, 76% of hotels will be closed. Domestic tourism, 75% of all tourism in OECD countries, is expected to rebound first, but the increase alone will be able to compensate for the loss of international tourist flows, especially in regions that are strongly dependent on international visitors are particularly relevant: for them, such a situation is likely to have significant macroeconomic effects (OECD 2020b).

Table 4 shows the concentration of above-mentioned risk factors in Italy and Spain, together with Greece, as compared with the EU-27 as a whole. Similar comparison is made in Table 5 with respect to decline in gross domestic product in the first and second quarters of 2020. It confirms the expectations that economic consequences in the southern countries are more severe than those experienced by member states in the remainder of the EU.

To conclude, the pandemic in Europe coincidentally hit hardest the very countries that were already particularly vulnerable, both fiscally and structurally. At the same time, they were the countries whose economic model was transitioning away from the demand-led growth sustained by high level of debt and had not yet completely

Table 4 Risk factors in selected countries

	Public debt (% GDP)	SMEs (% of employment)	Tourism (% GDP)
Italy	135	78.5	13
Spain	96	72	15
Greece	177	88	20
EU-27	n/a	67	10

Sources Greene (2020), Valero (2020a), and Eurostat

Table 5 Gross domestic product, % change in Q1 and Q2 2020

	2020-Q1	2020-Q2
Italy	−5.5	−12.8
Spain	−5.2 (p)	−18.5 (p)
Greece	−0.7 (p)	−14.0 (p)
EU-27	−3.2	−11.7

Flags (e) expected, (p) provisional
Source Eurostat

recovered from the previous crisis. Thus, the EU-wide debate on post-pandemic recovery should be seen as an attempt to contain the worst-case scenario where the economic recession translates into a quasi-permanent sovereign debt crisis similar to the one experienced by some countries of the Eurozone in the past. In 2020, the circumstances would be even more serious. The two particularly vulnerable countries—Italy and Spain—are both major economies, and the sheer volume of their debt is substantial (see Table 6).

Table 6 GDP and government debt in Italy, Spain, Portugal, Ireland and Greece. Gross domestic product at market prices; general government gross debt

	Gross Domestic Product (2019; million euro)	Government debt (2020-Q2, million euro)
Italy	1,787,664 (p)	2,431,077 (p)
Spain	1,245,331 (p)	1,224,161 (p)
Portugal	212,320 (p)	254,768 (p)
Ireland	356,051	213,792 (p)
Greece	187,456	329,296 (p)

Flags (p) provisional
Source Eurostat

5 The Recovery Package: "Next Generation EU"

In the light of these long-term divergences and vulnerabilities, the insufficiency of early measures becomes discernible. Aside the Commission's SURE and European Investment Bank's guarantees program (both specifically targeted), it was the European Central Bank's asset-purchasing programs and credit lines at the European Stability Mechanism that have been regarded as a means to deliver a general, macroeconomically significant stimulus. However, the instruments too have displayed serious limitations.

The ECB purchasing programs, limited as they are to purchasing government bonds on the secondary market, can only support the affected governments by helping to narrow the yield spreads between the bonds of more indebted countries and the German benchmark. They are certainly an important monetary policy tool, and when in the midst of the crisis the ECB President Lagarde hinted she did not consider "closing the spread" as the bank's purpose, she encountered immediate criticism and chose to take the statement back (Reuters 2020). Nevertheless, the ECB's PEPP program had been created to provide better conditions for further borrowing, yet for governments whose countries have already been burdened with high public debts, further loans are not a solution. In fact, Italy is the only country where, prior to the pandemic, the effective interest rate of the public debt was already higher than the estimated economic growth. It means that the debt-to-GDP ratio would continue growing even without additional borrowing. Even a small adverse fluctuation in growth or interest rates could make the debt unsustainable (Erce et al. 2020).

The same problem applied to the ESM credit lines, as proposed for example by Bénassy-Quéré et al. (2020). A "*Covid Credit Line*", with long duration and minimal conditionality, would provide governments with resources to deliver a large fiscal stimulus. This solution would be quick; the loans would be cheaper than those available through financial markets, and it would make use of the fact that ESM bonds already have an established market (ibid.; Erce et al. 2020).

However, in addition to being principally only another form of debt, there were other reasons why the ESM solution was controversial. The association of the instrument with humiliating conditionality provoked hesitancy on the part of recipient countries to undertake a similar dependency. The domestic pressure resultant from the health crisis deepened resistance as well as anxiety that such measure would lead to austerity in the near future (Erce et al. 2020).

In consequence, in the hopes of practically resolving debts, the debates within EU began to consider a "mutualization of debt": the EU member governments would authorize the European Commission to issue "coronabonds", jointly guaranteed and repaid by member countries. This solution would retain the advantage of collectively achieved superior credit rating by pooling the risks should a borrower-country fail to meet its obligations. It would have additional benefits of signifying a new progressive step in European integration and arguably also be an unprecedented show of solidarity.

This was the solution towards which the EU institutions and national governments worked. The result was the "*Next Generation EU*", an EU-wide recovery fund, built on a proposal put forward by the French and German governments, but officially presented by the President of the European Commission Ursula von der Leyen on May 27. It proposed that the European Commission be authorized to raise 750 billion euro on financial markets, which would be used to create a recovery fund supporting the most affected sectors and regions. According to the proposal, the major part of the fund 500 billion euro was to be distributed in the form of non-refundable grants. The borrowing was meant to be jointly backed by member governments—an important point making the consent of all a prerequisite for the scheme to work (Valero 2020b; Bayer et al. 2020).

The backing of the French and German governments added significant weight to the proposal. Further, the chances of its actualization were greatly increased by the coincidental occurrence that Germany held the EU 6-month rotational presidency in the second half of 2020. The German Chancellor thus had the formal standing to play a central role in negotiations. Most significantly, reversal of the traditional German position of opposing mutualization of debt that proved decisive in negotiating the measure.

Besides the German and French governments, the Italian and Spanish governments also strongly lobbied for the idea, arguing that jointly raised funds distributed in grants would embody the common European response to the health emergency as well as to the economic and social emergency (Gallardo and Barigazzi 2020).

However, resistance emerged as well, notably in the so-called "Frugal Four", comprising the Netherlands, Sweden, Denmark and Austria. Their leaders were the most vocal among those who criticized the principle of grants and argued for the "loans for loans" approach: the funds from the recovery package should be distributed in the form of loans to affected countries. The measure would still preserve the benefits of joint European borrowing, such as lower costs (Heikkila and Burchard 2020). The Frugal Four's position for loans parallels their long-term preference for resistance to expanding the EU budget, to which they contribute with significant net sums despite the fact that they are middle-sized countries. In fact, they actively promoted their preferences even before the pandemic started (Kurz et al. 2020) and they plan to continue their cooperation in future (Schulz and Grüll 2020).

Oppositions emerged also from another long-term platform. It concerned the countries of the Visegrad Group which comprises several Eastern EU members, namely Poland, Hungary, the Czech Republic and Slovakia, and unlike the Frugal Four is rather well institutionalized. With respect to the recovery fund, their governments found themselves in a "semi-frugal position". While Poland was in principle supportive of the Franco-German initiative, the governments of Czech Republic and Slovakia voiced a great deal of skepticism, claiming they were not in a position to be helping others (Ehl 2020; Euractiv 2020). The Hungarian Prime Minister Victor Orban described the Commission's proposal as "financing the rich from the money of the poor" and labelled it "absurd and perverse". What he opposed specifically was the idea that Hungarian taxpayers (whom he implied represented the poor) may need to take responsibility for repayment of "Greek, Italian or French debt" (quoted in Bayer 2020).

However, despite the difficulties, a consensus between leaders of the EU member countries was finally reached in July 2020 at an almost five-day long, face-to-face summit meeting. As a policy package, it represented a complex compromise. On the one hand, it made use of the regular, *Multiannual financial framework* (MFF), the EU long-term budget for 2021–2027, which would contain 1.074 trillion euro and was to be pro-growth and pro-recovery, while respecting some demands of the Frugal Four on its smaller size and limits on their contributions. On the other hand, the summit confirmed the "*Next Generation EU*" (NGEU) as a core instrument aimed at providing additional resources for short-term stimulus.

In the form negotiated during the "long summit" in July,[2] the "*Next generation EU*", will contain altogether 750 billion euro raised on financial markets through "coronabonds" with national governments' guarantees. Of this sum, 390 billion euro (down from 500 billion in the original Commission's proposal) will be distributed in grants, and 360 billion euro will be available as loans. Multiple specific instruments and programs will be used to distribute them, but a major part, comprising 312.5 billion euro in grants and 250 billion euro in loans, will be included in the *Recovery and Resilience Facility* (RRF). According to the agreement, the RRF grants will be distributed using two allocation keys. At first, 70% of the grants will be allocated in the years 2021 and 2022 based on a mix of criteria including a country's population, GDP per capita, and rate of unemployment in the period 2015–2019. The remaining 30% should be allocated in 2023 with the criterion of "the loss in real GDP observed over 2020 and by the cumulative loss in real GDP observed over the period 2020–2021" instead of the past unemployment rate (Bayer and Guàrdia 2020; Darvas 2020; European Commission 2020e).

It is notable that even without the conditionality traditionally associated with the ESM or IMF, the *New Generation EU* is not literally free money. For one, it needs to be ultimately repaid, an amount that, by inference, would be taken from future government revenues. Even grants are, therefore "repaid", even though on the basis of contributions to the EU budget, instead of directly as a debt repayment. The condition would, in effect, work to the detriment of Italy, which should be major receiver of recovery aid, but remains at the same time the third largest contributor to the EU budget (Roberts 2020).

Even more importantly, it was made clear that governments would be expected to make use of the funds in conformity with the EU-wide priorities. Specifically, they would have access to the money through "national recovery and resilience plans", submitted to and reviewed by the European Commission, and they should be defined "in line with the objectives identified in the European Semester, including the Green and Digital transformation, the Member States' national energy and climate plans, as

[2] As of the time of writing, its final approval is still in progress, and it requires member governments to give formal consent to an increase of their financial commitments as guarantees to the "coronabonds". This so-called Own Resources Decision needs to be taken in accordance with member countries' domestic constitutional requirements, typically involving a vote in national parliaments.

well as with the Just Transition plans" (European Commission 2020e). In other words, the European Semester, the EU framework for coordination of economic policies, will guarantee transparency and soundness of the way in which governments include the money in their fiscal policies. Together with the resilience these formulations imply a commitment of the countries who will seek support to avoid deepening their structural vulnerabilities. In the context of mainstream debates within economic and monetary union it means continuing emphasis on increasing competitiveness and flexibility of national social security and labor regulations.

The reference to the green, climate and digital policies is also significant. The post-pandemic recovery may represent an opportunity to achieve EU-wide economic transformation. As the Commission President von der Leyen stated, an already existing initiative for green transformation, the Green Deal, should serve as a "compass" to direct post-pandemic recovery (Simon 2020a). However, such optimism must be tempered with the notation that some voices, particularly from among eastern member countries, have resisted the ambitious climate policies as impediments to recovery. The Commission does not seem to accept these arguments (Simon 2020b).

6 Concluding Remarks

Considering the EU reaction to the pandemic with a view on economic recovery, several points seem to us worthy of attention.

First, the EU is characterized by diversity and divergencies that cannot be papered over by moralizing references to national selfishness and populism. They are rooted in member countries' histories and regional path-dependencies and are likely to emerge on the occasion of any crisis that requires intensive and long-term concerted recovery effort. The differing impact of the pandemic on member states is clearly a reflection of divergencies in institutions, economic performance and even circumstances of recovery from the post-2008 recession.

Second, in a serious crisis, the EU member states do not rely on the "community method" or supra-national decision-making. Instead, key decisions remain achievable via negotiations among heads of state and government, with a dominant mediating role played by the president of European Council, rather than the president of the European Commission. Even though the Commission has some leeway to take initiative or table proposals, the support from major countries' governments is decisive.

Third, such intergovernmentalism (Bickerton et al. 2015; Puetter 2014) does not mean that cooperation is being constrained. Neither does it aim at displacing functions of the EU on external platforms. As Puetter (2013) argues, the new intergovernmentalism does not indicate shallowness of cooperation but rather its depth: as the issues impinge on the core aspects of national sovereignty, coordinated actions require cooperation at the highest levels of government, a cooperation to which only the national leaders at the European Council can commit.

Finally, the EU reaction to the pandemic displays a degree of creativity. Instead of a purely defensive effort to protect employment and stabilize their economies, most national as well as EU-based elites seem determined to use the consensus over exceptional recovery measures to overcome the entrenched resistance to ambitious policies in energy transition, digitalization and combating climate change.

References

Amaro, S. (2020) Ryanair to cut up to 3,000 jobs; CEO O'Leary slams 'idiotic' quarantine periods. *CNBC,* May 18. Available at: https://www.cnbc.com/2020/05/18/ryanair-q4-2020-earnings-amid-coronavirus.html (Accessed 9 September 2020).

Bayer, L. (2020) EU recovery fund plan 'absurd,' Orbán says. *Politico Europe,* May 29. Available at: https://www.politico.eu/article/viktor-orban-eu-recovery-fund-plan-absurd/ (Accessed 13 September 2020).

Bayer, L., Burchard van der, H. and Smith-Meyer, B. (2020) France, Germany propose €500B EU recovery fund'. *Politico Europe,* May 18. Available at: https://www.politico.eu/article/france-germany-propose-e500b-eu-recovery-fund/ (Accessed 11 September 2020).

Bayer, L. and Guàrdia, A.B. (2020) The EU budget and recovery deal – in charts. *Politico Europe,* July 27. Available at: https://www.politico.eu/article/the-eu-budget-and-recovery-deal-in-charts/ (Accessed 13 September 2020).

Becker, J., Jäger, J. and Weissenbacher, R. (2015) Uneven and dependent development in Europe: The crisis and its implications. In: Jäger, J. and Springler E. (eds) *Asymmetric Crisis in Europe and Possible Futures: Critical Political Economy and Post-Keynesian Perspectives.* London and New York: Routledge, pp. 81–97.

Bénassy-Quéré, A., et al. (2020b) A proposal for a COVID Credit Line. In: Bénassy-Quéré, A. and Weder di Mauro, B (eds) *Europe in the Time of COVID-19.* London: CEPR Press, pp. 129–134.

Bickerton, C. J., Hodson, D. and Puetter, U. (eds.) (2015) *The New Intergovernmentalism: States and Supranational Actors in the Post-Maastricht Era.* Oxford: Oxford University Press.

Daianu, D. and Kumar, R. (2014) Introduction. In: Daianu, Daniel, et al. (eds) *The Eurozone Crisis and the Future of Europe: The Political Economy of Further Integration and Governance.* London: Palgrave Macmillan, pp. 1–8.

Darvas, Z. (2020) Having the cake, but slicing it differently: How is the grand EU recovery fund allocated? *Breugel.* Available at: https://www.bruegel.org/2020/07/having-the-cake-how-eu-recovery-fund/ (Accessed 14 September 2020).

ECDC. (2020) *COVID-19 Situation Update for the EU/EEA and the UK, as of 24 June 2020* [online]. Available at: https://www.ecdc.europa.eu/en/cases-2019-ncov-eueea (Accessed 26 July 2020).

Ehl, M. (2020) The other frugal four. *Visegrad Insight,* May 27. Available at: https://visegradinsight.eu/the-other-frugal-four-v4-eu-budget/ (Accessed 13 September 2020).

Erce, A. Pascual, A. G. and Marimon, R. (2020) The ESM can finance the COVID fight now. In: Bénassy-Quéré, A. and Weder di Mauro, B (eds) *Europe in the Time of COVID-19.* London: CEPR Press, pp. 135–146.

Euractiv. (2020) Visegrad leaders call for 'fair' EU recovery fund, June 12. Available at: https://www.euractiv.com/section/economy-jobs/news/visegrad-leaders-call-for-fair-eu-recovery-fund/ (Accessed 14 September 2020).

European Central Bank. (2020a) *Our Response to the Coronavirus Pandemic.* Available at: https://www.ecb.europa.eu/home/search/coronavirus/html/index.en.html (Accessed 30 August 2020).

European Central Bank. (2020b) *Pandemic Emergency Purchase Programme.* Available at: https://www.ecb.europa.eu/mopo/implement/pepp/html/index.en.html (Accessed 30 August 2020).

European Commission. (2020a) *Timeline of EU Action.* Available at: https://ec.europa.eu/info/live-work-travel-eu/health/coronavirus-response/timeline-eu-action_en (Accessed 26 September 2020).
European Commission. (2020b) *Overview of the Commission's Response.* Available at: https://ec.europa.eu/info/live-work-travel-eu/health/coronavirus-response/overview-commissions-response_en (Accessed 26 August 2020).
European Commission. (2020c) *Applying the Rules of the Stability and Growth Pact.* Available at: https://ec.europa.eu/info/business-economy-euro/economic-and-fiscal-policy-coordination/eu-economic-governance-monitoring-prevention-correction/stability-and-growth-pact/applying-rules-stability-and-growth-pact_en (Accessed 26 September 2020).
European Commission. (2020a) *Spring 2020 Economic Forecast: Press Release* [online]. Available at: https://ec.europa.eu/commission/presscorner/detail/en/ip_20_799 (Accessed 25 July 2020).
European Commission. (2020b) *Recovery Plan for Europe.* Available at: https://ec.europa.eu/info/live-work-travel-eu/health/coronavirus-response/recovery-plan-europe_en (Accessed 13 September 2020).
European Stability Mechanism. (2020) *ESM's Role in the European Response.* Available at: https://www.esm.europa.eu/content/europe-response-corona-crisis#:~:text=The%20ESM%20is%20the%20safety%20net%20for%20sovereigns,on%20the%20details%20attached%20to%20this%20credit%20line. (Accessed 11 September 2020).
Eurostat. (2019) *Eurostat Regional Yearbook.* 2019 Edition. Luxembourg: Publication Office of the European Union.
Fairhurst, J. (2016) *Law of the European Union.* Eleventh Edition. Harlow: Pearson.
Financial Times. (2020) Global recession already here, say top economists. *Financial Times* [online]. Available at: https://www.ft.com/content/be732afe-6526-11ea-a6cd-df28cc3c6a68 (Accessed 26 July 2020)
Flassbeck, H. and Lapavitsas, C. (2015) *Against the Troika: Crisis and Austerity in the Eurozone.* London: Verso.
Frieden, J. and Walter, S. (2017) Understanding the political economy of the Eurozone crisis. *Annual Review of Political Science,* 20, 371–390.
Gallardo, C and Barigazzi, J. (2020) Spain and Italy link arms ahead of EU summit on recovery plan. *Politico Europe,* July 8. Available at: https://www.politico.eu/article/spain-pedro-sanchez-and-italy-giuseppe-conte-link-arms-ahead-of-eu-summit-on-recovery-plan/ (Accessed 13 September 2020).
Greene, M. (2020) Get ready for a two-speed recovery. *Politico* (Europe), 15 May [online]. Available at: https://www.politico.eu/article/get-ready-for-a-two-speed-recovery/ (Accessed 16 May 2020).
Hall, D. and Soskice, P. (2001) *Varieties of Capitalism: The Institutional Foundations of Comparative Advantage.* Oxford: Oxford University Press.
Heikkila, M. and Burchard van der, H. (2020) "Frugal four" propose "loans for loans" approach to coronavirus recovery fund. *Politico Europe,* May 23. Available at: https://www.politico.eu/article/frugal-four-propose-loans-for-loans-approach-to-coronavirus-recovery-fund/ (Accessed 11 September 2020).
Horowitz, J. (2020) The global coronavirus recession is beginning. *CNN* (Media report) [online]. Available at: https://edition.cnn.com/2020/03/16/economy/global-recession-coronavirus/index.html (Accessed 26 July 2020).
ILO. (2020) *ILO Monitor: COVID-19 and the World of Work. 5th Edition: Updated Estimates and Analysis* [online]. Available at: https://www.ilo.org/wcmsp5/groups/public/@dgreports/@dcomm/documents/briefingnote/wcms_749399.pdf (Accessed 25 July 2020).
IMF. (2020) *World Economic Outlook Update* [online]. Available at: https://www.imf.org/en/Publications/WEO/Issues/2020/06/24/WEOUpdateJune2020 (Accessed 25 July 2020).
Jespersen, J. (2016) *The Euro: Why It Failed.* London: Palgrave Macmillan, pp. 1–8.
Jonung, L and Roeger, W. (2006) *The Macroeconomic Effects of a Pandemic in Europe–A Model-Based Assessment. ECOFIN Economic working paper No. 251* [online] Available at: https://ec.europa.eu/economy_finance/publications/pages/publication708_en.pdf (Accessed 27 July 2020).

Kurz, S. et al. (2020) The 'frugal four' advocate a responsible EU budget. Available at: https://www.government.se/opinion-pieces/2020/02/the-frugal-four-advocate-a-responsible-eu-budget/ (Accessed 14 September 2020).

Lagarde, C. (2020) Our response to the coronavirus emergency. European Central Bank. Available at: https://www.ecb.europa.eu/press/blog/date/2020/html/ecb.blog200319~11f421e25e.en.html (Accessed 29 August 2020).

Lane, P. R. (2020) The monetary policy package: An analytical package. In: Baldwin, R. and Weder di Mauro, B. (eds) *Mitigating the COVID Economic Crisis: Act Fast and Do Whatever It Takes.* London: CEPR Press, pp. 139–143.

McKibbin, W. J. and Fernando, R. (2020) The economic impact of COVID-19. In Baldwin, R. and Weder di Mauro, B. (eds) *Economics in the Time of COVID-19.* London: CEPR Press, pp. 45–51 [online]. Available at: https://www.researchgate.net/publication/339780440_The_economic_impact_of_covid-19 (Accessed 27 July 2020).

Mitchell, W. (2015) *Euro Dystopia: Groupthink and Denial on a Grand Scale.* Cheltenham and Northampton, MA: Edward Elgar Publishing.

Motta, M and Peitz, M. (2020a) EU state aid policies in the time of COVID-19. In: Bénassy-Quéré, A. and Weder di Mauro, B (eds) *Europe in the Time of COVID-19.* London: CEPR Press, pp. 73–77.

Motta, M and Peitz, M. (2020b) The EU recovery fund: An opportunity for change. In: Bénassy-Quéré, A. and Weder di Mauro, B (eds) *Europe in the Time of COVID-19.* London: CEPR Press, pp. 78–82.

Nölke, A. (2016) Economic causes of the Eurozone crisis: The analytical contribution of Comparative Capitalism. *Socio-economic Review,* 14(1), 141–161.

OECD. (2020a) *Corporate Sector Vulnerabilities During the COVID-19 Outbreak: Assessment and policy responses* [online]. Available at: http://www.oecd.org/coronavirus/policy-responses/corporate-sector-vulnerabilities-during-the-covid-19-outbreak-assessment-and-policy-responses-a6e670ea/ (Accessed 25 July 2020).

OECD. (2020b) *Tourism Policy Responses to the Coronavirus (COVID-19)* [online]. Available at: http://www.oecd.org/coronavirus/policy-responses/tourism-policy-responses-to-the-coronavirus-covid-19-6466aa20/ (Accessed 25 July 2020).

OECD. (2020c) *Evaluating the Initial Impact of COVID-19 Containment Measures on Economic Activity* [online]. Available at: http://www.oecd.org/coronavirus/policy-responses/evaluating-the-initial-impact-of-covid-19-containment-measures-on-economic-activity-b1f6b68b/ (Accessed 25 July 2020).

OECD. (2020d) *COVID-19 and International Trade* [online]. Available at: http://www.oecd.org/coronavirus/policy-responses/covid-19-and-international-trade-issues-and-actions-494da2fa/ (Accessed 25 July 2020).

OECD. (2020e) *COVID-19 and Global Capital Flows* [online]. Available at: http://www.oecd.org/coronavirus/policy-responses/covid-19-and-global-capital-flows-2dc69002/ (Accessed 25 July 2020).

OECD. (2020f) *Coronavirus (COVID-19): SME Policy Responses* [online]. Available at: http://www.oecd.org/coronavirus/policy-responses/coronavirus-covid-19-sme-policy-responses-04440101/ (Accessed 25 July 2020).

Parker, O. and Tsarouhas, D. (2018) Causes and consequences of crisis in the Eurozone periphery. In: Parker, Owen and Tsarouhas, Dimitris (eds) *Crisis in the Eurozone Periphery.* London: Palgrave Macmillan, pp. 1–27.

Pinder, J. (2008) *The European Union: A Very Short Introduction.* Oxford: Oxford University Press.

Puetter, U. (2013) The European Council – the new center of EU politics. *European Policy Analysis,* 16, pp. 1–14.

Puetter, U. (2014) *The European Council & the Council: The New Intergovernmentalism and Institutional Change.* Oxford: Oxford University Press.

Reuters. (2020) Italy furious at ECB's Lagarde 'not here to close spreads' comment. *Reuters,* March 13. Available at: https://www.reuters.com/article/us-ecb-policy-italy-minister-idUSKBN20Z3DW (Accessed 13 September 2020).

Roberts, H. (2020) Italy's coronavirus spending bonanza. *Politico Europe,* July 23. Available at: https://www.politico.eu/article/italy-coronavirus-spending-bonanza-economy/ (Accessed 14 September 2020).

Ryanair. (2020) Ryanair condemns €9 billion state aid to Lufthansa. *Ryanair Group,* May 26. Available at: https://corporate.ryanair.com/news/ryanair-condemns-e9-billion-state-aid-to-lufthansa/ (Accessed 9 September 2020).

Schulz, F. and Grüll, P. (2020) EU recovery deal: The summit that will cement Merkel's legacy. *Euractiv,* July 23. Available at: https://www.euractiv.com/section/future-eu/news/angela-merkel-der-gipfel-ihrer-karriere/ (Accessed 13 September 2020).

Simon, F. (2020a) Green deal will be 'our motor for the recovery', von der Leyen says. *Euractiv,* April 29. Available at: https://www.euractiv.com/section/energy-environment/news/green-deal-will-be-our-motor-for-the-recovery-von-der-leyen-says/ (Accessed 13 September 2020).

Simon, F. (2020b) Timmermans defends higher EU goals on climate change. *Euractiv,* September 2. Available at: https://www.euractiv.com/section/climate-environment/news/timmermans-defends-higher-eu-goals-on-climate-change/ (Accessed 13 September 2020).

Soskice, D. and Iversen, T. (2012) A structural-institutional explanation of the Eurozone crisis. Available at: http://www.people.fas.harvard.edu/~iversen/PDFfiles/Iversen&Soskice_euro2015.pdf (Accessed 6 September 2020)

Stiglitz, J. H. (2016) *The Euro: How a Common Currency Threatens the Future of Europe.* New York and London: W. W. Norton and Company.

Valero, J. (2020a) Commission to adopt broad summer package on 13 May. *Euractiv,* 7 May [online]. Available at: https://www.euractiv.com/section/economy-jobs/news/commission-to-adopt-broad-summer-package-on-13-may/ (Accessed 25 July 2020).

Valero, J. (2020b) Von der Leyen proposes €750 billion stimulus under member states' grip. *Euractiv,* May 27. Available at: https://www.euractiv.com/section/economy-jobs/news/von-der-leyen-proposes-e750-billion-stimulus-under-member-states-grip/ (Accessed 13 September 2020).

Wanat, Z. (2020) Poland set new presidential elections date. *Politico* (Europe), June 3 [online]. Available at: https://www.politico.eu/article/poland-sets-a-new-presidential-election-date/ (Accessed 26 July 2020).

Young, B. (2014) The power of ordoliberalism in the Eurozone crisis management. In: Daianu, Daniel et al. (eds) *The Eurozone Crisis and the Future of Europe: The Political Economy of Further Integration and Governance.* London: Palgrave Macmillan, pp. 126–137.

Government Emergency Responses During the COVID-19 Pandemic in the Context of Health Emergency and Disaster Risk Management: A Comparative Study

Johnston H.C. Wong

1 Introduction

On January 23, 2020 China responded to the first wave of COVID-19 by locking down the city of Wuhan, a city of more than 10 million residents. The National Health Commission of China (CNHC 23 January 2020) reported 571 confirmed cases of COVID 19 patients, 19 seriously ill and 17 deaths in Wuhan on January 22. The number of confirmed cases exploded between January 20 and February 6 and reached 32,583 with its peak on February 1. Centralized quarantine and treatment were found effective in leveling the curve of daily confirmed cases, although universal testing was not begun until February 17.

The World Health Organization (WHO) named the coronavirus on February 11, 2020 as COVID-19 and declared a pandemic on March 11, 2020. At that time, there was no vaccine to prevent infection and no proven therapeutics to treat the disease. Until February 7, 2021, the total number of confirmed cases has reached 105,745,975, and total number of deaths 2,309,000 (John Hopkins University, COVID-19 Map, 7 February 2021). No scientists ever envisaged that America would become the center of the pandemic.

The strategy adopted but not invented by China, is the "Social Distancing and Isolation Strategy". It is demonstrated by the lock down of Wuhan and the stopping of transportation, education, recreation, production and outside family social life for the whole of China. The WHO expert, Bruce Aylward, referred to such actions as an "Unprecedented Response", reported by Agnus Mcniece on China Daily (2020). It was often referred as the "Lock Down" or "Shut Down" policy.

J. H.C. Wong (✉)
Social Work and Social Administration (SWSA) Programme, Division of Humanities and Social Sciences, Beijing Normal University Hong Kong Baptist University United International College, Zhuhai, China
e-mail: johnstonhuang@uic.edu.cn

S.X.B. Zhao et al. (eds.), *COVID-19 Pandemic, Crisis Responses and the Changing World*, https://doi.org/10.1007/978-981-16-2430-8_7

The alternative approach promulgated by Boris Johnson, the Prime Minister of the United Kingdom, who claimed that he was advised by his health experts notably Sir Patrick Vallance, on the "Herd Immunity Strategy". Mills (2020), in discussing the strategies to contain COVID-19, differentiated two approaches: suppression and mitigation. Suppression means to reduce the basic reproduction number (Ro) to below 1 and thus reverse the growth of the coronavirus. Mitigation aims to slow down the spread of the epidemic but not reduce Ro below 1. The latter approach was recommended by the Imperial College COVID-19 Response Team to the British cabinet as the computational modeling showed that a collapse of the NHS could result from a hospital rush created by a suppression approach. Herd immunity was what they hoped to gradually flatten the curve.

The herd immunity strategy was openly endorsed in March 2020 by the UK. Sweden was generally considered to adhere to that approach but denied that it had adopted the herd immunity strategy. Peter Nilsson, a professor of internal medicine and epidemiology at Lund University argued that the deaths from COVID-19 would be far less than the deaths caused by societal lockdown when the economy was ruined (Sputnik 2020). The "flexible restrictive strategy" allowed Sweden to keep the economy afloat and avoid a spike in unemployment rates.

Herd immunity could be achieved either by actually having the majority of population infected by the coronavirus through widespread exposure and recover from it, or the same percentage of people receive safe and sufficient dosage of vaccine. However, herd immunity can only be reached when a critical percentage of the population becomes resistant to an infectious disease, and Grad (2020), estimated that the required percentage for COVID-19, according to its infectivity, would be around 60% of the world population. Later predictions, based on more knowledge about the strength of vaccines, suggested a vaccination rate as high as 90% (Fauci 2020).

Even in the UK more than 200 scientists have written a letter to warn about the stress it would create for the UK National Health Service (McMahon 2020). D'Souza and Dowdy (2020) commented that the herd immunity strategy for COVID-19 is not advisable because its death rate may be 10 times higher than general flu. Hoping that COVID-19 would become weaker is also probably unrealistic. The latest research has showed that while COVID-19 mutated from China to Italy to US, there is no evidence that it has turned weaker (Rose 2020). Rose (2020) suggested that the soonest date for the availability of a scientifically tested safe vaccine would be January 2021.

No country, including the United Kingdom, relied solely on the "let it go through" manner but practiced a mixed approach that imposed a certain degree of social distancing. How to mix the two approaches, in what ways, at what stages and for how long, was the question. No matter whether countries take a hard or soft approach in response, it is only part of the disaster management cycle that includes preparation, response, recovery and mitigation.

2 Health Emergency and Disaster Risk Management

2.1 WHO Health EDRM Framework

In May 2019, the World Health Organization published its Health Emergency and Disaster Risk Management (Health EDRM) Framework as the achievement of international research supported by the United Nations Office of Disaster Risk Reduction (Kayano et al. 2019). It pointed out that comprehensive management, multisectoral and multidisciplinary collaboration and a community centred approach are necessary to prepare for any major disaster including public health crises.

Dr. Tedros Adhanom Ghebreyesus, Director-General of the WHO, emphasized in the foreword of this Framework, of "the critical importance of prevention, preparedness and readiness, together with response and recovery, to save lives and protect health" (WHO 2019, p. v). The Health EDRM Framework pointed out that "communities" should be the "drivers of responses" (WHO 2019, Section 7.4, p. 16). It stressed that disaster will disproportionately affect the most vulnerable, the poorest, women and children, people with disabilities, older persons, migrants, refugees and displaced persons, and people with chronic diseases.

The Health EDRM Framework borrows from the concept of 'disaster management cycles', covering four major processes of "Preparedness, Response, Recovery and Mitigation" and applies it to the case of public health incidents. The Health EDRM involves a wide range of actors, those of emergency and disaster management, epidemic preparedness and response, social and psychological professionals, rescue responders, healthcare experts and government officials. Most importantly the WHO Health EDRM (WHO 2019) points to the need of the Whole-of-Government and Whole-of-Society strategy and regards it as a responsibility for governments.

2.2 Evaluating Preparedness

In October 2019, the John Hopkins University (2019), in collaboration with the Economist Intelligence Unit and the Nuclear Threat Initiative, launched the Global Health Security Index (GHSI). GHSI is the first of its kind aiming at measuring the capabilities and preparedness of a country to counteract a public health disaster. It was released on October 24, 2019. With this instrument, we can review whether countries performed during COVID-19 according to how well they were prepared. The United Kingdom and the United States are among the top performers according to the GHSI. Unfortunately, their actual response performances during the COVID-19 crisis have not lived up to their GHSI ranking.

2.3 Guiding Emergency Responses

As early as April 2020, the WHO recommended governments to take six categories of actions to minimize the threats of COVID-19 (WHO 2020c). The categories included:

To control COVID-19 transmission to a level of sporadic cases and clusters of cases.
To ensure that sufficient public health workforce and health system capacities are in place.
To minimize outbreaks in high-vulnerability settings.
To prevent outbreaks in workplaces.
To control exporting and importing cases from communities with high risks of transmission.
To engage communities in COVID-19 control measures.

To further elaborate, the WHO in April invited all governments to consider Public Health and Social Measures (PHSM) in a cautious and staged manner. PHSM includes international travel restrictions which were almost instantly imposed by major countries in different degrees. Internally it refers to movement restrictions, geographical area quarantine, and closure of schools and businesses.

Countries need to balance the benefits of these closures which may control the spread of the coronavirus against its potential harm to the economy which will certainly hit the most vulnerable hardest. If countries reopen schools and businesses prematurely, it may trigger a resurgence of COVID-19 cases and jeopardize people's health. However, if closure is prolonged, there must be sufficient financial assistance provided by governments or else those without work and daily means of living could not survive.

2.4 Documenting Government Responses

This brings our attention to the next step in the WHO Health EDRM, of "Public Health Outbreak Response". The taking of proper actions by governments becomes crucial in combating COVID-19, disregarding how well or poorly a country was prepared before the impact of the pandemic. In the past there was no instrument to measure Public Health Response. To fill the gap, Oxford University (2020a) immediately created a database platform to record government responses towards the pandemic, namely the Oxford Government Response Tracker, making comparisons of government policies and practices possible.

Recognizing the need to account for the actions taken by governments against COVID-19, the University of Oxford developed the Tracker and later a COVID-19 Government Response Stringency Index (GRSI) composed of 17 indicators, grouped under three Sub-Indices, namely:

Containment and Health Sub-Index: Public information campaign, testing policy, contact tracing, emergency investment in healthcare, and investment in Covid-19 vaccines.

Stringency Sub-Index: School closing, Workplace closing, Cancel public events, Restrictions on gathering size, Close public transport, Stay at home requirements, Restrictions on internal movement, Restrictions on international travel.

Economic Support Sub-Index: income support, debt/contract relief for households, fiscal measures, and giving international support.

Putting it in the Health EDRM Framework, the GSRI provided an assessment tool to evaluate response policies and practices of governments, that reflected to a certain extent the Whole-of-Government and Whole-of Society approaches, which will enhance "Community Resilience and Capacity Building" advocated by the WHO Health EDRM.

2.5 *Objectives of This Study*

It is the aim of this chapter to review and compare the response actions of various governments internationally in terms of the Health EDRM and discuss whether these actions could lead to positive health outcomes. The entire four phases of the Health EDRM has not been covered as COVID-19 exerts long term impact, and it remains premature, as well, to discuss Recovery and Mitigation work. Therefore, this paper will focus on the Emergency Response stage in relation to the state of preparedness.

This is only an exploratory study for the first year of health emergency actions. This was not without difficulties because government actions were interfered with by behaviors of its people which are shaped by their historical and cultural backgrounds and their social and economic structures. Actions governments took were also restricted by the financial situations of the governments and health service capacities of the countries. Nevertheless, these limitations exist for all international comparisons. Keeping limitations in mind this chapter hopefully could shed light on what were the more effective interventions to contain the spread of the coronavirus. Being an exploratory study, this chapter raises more questions than it provides definite answers on most effective actions.

To summarize, the objective of this chapter is to identify, through reviewing global tracking data made available by reputable medical and humanitarian sources of selected countries, those measures that appeared to be useful in combating COVID-19 in the year 2020. Its findings hopefully will lead to more conclusive comparisons and experimental studies.

3 Methods

3.1 Major Aspects of Study

This paper analyzes the Response Actions of governments during the COVID-19 pandemic that aimed to contain the communicable disease, and consequently how these actions were related with health outcomes. Actions included medical interventions in treating the confirmed cases and the introduction of testing to identify potential cases. It also involved public policies and practices to track potential cases, isolate the suspected cases, and enforce social distancing.

Health Outcomes included the crude death rate, number of deaths per million of population, and the sickness death rate; the number of patients who died among the confirmed cases.

Preparedness of the country was considered as the antecedent variable that shaped government response actions. To what extent these countries were prepared for a major public health outbreak will also be examined.

3.2 Data Collection and Analysis

Secondary data analysis was conducted on reliable sources including reports from the WHO, World Bank, governments' Centers of Disease Control and informatics from major universities including the John Hopkins University, Oxford University and the University of Washington.

3.3 Selection of Countries

Since it is impossible to compare the situations of too many countries, a sample of 14 countries has been strategically chosen based on economic development as reflected by GDP, population size and geographic location.

On October 7, 2020, figures provided by John Hopkins University Coronavirus Resource Center, showed 35,832,271 of confirmed cases and 1,050,115 number of deaths globally (John Hopkins University 2020). Thirty-five million persons, if not more, and their families were affected.

Countries ranked highest in death tolls were the United States, India, Brazil, Russia, Colombia, Peru, Spain, Argentina, Mexico, South Africa, France, and the United Kingdom, in that order. COVID-19 left no region and no corner of the globe safe. It affected developed countries as well as underdeveloped countries. It spread in climates featuring cold temperatures, as well as high temperatures. Scientists, unfortunately, need more time to study its characteristics.

Some observations suggested that COVID-19 has an urban-centric character, as more than 1,430 cities are affected by the pandemic in 210 countries and well above 95% of the total cases are located in urban areas (UN-Habitat 2020). However, cities are supposed to have the best healthcare facilities and disease related mortality rate may be lower than those in the rural areas. Studying COVID-19 in cities alone therefore cannot provide a comprehensive picture.

A more diversified selection of countries could provide a more comprehensive picture. The strategical selection should include countries which are:

Different in population sizes.
Different in numbers of deaths caused by COVID-19.
At different stages of economic development.
Different in resourcefulness in health care facilities.
Different in geographical locations from different continents of the globe.

The following countries: Brazil, China, Denmark, India, Germany, Philippines, Mexico, Rwanda, South Korea, Thailand, the United Kingdom (UK), the United States (US), Venezuela and Zambia were included in this study. The selection has considered several factors. First in terms of geographical locations countries should cover America, Africa, Asia, Europe and Southeast Asia. Secondly it aimed to cover high income, middle income and low income countries as classified by the World Bank. To study the factor of Public Health Crisis Preparedness as ranked by GHSI, countries which are most prepared, more prepared and least prepared were included.

3.4 Demographic Characteristics of the 14 Selected Countries

The demographic data of the selected 14 countries is listed in Table 1.

In terms of geographical locations, it covers different parts of Asia, Eastern Africa, South and North America, as well as Western and Northern Europe. It is realized that Australia has not been included in the list. However, Australia is to a great extent an isolated continent which has found it easier to keep itself outside the influence of the pandemic. It is also true that Middle East countries are not represented. In the selection process, it is also important to avoid countries which are engaged in other disastrous incidents like civil wars because this will affect their health performance.

The two most populated countries China and India were included both for comparison between them and to increase the overall representation of this study. World population in 2020 is calculated at 7,794.8 million; whereas China, India and United States add up to 3,150.331 million. Therefore, the total of 14 countries or 3,939.707 million may represent 50.5% of the total population of the world. On the other end Denmark has a rather tiny population of only 5.792 million. Rwanda, Zambia and Venezuela have tiny populations of below 50 million. South Korea, Thailand, United Kingdom, and Germany can be regarded as small countries in terms of population size ranging from 50 to 100 million. Mexico, Brazil and America have larger population sizes ranging from 100 to 300 M.

Table 1 Demographic data of selected countries (2020)[a]

Country	Region	Population (Million)	GDP (USD) per capita	% of age (0–14/60+)	Physicians/1000 persons
Brazil	South America	212.559	8,920.7	20.07/14.00	2.2
China	Eastern Asia	1,439.324	9,531.9	17.7/17.4	2
Denmark	Northern Europe	5.792	61,833.7	16.3/26.1	4
Germany	Western Europe	83.784	47,513.7	14.0/28.6	4.2
India	Southern Asia	1,380.004	2,054.8	26.2/10.1	0.9
Mexico	Central America	128.933	9,694.9	25.8/11.2	2.4
Philippines	South Eastern Asia	109.581	3,102.7	30.0/8.6	0.6
Rwanda	Eastern Africa	12.952	773	39.5/5.1	0.1
Republic of Korea	Eastern Asia	51.269	33,621.9	12.5/23.2	2.4
Thailand	South Eastern Asia	69.800	7,273.6	16.6/19.2	0.8
United Kingdom	Northern Europe	67.886	42,526.4	17.7/24.4	2.8
United States	Northern America	331.003	62,917.9	18.4/22.9	2.6
Venezuela	South America	28.436	7,212.2	27.3/12.1	Missing
Zambia	Eastern Africa	18.384	1,572.3	44.0/3.4	1.2

[a]All information derived from UN Data http://data.un.org/en/index.html; GDP data derived from World Bank (2018)

In terms of income per capita of these countries the lowest is Rwanda's, of only US$773. The highest is that of the United States of US$62,917.9. The former is only 1.22% of the latter. In terms of age, Rwanda and Zambia have youngest populations. As older people are more vulnerable to COVID-19, having a larger percentage of population over 60 years of age, in the case of those highly developed countries, is an obvious risk factor.

Most countries recorded 2 or more physicians per thousand population. It is an indirect indicator for the level of health services in a country. The highest number of doctors were found in Denmark and Germany. The status of India, Thailand and Zambia are unsatisfactory while Rwanda has a negligible number of 0.1/1000 and Venezuela did not provide an entry to this section of UN-DATA.

From the above dimensions of regional location, population size, income per capita, age profiles and number of physicians per population, it is evident that the 14 countries have very diverse profiles and represent over half of the world population.

Their responses to COVID-19 warrant our scrutiny and their lessons should be valuable for other countries of similar size, similar stage of economic development and which are similarly limited in terms of medical and health facilities.

3.5 Timing of Comparisons

As the COVID-19 crisis prolonged for more than a year since January 2020, countries have modified their disease control strategies significantly. For example as of April 2020 China has resumed social and economic activities while the United Kingdom has stepped back from herd immunity and opted for more stringent control. This study took a snapshot of the performance of selected governments in October 2020, and provided an update of health outcomes in January 2021.

3.6 Measurements

Measurement of health outcomes were based on data provided by the John Hopkins COVID-19 Tracker. Numbers of total confirmed cases and total deaths in each country were updated daily. The same data could be found on the WHO tracker; In any case we have to rely on available data and the John Hopkin's statistics will be used to examine the number of confirmed cases, the number of deaths, the case fatality rate (the ratio of deaths per 1000 confirmed cases of COVID-19) and the cause-specific mortality rate (the ratio of deaths caused by COVID-19 among the total population of the country). Both rates are counted within the same given period of time.

To measure Preparedness, the Global Health Security Index (GHSI) was used. Formulation of the GHSI is based on six aspects, namely Prevention, Detection and Reporting, Rapid Response, Health Systems, Compliance to International Norms and Risk Environment (Global Health Security Index 2020). So far there is no other index internationally available to estimate a country's preparedness for public health incidents.

Measuring government responses during COVID-19, Oxford University developed the Oxford Government Response Tracker (OxCGRT) and an Index of Stringency. It recorded the measures introduced by governments to control the spread of COVID-19 and financial assistance to people when workplaces were locked down. The indicators under the category of "Containment and Closure" include "School Closing", "Workplace Closing", "Cancel Public Events", "Restriction on Gathering Size", "Close Public Transport", "Stay at Home Requirements", "Restrictions on Internal Movement" and "Restrictions on International Travel".

3.7 Analysis of Data

To scientifically examine the relationships between Preparedness, Responses, and Health Outcomes it is possible to use quantitative methods as all indices were provided as interval scales. Health outcomes counted included Attack rates (number of confirmed cases among the population), Fatality rates (number of deaths among confirmed cases) and crude death rates (number of deaths among the population) were all interval data. However, using a purely mathematical model might not allow us to imagine and explain variations between countries at the exploratory stage. Therefore a more common mode of international comparisons of percentages and trends illustrated by tables and graphs will be used.

3.8 Limitations

One limitation this study faced is the presence of unidentified, unreported and undiagnosed cases and consequently inaccurate health outcomes.

The number of confirmed cases can be under-reported. A research report released in April by the University Hospital of Bonn using serological antibody tests to collect a representative sample in the community of Gangelt, found that people infected by COVID-19 were undetected, representing 20% more than the reported cases. The study showing the actual number of infected cases as larger than that of reported cases, suggested a lower fatality rate (the Infected Fatality Rate is differentiated from Case Fatality Rate), of 0.37%, as compared to 3.4% calculated by WHO.

Meanwhile, the number of deaths can also be under-reported. There is no comprehensive testing capacity in poorer countries therefore people who died without a test would not be counted as COVID-19 related deaths. Even in developed countries like the United States many older people may have died in their homes without the chance to take any tests or medical examinations.

Another limitation of this study is the reliance on secondary data mainly provided by informatics instruments recently developed to track the information of COVID-19. These instruments need time to be refined for its validity and reliability. For example, the GHSI of John Hopkins University, though designed for public health incidents, is not modified timely to suit the special features of COVID-19. A higher ranking in GHSI means that the country has a lot of ICU beds, but it cannot tell whether people would wear face masks. Analysis for this paper can only be based on available data and indices.

4 Findings

4.1 Finding 1: Number of Reported Cases and Deaths

The health outcomes of the 14 selected countries in October 2020 are presented in Table 2. Data includes population size, number of confirmed cases, number of deaths, case fatality rate, cause-specific mortality rate expressed in number of deaths among 10,000 persons in population and were derived from WHO's COVID-19 country situations report (WHO 2020b). Population size extracted from UN-DATA shown in Table 1, was added to relate demographic data with health outcomes.

If death rate by population is concerned Thailand has done a superb job up until October 2020. Its population death rate was only 0.008 per 10,000. At the other end of the spectrum are Brazil (6.898 per 10,000), the United States (6.308 per 10,000), the United Kingdom (6.252 per 10,000) and Mexico (6.148 per 10,000). The data certainly upset our general assumption that more developed countries would perform better than less developed countries which have less resources and experience in dealing with communicable diseases. Population size cannot explain the differences as Thailand and the United Kingdom have similar size of population, respectively 69.800 and 67.886 M, but a differing death rate of 0.008 and 6.252 per 10,000

Table 2 Health outcomes of the 14 selected countries (October 2020)[a]

Country	Population (millions)	Number of confirmed cases	Number of deaths	Attack rate	Case fatality rate	Number of deaths per 10,000
Brazil	212.559	4,927,235	146,615	2.32	2.976	6.898
China	1,439.324	91,188	4,746	0.01	5.205	0.033
Denmark	5.792	30,379	663	0.52	2.182	1.145
Germany	83.784	306,086	9,562	0.37	3.124	1.141
India	1,380.004	6,757,131	104,555	0.49	1.547	0.758
Mexico	128.933	765,082	79,268	0.59	10.361	6.148
Philippines	109.581	326,833	5,865	0.30	1.794	0.535
Rwanda	12.952	4,783	29	0.04	0.606	0.022
S. Korea	51.269	24,353	425	0.05	1.745	0.083
Thailand	69.800	3,615	59	0.01	1.632	0.008
UK	67.886	530,117	42,445	0.78	8.007	6.252
US	331.00	7,380,326	208,787	2.23	2.829	6.308
Venezuela	28.436	79,796	665	0.28	0.833	0.234
Zambia	18.384	15,224	335	0.08	2.200	0.182
World		35,659,007	1,044,269	2.928		

[a]All information derived from WHO (7 October 2020), https://covid19.who.int/ except population size is derived from UN Data http://data.un.org/en/index.html

respectively. Strangely differences can neither be explained by wealth. Rwanda, the poorest among the 14 selected countries with a GDP per capita of only US$733 recorded the death rate of 0.022 per 10,000; while the United States, richest of the list enjoying income per capita of US$62917.9, recorded a death rate of 6.308 per 10,000. Another country which is equally rich, Denmark, has a death rate of only 1.145 per 10,000.

Since early 2020, UN experts worried that the least developed countries where people lived in crowded housing with no proper water supply and were incapable of home quarantine would be seriously affected by COVID-19.

However, from the data shown in Table 2, the least developed countries like Rwanda and Zambia, did not report a particularly high Attack rate (ratio of confirmed cases to the population) and Crude Fatality rate (ratio of disease related deaths to the population). Accuracy of these figures may be questionable as countries vary in detection and treatment facilities. Nevertheless, comparisons are meaningful, for example among high-income countries, namely the UK, US, South Korea, Denmark and Germany, there existed big variations in terms of health outcomes. The Attack rates ranged from 0.05 of South Korea to 2.23 of the US and Crude Fatality rates ranged from 1.76 of South Korea to 7.24 of the UK. South Korea achieved the best records among the five high income countries. There was no uniform pattern among the 5 Upper middle income countries including Brazil, China, Mexico, Thailand and Venezuela. In short high-income countries were not spared by the Pandemic. On the contrary because of stronger commercial linkages and travel connectedness, richer countries are more exposed to international transmission of the disease.

Evidently the number of infected cases were under-reported, but at the same time deaths caused by COVID-19 were also under-reported, and death tolls continued to rise. According to the Johns Hopkins University's COVID Case Tracker, the milestone of one-million deaths was hit on September 28, 2020. Researchers from the International Health Metric and Evaluation Center, University of Washington, warned in October 2021 that the actual number of people who have died from COVID-19 was grossly underestimated (Reiner et al. 2020). In the worst-case scenario, if existing social distancing measures were eased, the number of deaths could exceed 2.5–3 million people by January 2021 (University of Washington 2020). If the current control of social distancing is maintained the number of deaths could be reduced to 2.2 million whereas if universal masking were enforced, the global death toll could be further reduced by 1.5 million. The projection unfortunately was very close as the total number of deaths stood at 2,309,000 on February 7, 2021 according to the John Hopkins Tracker.

4.2 *Finding 2: Preparedness (GHSI)*

The Global Health Security Index (GHSI) was developed and announced in 2019. The GHSI (2020) measured 6 components of Prevention, Detection, Response, Health, Norms and Risk, with 34 indicators. The highest score for GHSI as well as its 6

Table 3 Global Health Security Index (2020)

Country	GHSI	GHSI country rank	GHSI category
Brazil	59.7	22	More prepared
China	48.2	51	More prepared
Denmark	70.4	8	Most prepared
Germany	66	14	More prepared
India	46.5	57	More prepared
Mexico	57.6	28	More prepared
Philippines	47.6	53	More prepared
Rwanda	34.2	117	More prepared
South Korea	70.2	9	Most prepared
Thailand	73.2	6	Most prepared
UK	77.9	2	Most prepared
US	83.5	1	Most prepared
Venezucla	38.2	164	Least prepared
Zambia	44.2	141	Least prepared

Note Information extracted from GHSI, Johns Hopkins University, EIU & NTI, 2019. Range 0–100, the higher the better prepared

sub-indices is 100, the higher the better. Rank of the country is given according to its score among 195 countries. The Index rating, ranking and category of the selected 14 countries is presented in Table 3.

The GHSI ranked United States number one in total score while Venezuela, lowest among the 14 sampled countries, ranked 164. The sample covered a considerably wide range of countries in terms of GHSI as there were a total of 195 countries enlisted. Countries of the sample categorized as most prepared (Table 2) included the United States (1st), United Kingdom (2nd), Thailand (3rd), Denmark (8th), and South Korea (9th). Only two countries were regarded as least prepared, they were Zambia (141st) and Venezuela (164th).

In Table 4, the breakdown of 6 sub-indices with their sub-ranking in bracket were presented.

To determine as to what extent "Preparedness" as reflected by GHSI determined "Health Outcomes" during COVID-19 it is important not only to count the overall index scores. It would be more meaningful also to investigate whether sub-indices were better related with health outcomes. For example, the Index of Norms, assessing the willingness of governments to follow international standards and commitment to further improve risk management structures, may allow countries to follow more closely the advice of WHO to contain the coronavirus. On the other hand, the Index of Health may reflect the capacity and qualities of health care of the country to lower death rates and minimize the loss of lives. The Index of Respond could indicate government capacity to mobilize multisectoral resources in times of public health crisis.

Table 4 Sub-indices of GHSI of the 14 selected countries in 2019

Country	Prevent	Detect	Respond	Health	Norms	Risk
Brazil	59.2(16)	82.4(12)	67.1(9)	45.0(33)	41.9(135)	56.2(94)
China	45.0(50)	46.5(64)	48.6(47)	45.7(30)	40.3(141)	64.4(58)
Denmark	72.9(5)	86.0(7)	58.4(19)	63.8(5)	62.6(28)	80.3(17)
Germany	66.5(13)	84.6(10)	54.8(28)	48.2(22)	61.9(29)	82.3(11)
India	34.9(87)	47.4(67)	52.4(32)	42.7(36)	47.7(100)	54.4(103)
Mexico	45.5(49)	71.2(32)	50.8(39)	49.6(24)	73.9(6)	57(89)
Philippines	38.5(71)	63.6(41)	43.8(68)	38.2(47)	49.8(84)	50.3(124)
Rwanda	33.8(90)	36.0(111)	31.9(117)	24.1(89)	38.0(148)	43.6(144)
S. Korea	57.3(19)	92.1(5)	71.5(6)	58.7(13)	64.3(23)	74.1(27)
Thailand	75.7(3)	81.0(15)	78.6(5)	70.5(2)	70.9(12)	56.4(93)
UK	68.3(10)	87.3(6)	91.9(1)	59.8(11)	81.2(2)	74.7(26)
US	83.1(1)	98.2(1)	79.7(2)	73.8(1)	85.3(1)	78.2(19)
Venezuela	23(176)	23.5(140)	8.7(182)	19.7(180)	12.9(141)	42.2(132)
Zambia	28.7(152)	24.5(132)	21.9(151)	28.6(134)	20.3(106)	38.0(148)

Note Information extracted from GHSI, Johns Hopkins University, EIU, NTI, 2019

4.3 Finding 3: Stringency of Government Responses

Table 5 provides information about the Oxford GRSI for the 14 selected countries, showing the average monthly score of the Overall Government Response Index from January to September 2020, as well as the average monthly scores of the Stringency Sub-Index, Containment & Health Sub-Index, and the Economic Support Sub-Index.

It seems that the variation of stringency among the 14 countries was not as large as expected. Zambia has the lowest score in GRSI of 35, and Rwanda the second lowest, 41. China has the highest score in GRSI of 66, and Mexico second highest of 63. The United Kingdom scored 48, Philippines 51 and the United States 52. But Germany and Denmark also have a low GRSI score of 50.

One factor not to be neglected was change of government policies over time. For example, India reported the first coronavirus positive patient on January 30, a medical student studying in Wuhan, China. Two of her classmates also turned positive but all three of them recovered (Indiatimes 2020). Another source of early identified COVID-19 carriers for India were 16 Italian nationals. By March 20 the number of confirmed cases rose to 199, leaving the Indian Prime Minister Narendra Modi no choice but to announce on March 22 self-imposed public curfew and the banning of international flights. Then for a period of time India seemed unaffected by the coronavirus disease as the number of confirmed cases remained low. Unfortunately, the initially extremely insignificant number of 199 exploded in mid-May into 6,000,000 by late September with 94,500 lives lost (John Hopkins 2020). As shown in Tables 6 and 7, India has relaxed its containment and stringency measures since July and August of 2020. This should not be interpreted as coincidence.

Table 5 Mean of monthly government Response Stringency Index from January to September 2020

Country	Containment and Health Index	Stringency and Policy Index	Economic Support Index	Overall Government Response Index
Brazil	51	56	34	49
China	74	70	20	66
Germany	52	48	36	50
Denmark	49	45	58	50
India	52	53	71	55
Mexico	65	62	54	63
Philippines	54	47	35	51
Rwanda	49	53	0	41
South Korea	66	64	18	58
Thailand	61	57	25	55
UK	46	43	59	48
US	54	52	43	52
Venezuela	56	62	38	53
Zambia	38	37	17	35

Note Information from GHSI, Johns Hopkins University, EIU, NTI, 2019

Table 6 OxCGRT Containment and Health Index January to September (Oxford University 2020)[a]

Country	January	February	March	April	May	June	July	August	September
Brazil	1	8	39	64	70	69	71	69	75
China	29	77	80	67	79	84	85	85	79
Germany	5	20	50	71	66	66	65	66	59
Denmark	0	1	50	67	69	65	63	60	59
India	3	21	36	68	66	73	69	70	64
Mexico	3	20	57	97	85	80	78	80	80
Philippines	2	45	69	73	54	65	60	60	63
Rwanda	0	0	21	74	75	66	66	67	66
S. Korea	3	32	68	97	92	81	83	72	61
Thailand	4	15	54	92	77	67	74	79	81
UK	0	0	37	73	77	67	55	53	50
US	2	9	50	73	73	71	69	69	66
Venezuela	0	3	46	70	77	75	80	79	77
Zambia	0	4	23	59	53	47	54	53	52

[a] All information derived from Oxford University COVID-19 Government Response Tracker. Range 0–100, the higher the more stringent

Table 7 Oxford Stringency and Policy Index January to September 2020[a]

Country	January	February	March	April	May	June	July	August	September
Brazil	1	6	44	75	81	77	80	74	73
China	22	77	80	60	75	80	82	82	74
Germany	1	10	49	77	64	61	57	58	50
Denmark	0	1	53	70	64	57	55	51	50
India	2	11	37	80	74	71	65	68	66
Mexico	2	10	55	99	82	76	77	80	79
Philippines	0	36	63	67	44	57	51	51	54
Rwanda	0	0	20	82	82	72	71	72	72
S. Korea	3	24	65	100	95	81	80	70	56
Thailand	4	14	49	91	72	60	69	75	77
UK	0	0	36	76	75	63	49	47	43
US	0	5	46	73	73	71	68	67	64
Venezuela	0	1	52	82	84	81	87	85	82
Zambia	0	5	24	58	50	42	51	50	49

[a]All information derived from Oxford University COVID-19 Government Response Tracker. Range 0–100, the higher the more stringent

Hale et al. (2020a) in their report on the Lockdown Roll Back Check List based on the GSRI, suggested that "The biggest variation in well-performing countries is around testing and tracing, likely a reflection of different testing levels" (Hale et al. 2020b, BSG Working Paper, V10.0, p. 12). In their September 2020 Report, version 10, Hale discovered that some countries, like China, France, Italy and South Korea, imposed more stringent measures as reflected in the GRSI after the report of 100 cases. Other countries were slow to raise their stringency measures even after 100 recorded cases, including the United Kingdom and United States (please refer to Tables 6 and 7).

Table 6 showed that in terms of containment, covering the indicators of public information campaign, testing policy, contact tracing, emergency investment in healthcare, and investment in Covid-19 vaccines, the highest scores were recorded in April 2020 for Mexico at 97, South Korea also at 97 and Thailand at 92. On the other hand, China's score reached 85 only in July and August of 2020. There is a misconception that China was tracking the suspected patients in a more authoritarian manner than some democracies.

Table 7 reveals some important messages as it presents Stringency of Government Responses of the 14 countries over time. China has scored highest in average monthly GSRI, but it didn't always impose the most stringent measures. For example, South Korea in April 2020 was given a 100 Stringency score by OxCGRT, and in May 2020 the score only dropped for 5 points to 95. In April 2020, both Thailand and Mexico imposed stringent measures and scored over 90.

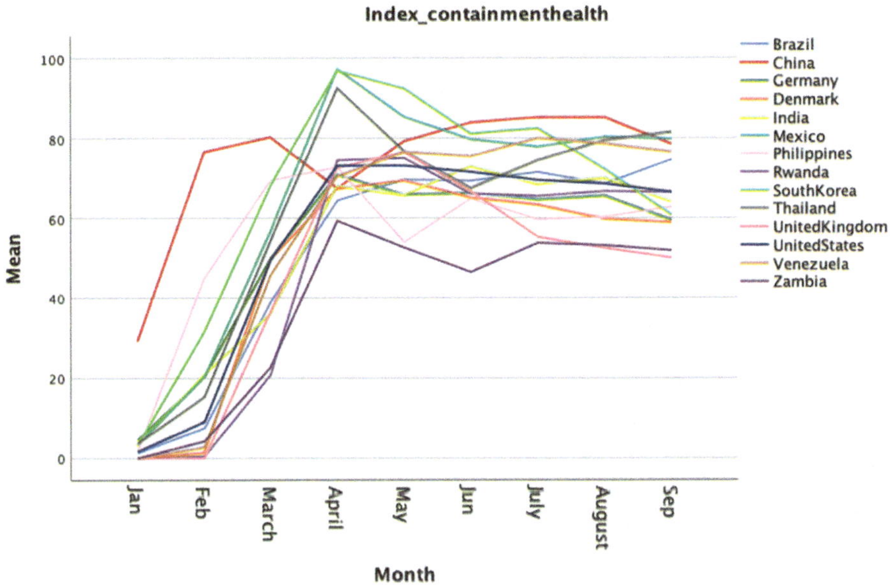

Diagram 1 OxCGRT Containment and Health Index of 14 selected countries (Oxford University 2020a)

Three graphs are presented to show the trends of Government Responses of the 14 countries about containment, stringency and economic assistance one by one (Diagrams 1, 2 and 3).

Diagram 1 demonstrated that China has maintained a relatively high containment score all through the months of summer 2020. For other countries stringency scores rose sharply in March, peaked in April but declined gently since June of 2020 before the curves plateaued.

Referring back to Table 5, some less "Stringent" countries as reflected by the average Stringency and Policy Index (India = 53, UK = 43, Denmark = 45, US = 52) actually provided more assistance as revealed in Diagram 3 by the Economic Support Index (India = 71,, UK = 59, Denmark = 58, US = 43). On the contrary, in Diagram 2, China scored 70 and South Korea 64 in the Stringency Index but recorded only 20 and 18 respectively in the Economic Support Index, ranking lowest among the 14 countries with the exception of the two least developed countries of Rwanda and Zambia. Rwanda provided no assistance at all and Zambia's score in Economic Support Index was merely 17.

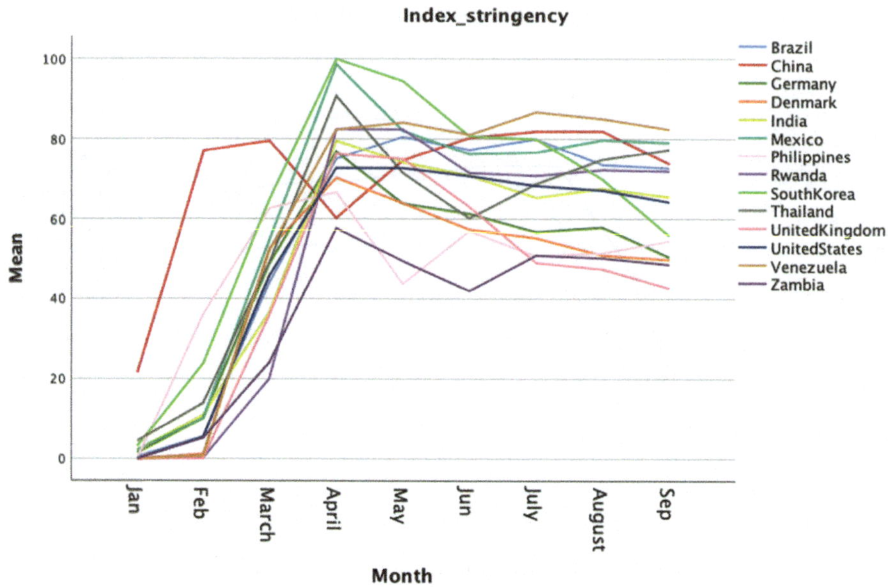

Diagram 2 OxCGRT Stringency and Policy Index of 14 selected countries (Oxford University 2020b)

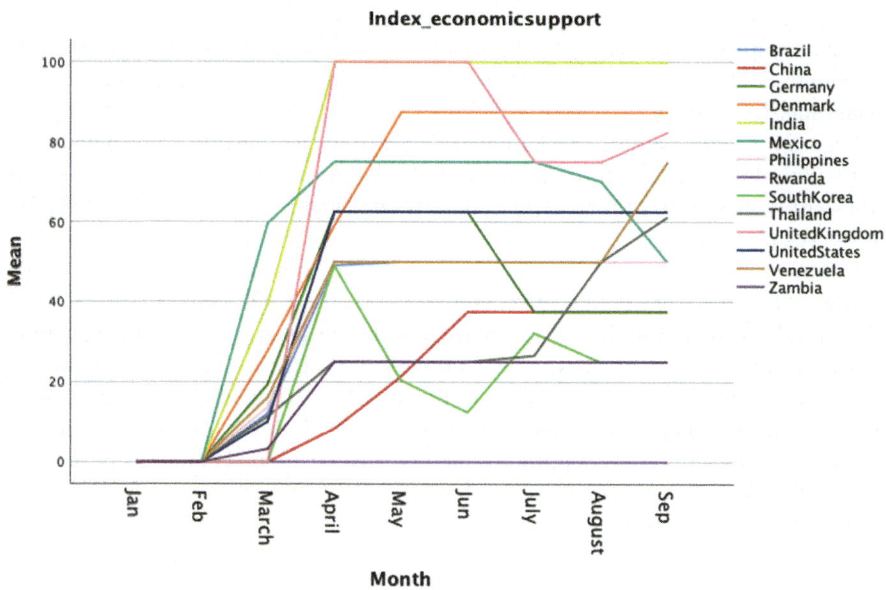

Diagram 3 OxCGRT Economic Support Index of 14 selected countries (Oxford University 2020a)

Table 8 Preparedness and health outcomes (JHU, WHO 2020)

Country	GHSI	Respond	Health	Case fatality rate (%)	Death/10,000	Rank by death rate among 14 countries
Brazil	59.7(22)	67.1(9)	45.0(33)	2.976	6.898	14
China	48.2(51)	48.6(47)	45.7(30)	5.205	0.033	3
Denmark	70.4(8)	58.4(19)	63.8(5)	2.182	1.145	10
Germany	66(14)	54.8(28)	48.2(22)	3.124	1.141	9
India	46.5(57)	52.4(32)	42.7(36)	1.547	0.758	8
Mexico	57.6(28)	50.8(39)	49.6(24)	10.361	6.148	11
Philippines	47.6(53)	43.8(68)	38.2(47)	1.794	0.535	7
Rwanda	34.2(117)	31.9(117)	24.1(89)	0.606	0.022	2
S. Korea	70.2(9)	71.5(6)	58.7(13)	1.745	0.083	4
Thailand	73.2(6)	78.6(5)	70.5(2)	1.632	0.008	1
UK	77.9(2)	91.9 (1)	59.8 (11)	8.007	6.252	12
US	83.5(1)	79.7(2)	73.8 (1)	2.829	6.308	13
Venezuela	38.2(164)	8.7(182)	19.7(180)	0.833	0.234	6
Zambia	44.2(141)	21.9(151)	28.6(134)	2.2	0.182	5

4.4 Finding 4: Preparedness and Health Outcomes

In Table 8, the GHSI, Respond Sub-index and Health Sub-index are presented and the health outcomes of Fatality Rate and Death Rate per 10,000, are listed for comparison.

From Table 8, no relationship was found between overall GHSI and death rate in population. For example, the United States and United Kingdom ranked number one and two in the GHSI, but ranked 12th and 13th in number of deaths in population, only better than Brazil, the worst of all 14 countries. On the other end Venezuela ranked 164 and Zambia ranked 141 in GHSI, won the 5th and 6th place in terms of low death rates. Surprisingly, they even outperformed Denmark and Germany. The country with the lowest income per capita, Rwanda, has a very low death rate of 0.022 per 10,000, or second lowest among the 14 countries. Though the ranking of countries in overall GHSI scores may be different from that of the Respond sub-index and Health sub-index, there is no relationship between the two subs-indices and death rate in population.

4.5 Finding 5: Stringency and Health Outcomes

In the following Table 9, the Government Response Stringency Index developed by Oxford, its Containment sub-index and Stringency sub-index were presented. Performances of the 14 countries in fatality and death rates were shown together in

Table 9 Stringency and Health Outcomes (Oxford University 2020a; WHO 2020b)

Country	GRSI	Containment	Stringency	Case fatality rate (%)	Death/10,000	Rank by death rate among 14 countries
Brazil	49	51	56	2.976	6.898	14
China	66	74	70	5.205	0.033	3
Germany	50	52	48	2.182	1.145	10
Denmark	50	49	45	3.124	1.141	9
India	55	52	53	1.547	0.758	8
Mexico	63	65	62	10.361	6.148	11
Philippines	51	54	47	1.794	0.535	7
Rwanda	41	49	53	0.606	0.022	2
South Korea	58	66	64	1.745	0.083	4
Thailand	55	61	57	1.632	0.008	1
UK	48	46	43	8.007	6.252	12
US	52	54	52	2.829	6.308	13
Venezuela	53	56	62	0.833	0.234	6
Zambia	35	38	37	2.200	0.182	5

this table such that the relationship between stringency and health outcomes could be identified.

Examining the relationship between GRSI and Ranking by Death in population, there was no definite conclusion. It is true that in those countries reporting a high death rate like Brazil, the United States and United Kingdom, their overall GRSI scores were relatively low, around 50. However, there were counter examples like Mexico, ranking 11th in Low Death Rate, which was much more stringent than the US and UK. While Zambia, with only 35 points in GSRI, and Rwanda with 41, the two lowest in terms of stringency among the 14, did not have a high death rate. In other words, the relationship between Stringency and Health Outcomes may not be linear and there are other antecedent or intermediate factors that might affect the outcomes of government actions.

4.6 Finding 6: Preparedness, Response and Health Outcomes

To recap, the aim of this paper is to review the Health EDRM mechanism of the selected countries with the hope of finding effective approaches and lessons to be learned from the experiences of combating COVID-19. Seemingly, the results so far are rather inconsistent and therefore a clear pattern of effective measures is not apparent. First of all, the preparedness of countries measured by GHSI failed to

Table 10 Preparedness, response and health outcomes (JHU, Oxford, WHO)

Country	GHSI	GHSI rank	GRSI	GRSI rank	Deaths/10,000	Rank by death rate among 14 countries
Brazil	59.7	7	49	11	6.898	14
China	48.2	9	66	1	0.033	3
Germany	70.4	4	50	9	1.145	10
Denmark	66	6	50	9	1.141	9
India	46.5	11	55	4	0.758	8
Mexico	57.6	8	63	2	6.148	11
Philippines	47.6	10	51	8	0.535	7
Rwanda	34.2	14	41	13	0.022	2
Korea	70.2	5	58	3	0.083	4
Thailand	73.2	3	55	4	0.008	1
UK	77.9	2	48	12	6.252	12
US	83.5	1	52	7	6.308	13
Venezuela	38.2	13	53	6	0.234	6
Zambia	44.2	12	35	14	0.182	5

Note There were two countries ranked as 4 and two others ranked as 9, because of having the same score on GRSI

predict successful reduction of confirmed cases and consequent deaths. Moreover, Government Responses measured by Oxford GRIS did not show any clear relationship with health outcomes. Table 10 shows the data of Preparedness, Response and Health Outcomes together for easy reference.

As mentioned earlier, Preparedness did not predict health outcomes. In the case of Response, it seemed more Stringency was related to lower crude death rates though it might not lead to lower fatality rate. For example, China, South Korea, Thailand and Venezuela, which imposed stringent controls, reported a lower death rate than Brazil, United Kingdom and the United States. The exception is Mexico, which was ranked as the second most stringent country, but recorded a high death rate of 6.148 per 10,000 people. The two African countries Zambia and Rwanda astonished the world with their low death rates while their responses were rather relaxed and health resources were understood as inadequate. With these findings that Preparedness was not predictive of health outcomes and Responses relationship with death rates was inconclusive, it seemed that the search for effective measures to combat COVID-19 should be expanded to a larger social and cultural context.

5 Discussions

5.1 Attack Rate: To Control or not to Control?

Effective tracking, testing and isolating of suspected cases helped to reduce attack rate. Countries capable of minimizing the number of people contracting the disease happened to be those that adopted lock down measures soon after the first 100 cases were reported. China, with an attack rate of 0.01, Thailand (0.01), Rwanda (0.04) and South Korea (0.05) all adopted early lock down. As of October 2020, in China 4,746 people have died because of COVID-19. In the United States by this time there were 208,787 deaths, in Brazil 146,615, India 104,555, Mexico 79,268 and the United Kingdom 42,445, representing high attack rates in relatively large populations. China has a much higher crude fatality rate (5.2%) than the US (2.80) and Brazil (2.96), but its attack rate was only 0.01, comparing to 2.23 and 2.32% of the latter two countries.

Low attack rates were found in Rwanda (0.04), and Zambia (0.08). These two countries were actually "protected naturally" against COVID-19, because of their young populations, with age group over 60 composing only 5.1 and 3.4% of their populations respectively. The two least developed countries of our sample were least vulnerable, as compared to the more developed countries which have aging populations. The Indian population has only 10.1% who were above 60, but it is a huge size to worry about. China's population is aging as 17% of them were over 60. This explains why China had no choice but to impose lockdown policies as soon as possible. In the case of the UK, where 24.4% of population is aged over 60, not to control the attack rate is not advisable.

5.2 Does Stringency Work?

Social distancing, or even isolation, is one of the standard and oldest measures in communicable disease control. Isolation was first introduced in 1377 in Dubrovnik on Croatia's Dalmatian Coast (Tognotti 2013). The first permanent lazaretto, or plague hospital, was opened in 1423 on the small island of Santa Maria di Nazareth, by the Republic of Venice. Later this approach was also called the Venetian Model. During SARS in 2003, China followed international advice to employ quarantine measures which aimed to identify the infected patients as soon as possible and isolated them temporarily from the society for treatment. For this purpose, the Chinese Government built isolated treatment facilities from scratch.

Constructing cabin hospitals to provide medical rescue to Wuhan citizens was exactly what the Chinese medical professionals learned from the hard lessons of SARS, 17 years ago. Soon after the outbreak health experts knew that isolating only confirmed patients was not adequate to stop the disease from spreading because it was very contagious before noticeable symptoms were shown (WHO 2020c). The strictest kind of quarantine or shut down of whole community seemed unavoidable.

Even in the United Stated strong measures of social distancing in March and April 2020 was found effective to stop COVID-19 spreading (Courtemanche et al. 2020). The US has banned large social gatherings and closed schools, gyms, bars and dining areas. Shelter-in-place was ordered in some states. The researchers studied the effect of these measures across the US in March and April, 2020, and found that government-imposed social distancing measures did reduce the daily number of confirmed cases by 5.4% after 1–5 days, and 9.1% after 16–20 days. Their results implied that COVID-19 spread would be 10 times greater or reaching 10 million cases without shelter-in-place orders alone.

5.3 Could Shut Down Policy Stand Alone?

If shut down continues it will bring the economy particularly the stock market to a melt-down. Perhaps some economies cannot wait until January 2021 and have no choice but relaxing city shut down. Seemingly those countries that did not impose stringent measures were later forced to provide more economic assistance to individuals and business vendors. Referring to Table 3, the top few countries in providing financial assistance were India (71), United Kingdom (59), Denmark (58), and Mexico (54). Their respective Stringency Sub Index scores were 53 for India, 43 for United Kingdom, 45 for Denmark and 62 for Mexico.

In the case of the US tremendous amounts of money were injected into the system, and Wall Street became the major beneficiary though one could argue that saving the stock market was saving enterprises and employment. However according to the Oxford GRSI Assistance Sub-index, the score for US was only 43, rather low. The United States seemed to have adopted a double "NO" approach, no Stringency and no Assistance, with a price tag of over 250,000 lives even in September 2020.

5.4 Could Herd Immunity Prevent Healthcare Systems from Collapse?

At the beginning of the pandemic the UK argued that by adopting a herd immunity strategy, it would save the NHS from collapsing because people would run on the hospitals and squeeze healthcare resources. This theory was not supported by the results of China, South Korea and Germany, which carried out effective tracing, tracking, separating and treating of confirmed patients. By controlling the spread and bringing down the number of confirmed cases and serious cases, medical resources of these countries, which were less abundant than the US and UK, became sufficient to reduce the number of deaths caused by COVID-19.

5.5 *Could Stringency Be Applied to Democracies?*

Yan et al. (2020) in the analysis of COVID-19 country situations in China, Japan, France and Sweden, proposed that there are two contextual factors which affect the responses or stringency of governments, namely: (a) centralized versus decentralized government authority and (b) loose versus tight society culture. Their data were also derived from OxCGRT. To consider this question Tables 5 and 6 showed clearly that all countries including the United States, United Kingdom, Denmark and Germany have implemented very stringent measures.

5.6 *Does Herd Immunity Save the Economy?*

Contrasting Sweden with Denmark in handling the COVID-19 challenge, Zuesse (2020), wrote that the herd immunity strategy did not save the economy of the former as Peter Nilsson had hoped. The unemployment rate in Sweden rose from 6% in December 2019 to 9% in May 2020. Denmark, which has imposed more stringent measures, had seen its unemployment rate rise from 3.7% in February 2020, to only 5.4% in April 2020. Zuesse coined the term "Socialistic approach" for Denmark and countries like China and South Korea, and the term "Libertarian approach" for Sweden and countries like United Kingdom (Zuesse 2020). For Sweden by February 2020 the number of deaths had accumulated to 12,188, versus that of Denmark's 2,215; its death rate was 12.02 per 10,000, as compared to 3.8 of Denmark. Stavrou (2020) argued that in adopting a "soft" approach Sweden aimed neither to save the economy nor its health services. Sweden's approach was rooted in their traditions and cultures that favored individual liberty. Sweden was defeated by its failure to protect its older people and preventing them from contracting the disease when stringent isolation of old aged homes was necessary. The Sweden health model has failed to deliver its earlier promises.

5.7 *Could Healthcare Budgets Afford Treatments of COVID-19 Patients?*

Zuesse (2020) rightly pointed out that the highest costs for fighting COVID-19 to governments would be health costs not unemployment benefits. The United Kingdom has earned a good reputation for its equal access to health with its National Health Service (NHS) which is free to its citizens supported by taxpayers' money. However, in previous decades the UK Government has cut spending on NHS leaving it very fragile under the threats of COVID-19. The United States left the financial burden of illness treatments mainly to the individuals who have to purchase private insurances. Its hospitals and doctors are mainly private businesses and private practitioners.

The US health services, consuming 17% of GDP, left 30% of US citizens without insurance coverage of any kind (WHO 2020?). This explained why the UK had a high case fatality rate (7.24) and crude death rate (6.252) and the US had a high attack rate (2.23) as well as high crude death rate (6.308). Germany and China have their own healthcare financing models, Bismarkian and Chinese Socialistic, which provide the best protection for their people and relatively very low crude death rates (1.141 and 0.033 deaths per 10,000 people respectively) during COVID-19.

What is the best time to lift stringency measures?

Streeck et al. (2020) recommended a four steps approach to open up lockdown:

Phase 1: Social quarantine with the aim to contain and slow down the pandemic spread and avoid overloading the health care system.
Phase 2: Withdraw quarantine while ensuring hygienic behavior.
Phase 3: Remove quarantine while maintaining hygienic framework.
Phase 4: Return to public life as it was before the COVID-19 pandemic.

These recommendations are referred to as the German Approach or the "Heinsberg Protocol" of "gradual relaxation". The best timing for leaving one phase and moving into another, such that a second wave can be prevented, and that the effectiveness of community shut down could be maximized, was somehow unanswered.

The Oxford Government Response Tracker scientists recommended that each country should decide its best timing to reopen the economy without underestimating the risks of the second wave of COVID-19. Exhaustion in material and emotional strengths might lead to overall system collapse in the form of multiple disasters in the second wave. Unfortunately, a second wave having an even higher spike than the first has arrived (see Diagram 4).

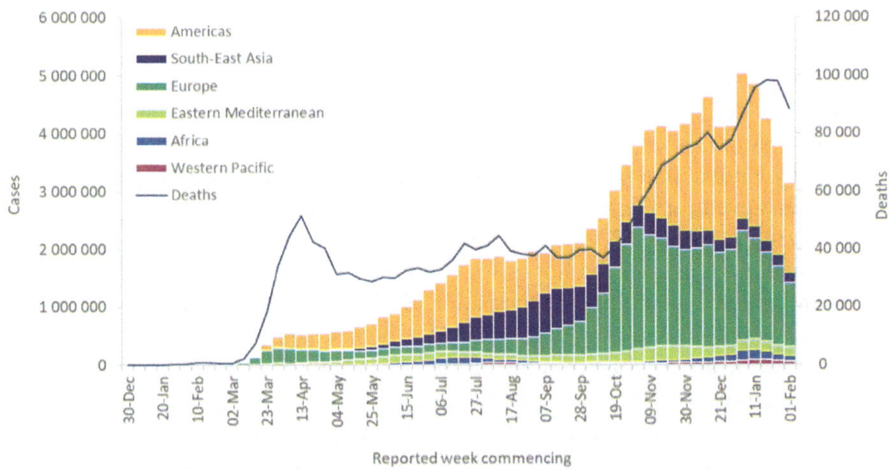

Diagram 4 Second wave shown by WHO data (February 7, 2021)

6 The Second Wave

The number of daily confirmed cases for Italy recorded on July 17 was 10,925, while the spike of the first wave, on March 22, was 6,557; for Spain on October 15 the daily increase was 11,970 with the spike of the first wave, recorded on March 31, at 9,222; Germany's daily increase on October 15 was 5,604, and the spike of the first wave was recorded on March 28, at 10,129; for France on October 15 the daily increase was 43,920, the spike of the first wave was recorded on April 5, at 7,832; in the UK on October 15 the daily increase was 12,874, and the spike of the first wave occurred on April 12 at 5,332; in Sweden on October 13 there were 2,203 new cases, and the spike of the first wave occurred on June 22, at 2,889. The arrival of the second wave of COVID-19 in Europe is obvious and there is no evidence that COVID-19 has become weaker over time (Rose 2020).

Diagram 4 shows that in Europe, the curve has been flattened by April 2020 and then dropped. Then there was a gradual growth until September 2020 when the growth became uncontrollable. In the United States, it was a continuation of the First Wave since its curve never flattened.

Referring to Diagram 2, many countries (the UK, Germany, and India) started from June or July of 2020 to loosen containment and closure measures as reflected by the monthly average Stringency Index. With the surge of the second wave the price tag of premature relaxation is now evident. In contrast China, South Korea and Venezuela kept their Stringency Index continually above 80. It shows that the lockdown strategy is applicable to less developed countries as it may save resources from expenditures on economic support while the cost for economic downturn must also be taken into account.

The Impact of COVID-19 including that of the second wave for the 14 selected countries is presented in Table 11.

Comparing the deaths per 10,000 persons a direct observation is that most countries have worse figures in January 2021 than in October 2020 with the exception of China, changing from 0.033 to 0.034 deaths per 10,000 of population. Notably the United Kingdom recorded the highest deaths per 10,000 of population (16.511) followed by United States (13.768), Mexico (12.743) and Brazil (10.822). The statistics look bad even for Germany, where death rates had risen from 1.141 in October 2020 to 7.343 in January 2021; and Denmark from 1.145 to 3.826.

Vaccination carries all the hopes for a full recovery, even though Fauci (2020) has recently raised the effective vaccination rate to 90%. Director-General of WHO Tedros lamented on January 19, 2021 that a poor country on average received a mere 25 vaccine doses while over 39 million doses have been administered in nearly 50 richer nations. The vaccine supply will not be equally accessible because of its cost, transportation in cold temperatures, and medical facilities requirements (WHO 2021). Vaccines alone cannot save the world and the Stringency Strategy becomes a necessary tool to deal with the Second wave. In China, the terms, "accurate control"

Table 11 Health outcomes as at January 2021[a]

Country	Population (million)	Number of confirmed cases	Number of deaths	Case fatality rate	Crude death rate October 7, 2020	Crude death rate February 7, 2021
Brazil	21,256	9,447,165	230,034	2.435	6.898	10.822
China	1,439,32	101,272	4,831	4.770	0.033	0.034
Denmark	579	201,186	2,215	1.101	1.145	3.826
Germany	8,378	2,284,010	61,517	2.693	1.141	7.343
India	138,000	10,826,363	154,996	1.432	0.758	1.123
Mexico	12,893	1,912,871	164,290	8.589	6.148	12.743
Philippines	10,958	535,521	11,110	2.075	0.535	1.014
Rwanda	1,295	16,337	217	1.328	0.022	0.168
S. Korea	5,127	80,896	1,471	1.818	0.083	0.287
Thailand	6,980	23,371	79	0.338	0.008	0.011
UK	6,789	3,929,839	112,092	2.852	6.252	16.511
US	33,100	26,547,977	455,735	1.717	6.308	13.768
Venezuela	2,844	129,231	1,223	0.946	0.234	0.430
Zambia	1,838	61,427	839	1.366	0.182	0.456

[a]All information derived from WHO (7 February 2021), https://covid19.who.int/ except population from UN Data http://data.un.org/en/index.html

and “flexible stringency,” have been invented to refine the modifications in containment and social distancing, as practiced recently in Shanghai, in February 2021. Evaluation of its effectiveness will probably have to take another 6 months.

7 Preliminary Observations

Questions were raised about whether stringency worked, whether it could be implemented without financial assistance to the poor and when would be the best time to end stringency or how stringency could be relaxed. There were no definite answers to these questions from the review. Nevertheless, this study illustrated that in combating COVID-19:

1. Preparedness of a country, though important, did not necessarily lead to better health outcomes.
2. Stringency, on the other hand, if persistent, contributed to better health outcomes. Most countries that were successful in minimizing serious sickness and deaths imposed stringent measures persistently.
3. A few stringent countries did not get good results. In other words, stringency is a necessary but not sufficient condition for stopping the spread of COVID-19.

4. Meanwhile, enforcement of a Stringency Strategy requires a health governance that is based on trust of the citizens towards the health advice of their governments. Having prior legislation in place like South Korea will make stringency easier to enforce.
5. A Stringency Strategy must be supplemented by other financial assistance and community support.
6. A Stringency Strategy may have to be imposed for a long period of time even after safe vaccines have been developed because a lot of poorer countries cannot afford to purchase these vaccines.

Supported by the observations of this paper, employing the Stringency Strategy, be it called Suppression approach (Mills 2020) or Socialistic Model (Zuesse 2020), is necessary in flattening the curve of new cases of disease and deaths, in all countries. The Herd Immunity Strategy, Mitigation Approach (Mills 2020) or the Libertarian Model (Zuesse 2020), were related with negative health outcomes.

The Imperial College Team, while recommending Herd Immunity Strategy to the British government, also considered that social distancing was necessary, even adopting the Mitigation approach for 12 months as a vaccine would not have been ready within 18 months. Unfortunately, governments could not wait that long and economies were reopened in June and July, as illustrated by the analysis of GRSI in Diagram 2. Early relaxation of stringency has facilitated the second wave, even if it didn't cause it.

A "Scaled-up Health Services Delivery" through pulling all medical human resources available in the community must be mobilized to meet any major public health crisis. In China, the state was the mobilizer, in the UK and US, voluntarism came to assistance as many retired medical staff joined in the fight.

However, stringency is not a pure health science. It is more a behavioral science. Whether wearing a mask is acceptable, meeting friends and visiting families should be allowed, or schools and entertainment venues should be closed, are all social and cultural issues.

Suppression, in the form of Stringent Government Response as suggested by Mills (2020), cannot be a stand-alone measure. It must be accompanied by effective emergency health responses, strong community support and public financial aids. Comprehensive testing with efficient laboratories, centralized quarantine provided with increased bed capacity in temporary hospitals, community support services for the needy disabled persons and older people, plus social and financial aids for the poorer sectors are required to build up a "health and living and income safety net" (Mills 2020, pp. 71–79). Whether the "multi-sectoral, multi-disciplinary, whole-of-government and whole-of-society" approach was mobilized to its fullest strength, by governments as well as communities, determines success or failure in Disaster Response against COVID-19. The theoretically proper approach to handle any pandemic was outlined in the WHO 2019 Health—Emergency and Disaster Risk Management Framework, in full details; the question is whether the world can implement them.

It is impossible to predict how the Second Wave will developed in the coming months. Fortunately, in the latest update the WHO (2021) stated on February 9, 2021, that:

For the fourth week in a row, the number of global new cases reported fell, with 3.1 million new cases last week, a 17% decline compared to the previous week. This is the lowest figure since the week of 26 October 15 weeks ago. Although there are still many countries with increasing numbers of cases, at the global level, this is encouraging. The number of new deaths reported also fell for a second week in a row, with 88,000 new deaths reported last week, a 10% decline as compared to the previous week. All WHO regions reported a decline in new cases, with five out of six regions reporting more than 10% decreases (WHO 2021, Weekly epidemiological update, p. 1) (see Diagram 4).

This development hopefully signaled the flattening of the Second Wave on a global level even without the full implementation of vaccines. Or else, the battle against COVID-19 would be prolonged until satisfactory rate of vaccinations was achieved.

Tracing back even earlier, health scientist Rubin (2011) from the University of Pennsylvania in his report to the OCED entitled "the Future Global Shock of Pandemic" projected that if case fatality ratio was higher than 2.0, classified in the report as Category 5, then there would be 1.8 million deaths in the United States. His prediction sadly has come true. For Category 5 of his Pandemic Severity Index, he recommended stringent mitigation measures by closing down all workplaces, schools and public facilities. Home isolation, though voluntary, was recommended. It sounds familiar. Let these words of Rubin be remembered:

The daunting challenge of tracking, detecting, preventing and treating infectious diseases is the arms race of the 21st century. The race is not between states; the race is between the global community and pathogens found in nature or pathogens nefariously disseminated. The challenge calls for new solutions that integrate basic science, technology, and social, political, legal and economic realities. The solution should optimize tradeoffs in the interplay of international security, global health, the creation and open dissemination of new knowledge and the maintenance and enhancement of the positive role of modern molecular biology on the economy of the developing world (Rubin 2011).

References

Courtemanche, C., Garuccio, J., Pinkston, J., & Yelowitz, A. (2020) Strong Social Distancing Measures in the United States Reduced the COVID-19 Growth Rate. *Health Affairs, 39*(7). Available at: https://www.healthaffairs.org/doi/full/10.1377/hlthaff.2020.00608.

D'Souza, G., & Dowdy, D. (2020) What Is Herd Immunity and How Can We Achieve It with COVID-19? John Hopkins University. *School of Public Health Expert Insights*, April 10, 2020. Available at: https://www.jhsph.edu/covid-19/articles/achieving-herd-immunity-with-covid19.html.

Fauci, A. (2020) Fauci Says Herd Immunity Could Require Nearly 90% to Get Coronavirus Vaccine. GMA Network, December 25, 2020 2:41 am. Available at: https://www.gmanetwork.

com/news/news/world/769337/fauci-says-herd-immunity-could-require-nearly-90-to-get-coronavirus-vaccine/story/.
Global Health Security Index (2020). Why is the GHS Index Needed? Available at: https://www.ghsindex.org/about/#Developing-the-GHS-Index.
Grad, Y. (2020) Coronavirus COVID-19: Press Conference. Harvard TH Chan School of Public Health, 09/25/20. Available at: https://www.hsph.harvard.edu/news/features/coronavirus-covid-19-press-conference-with-yonatan-grad-09-25-20/.
Hale, T., Phillips, T., Petherick, A., Kira, B., Angrist, N., & Webster, S. (2020a) Lockdown Rollback Checklist: Do Countries Meet WHO Recommendations for Rolling Back Lockdown? *Blavatnik School Working Paper Version 4.0.* University of Oxford, Blavatnik School of Government, June 1, 2020. Available at: https://www.bsg.ox.ac.uk/sites/default/files/2020-06/Lockdown%20Rollback%20Checklist%20v4.pdf.
Hale, T., Angrist, N., Boby, T., Blake, E. C., Hallas, L., Kira, B., Majumdar, S., Petherick, A., Phillips, T., Tatlow, H., & Webster, S. (2020b) Variation in Government Responses to COVID-19. *Blavatnik School Working Paper Version 10.0.* University of Oxford, Blavatnik School of Government, May 25, 2020. Available at: https://www.bsg.ox.ac.uk/research/publications/variation-government-responses-covid-19.
Indiatimes. (2020) COVID-19 Count Reaches 39 in India. Available at: https://economictimes.indiatimes.com/news/politics-and-nation/covid-19-count-reaches-39-inindia/articleshow/74538233.cms?utm_source=contentofinterest&utm_medium=text&utm_campaign=cppst.
Johns Hopkins University. (2019) Bloomberg School of Public Health. *Inaugural Global Health Security Index Finds Significant Gaps in Preparedness for Epidemics and Pandemics.* October 24. Available at: https://www.jhsph.edu/news/news-releases/2019/inaugural-global-health-security-index-finds-significant-gaps-in-preparedness-for-epidemics-and-pandemics.html.
John Hopkins University. (2020) COVID-19 Map. Coronavirus Resource Center. Available at: https://coronavirus.jhu.edu/map.html.
Kayano, R., Chan, Y. Y., Murray, V., Abraham, J., & Barber, S. L. (2019) WHO Thematic Platform for Health Emergency and Disaster Risk Management Research Network (TPRN): Report of the Kobe Expert Meeting. *International Journal of Environmental Research and Public Health, 16*(7), 1232. Available at: https://doi.org/10.3390/ijerph16071232.
McMahon, A. (2020) Coronavirus: UK Government's 'Herd Immunity' Plan Sparks Fear and Fury. *New Zealand Herald,* March 17. Available at: https://www.nzherald.co.nz/world/coronavirus-uk-governments-herd-immunity-plan-sparks-fear-and-fury/ARQ3BOD4IGBLSM3WEQXAYBMGYI/.
Mills, S. (2020) COVID-19, Public Health Measures, Legal Considerations: A Medical Perspective. *Judicial Review, 25*(2), 71–79. Available at: https://doi.org/10.1080/10854681.2020.1760575.
Oxford University. (2020a) Coronavirus Government Response Tracker. Available at: https://www.bsg.ox.ac.uk/research/research-projects/coronavirus-government-response-tracker.
Oxford University. (2020b) Government Response Stringency Index. Available at: https://www.bsg.ox.ac.uk/research/research-projects/coronavirus-government-response-tracker.
Reiner, R. C., Barber, R. M., & Murray, C. J. L. (2020) Modeling COVID-19 Scenarios for the United States, IHME COVID-19 Forecasting Team, University of Washington. *Nature Medicine, 27*, 94–105. Available at: https://doi.org/10.1038/s41591-020-1132-9.
Rose, J. (2020) COVID-19 Will Mutate What Does It Mean to a Vaccine? Healthline. Available at: https://www.healthline.com/health-news/what-to-know-about-mutation-and-covid-19.
Rubin, H. (2011) Future Global Shocks: Pandemics, Organization for Economic Cooperation and Development (OCED), International Future Shock Project. Available at: http://www.oecd.org/governance/risk/46889985.pdf.
Sputnik. (2020) Swedish Model: Ruined Economy Will Cause More Deaths Than Coronavirus, May 7. Available at: https://www.sott.net/article/434004-Swedish-Model-Ruined-economy-will-cause-more-deaths-than-coronavirus-Prof [05:00].
Stavrou, D. (2020) Sweden Is the Key Coronavirus Test Case in Preparing for a Second Wave. *Haaretz*, June 6. Available at: https://www.haaretz.com/misc/writers/WRITER-1.5601908.

Streeck, H. et al. (2020) Infection Fatality Rate of SARS-CoV2 in a Super-Spreading Event in Germany. Nature Communications, November 17. Available at: https://www.nature.com/articles/s41467-020-19509-y#rightslink.

Tognotti, E. (2013) Lessons from the History of Quarantine, from Plague to Influenza A. *Emerging Infectious Diseases, 19*(2), 254–259. Available at: https://dx.doi.org/10.3201/eid1902.120312.

UN-Habitat. (2020) COVID-19 Response Plan. Available at: https://unhabitat.org/sites/default/files/2020/04/final_un-habitat_covid-19_response_plan.pdf.

University of Washington. (2020). COVID-19 Projections. Institute of Health Metric and Evaluation, October 15. Available from: https://covid19.healthdata.org/global?view=total-deaths&tab=trend.

World Bank. (2018) New Country Classifications by Income Level: 2018–2019. World Bank Data Team. Available at: https://blogs.worldbank.org/opendata/new-country-classifications-income-level-2018-2019.

World Health Organization. (2019) Health Emergency and Disaster Risk Management Framework, Section 7.1. p. 15, Geneva: License: CC BY-NC-SA 3.0 IGO. Available at: https://apps.who.int/iris/bitstream/handle/10665/326106/9789241516181-eng.pdf?sequence=1&isAllowed=y.

World Health Organization. (2020a) Coronavirus Disease 2019 (COVID-19) Situation Report—40. Available at: https://www.who.int/docs/default-source/coronaviruse/situation-reports/20200229-sitrep-40-covid-19.pdf?sfvrsn=849d0665_2.

World Health Organization. (2020b) WHO Coronavirus Disease (COVID-19) Dashboard. Available at: https://portal.who.int/report/eios-covid19-counts/#display=Countries_and_Territories&nrow=2&ncol=3&arr=row&pg=1&labels=cur_death_who&sort=cur_death_who;desc&filter=&sidebar=4&fv=cur_death_who.

World Health Organization. (2020c) Considerations in Adjusting Public Health and Social Measures in the Context of COVID-19 Interim Guidance. Available at: https://apps.who.int/iris/bitstream/handle/10665/331773/WHO-2019-nCoV-Adjusting_PH_measures-2020.1-eng.pdf.

World Health Organization. (2021) Weekly Epidemiological Update, 9 February 2021. Available at: https://www.who.int/publications/m/item/weekly-epidemiological-update—9-february-2021.

Yan, B., Zhang, X. M., & Wu, L. (2020) Why Do Countries Respond Differently to COVID-19? A Comparative Study of Sweden, China, France, and Japan. *The American Review of Public Administration, 50*(6–7), 2020. Available at: https://journals.sagepub.com/doi/full/10.1177/0275074020942445.

Zuesse, E. (2020) Herd Immunity Is a Failed Response to Coronavirus. *Duran*, 06-29. Available at: https://theduran.com/herd-immunity-is-a-failed-response-to-coronavirus.

Country Reports and Comparative Studies

Experiences of and Responses to COVID-19 in East Asia: The Cases of Japan and Korea

Yong Xin Ruan and Charles T. L. Leung

Abstract Although the outbreak of COVID-19 has spread around the globe to become a pandemic, differences between the West and the East are observed. In the case of East Asia, represented by Japan and Korea, relatively low prevalence and death rates are reported. This chapter therefore aims to explain the phenomenon with reference to the knowledge of social sciences, with specific focus on the health-care measures and initiatives on the older adults. Possible reasons of the effectiveness would also be illustrated. It is expected that this chapter may provide a lesson learned in these two East Asian countries fighting against the epidemic situation.

Keywords COVID-19 · East Asia · Healthcare · Older adults · Social sciences

1 Introduction

According to the official data released by the World Health Organization [WHO] (2020a), up to the beginning of September 2020, total global cumulative cases of COVID-19 have reached more than 27 million in which more than 3% death rate (almost 891 thousand cases) were reported. Despite the spread of COVID-19 around the globe, differences among the countries are explicitly revealed. When compared the situation across the regions divided by WHO, it is found that the number of confirmed cases ($n = 522{,}080$) and that of death cases ($n = 1{,}353$) in the region of West Pacific are the lowest (WHO 2020a). Located in West Pacific, Japan has 72,234 cumulative total cases while the Republic of Korea [Korea] has 21,423, an aggregate significantly lower than other western countries like the U.S. ($n = 6{,}222{,}974$) and the U.K. ($n = 350{,}104$) (WHO 2020b).

Y. X. Ruan
The Chinese University of Hong Kong, Hong Kong, China

C. T. L. Leung (✉)
Beijing Normal University-Hong Kong Baptist University United International College, Zhuhai, China
e-mail: charlestlleung@uic.edu.cn

S.X.B. Zhao et al. (eds.), *COVID-19 Pandemic, Crisis Responses and the Changing World*, https://doi.org/10.1007/978-981-16-2430-8_8

In view of the two well-performing countries, this chapter attempts to explore their experience on case control, with a focus on older adults. The authors firstly review the situations of both countries affected by the epidemic outbreak. They then highlight those effective initiatives of healthcare on older adults against the infection of COVID-19 in Japan and Korea. The reasons of effectiveness are then examined. Last but not least, the experiences of East Asia drawn from these two countries are further deliberated and discussed so as to provide insights to other regions and countries also facing a "new normal".

2 Historical Review of the Outbreaks in Japan and Korea

According to Tashiro and Shaw (2020), in Japan, the beginning of the COVID-19 pandemic in Japan can be traced back to possibly January 10–15, 2020. Since then, Japanese government promptly carried out Infection Disease Control Law in handling of the epidemic situation (Tashiro and Shaw 2020). Following the first confirmed case, infection occurred in the Diamond Princess cruise ship. Later, there was a local outbreak in February, and the number of new cases continuously rose from February to March (Wake et al. 2020). To control the rate of infection, the government strengthened their medical capacities as well as carried out basic countermeasure policies during this period (Tashiro and Shaw 2020). Later, the government of Japan decided to declare a state of emergency on April 7. The number of new cases declined immediately afterward. In May, the state of emergency was gradually eased and finally lifted on May 25. Later, the government proactively implemented testing in night-life settings and screened out the confirmed cases. Hence, since June, there was an increase in the number of daily new cases (Oshitani 2020) (Fig. 1).

In Korea, the first case of COVID-19 was reported on January 20, 2020 (Ministry of Science and ICT [MSI] 2020). The government reacted rapidly by establishing an emergency response committee and prepared for massive testing (Our World in Data 2020). The outbreak was identified when an infected patient was discovered to have attended a number of gatherings while travelling the approximately 240 km between Daegu and Seoul, the capital city. On March, the number of new cases firstly declined, followed by a drop to well below 200 cases daily from March 12 to August 15. During this time, the government carried out different arrangements for patients based on the severity of individual case in order to reduce burden of healthcare system and implemented strict rules on social distancing (The Government of the Republic of Korea 2020). On August 16, the number of new cases rose above 200, with the primary source being an outbreak in Sarang Jeil Church (Korea Centers for Disease Control & Prevention 2020). Before September, there was a fluctuating increase in the daily number of new cases and the amount of new cases were over 200 daily. Most of the new cases were related to church gatherings (Korea Centers for Disease Control & Prevention 2020). Since 15 August, mandatory infection control measures were implemented in church, and later social distancing level 2 were effective (Korea

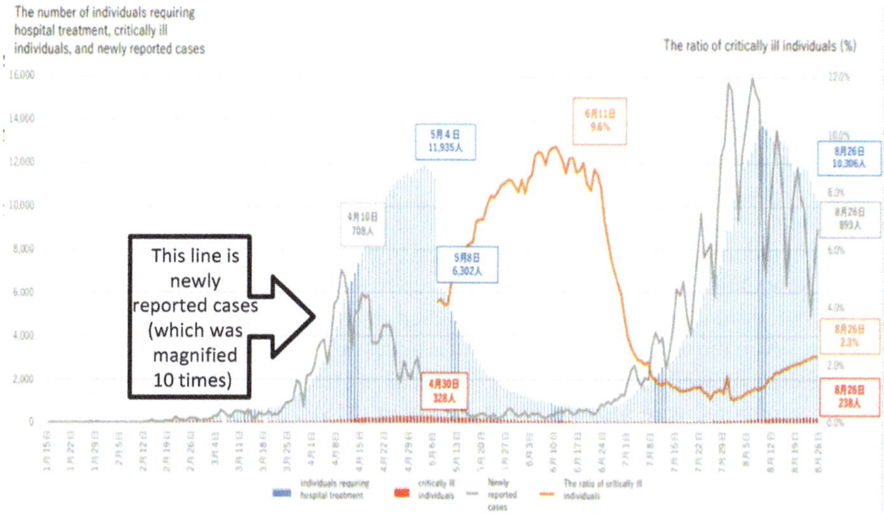

Fig. 1 The number of individuals requiring hospital treatment, critically ill individuals, and newly reported cases (January–August) (*Source* https://www.mhlw.go.jp/content/10900000/000666371.pdf)

Centers for Disease Control & Prevention 2020). On September, the amount of daily new cases dropped below 200 (Fig. 2).

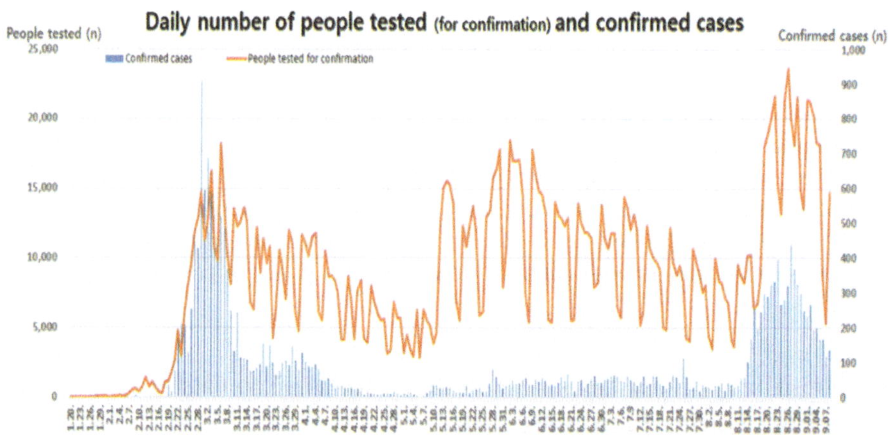

Fig. 2 The daily number of confirmed cases and people tested (January–September) (*Source* http://www.kdca.go.kr/board/board.es?mid=a30402000000bid=0030)

3 Overview of the Impacts on Citizens

Various issues affecting the daily life of citizens in both countries are observed. In Japan, the information released by the Ministry of Health, Labour and Welfare has shown that the provision of childcare and after-school services were reduced and temporarily closed (Wake et al. 2020). The number of consultations reported for mental health services were dramatically increased almost three times in April (n = 4946) when compared with the data between February and March (n = 1739) (Jijitsushin New Online 2020). According to a report of Wake et al. (2020), the number of cases of child abuse and domestic violence on women has increased. Numerous Japanese, even those with property, found it necessary to apply for public assistance. The infected as well as the attending medical professionals faced discrimination. Similar situations were also observed in Korea (MSI 2020). It has been observed that mental health issues such as anxiety, depression and sleep disorder increase in prevalence. Therefore, they are in need of psychological support services (Park and Yu 2020). It is also reported that spiritual needs for religious services are highlighted (MSI 2020).

Among the individuals suffering from the pandemic, older adults comprise the most vulnerable population. There were 11,590 patients over 60 years old by August 26, 2020 in Japan. Though patients aged from 20–29 years old (n = 18,601) had the highest number of cases compared with other age groups, the amount of deaths of older patients outnumbered other age groups (Statista 2020a). In Korea, a similar situation was observed. The 20–29 age group occupied the highest percentages of case number (23.52%) while people from 60–69 years old occupied the third largest percentages of case number (14.05%) by August 21, 2020. However, the fatality rate increases with the increase of age and it accelerates after 60 years old (Statista 2020b).

A cause for the high percentage of cases in the 20–29 age group may be traced to the tendency in that group to being more socially active (Korean Society of Infectious Disease et al. 2020). However, the fatality rate of older adults remains higher than other age groups because older adults will have more serious outcomes when becoming infected (Shahid et al. 2020). The following paragraphs will introduce how the governments in both countries to protect this group of people.

4 Healthcare Measures and Policies Related to Older Adults Under Pandemic

Healthcare measures and policies carried out by the governments in both countries pay special attention to vulnerable groups of people such as older adults under the pandemic.

In Japan, regarding medical care, call-center-based consultation systems are established for healthcare seeking and referral. Individual in need of medical attention are required to consult the call-centers before seeking medical care, which can ease the burden of healthcare delivery system as well as providing an overview of epidemic scale (Gai and Tobe 2020). However, during the consultation, older patients are encouraged to seek medical care because of their vulnerability, so they are given priority in healthcare delivery. Also, necessary cares are guaranteed for older adults. They can receive the care via phone call without visiting medical institutions (Ministry of Health, Labour and Welfare, [MHLW] 2020).

In term of long-term care facilities, which have high risks of infections, thorough infection control measures are required to be taken including personal hygiene measures such as washing hands and wearing masks, prohibiting visitors, measures to prevent workers to become source of infection, and isolating suspected patients and implementing counter-infection measures (MHLW 2020).

Apart from that, some policies not specific to but having influence on the conduct of the older adults, have also been included. Firstly, to reduce chances for infection, the Japanese government requires citizens to stay at home, exemption is given for necessary activities such as going to the hospital and buying food. Also, citizens are requested to avoid the "3Cs" setting (closed spaces, crowded places, and close-contact setting) both indoors and outdoors. Apart from that, the government would provide accurate and updated information about the situation of pandemic, counter-infection measures, guidelines for healthcare seeking, etc. through social media vehicles such as the government website and appropriate YouTube channels in order to raise public awareness with the objective of changing behaviour and reducing panic (MHLW 2020).

In Korea, similar measures and policies were carried out. Older patients were given priority to be hospitalized as well. Especially, comprehensive measures were taken in long-term care institutions (LTCI) to prevent the infections. Firstly, the government provides reimbursement guidelines for LTCI to help them to deal with staff shortages and order masks for care workers. Secondly, strict monitoring was implemented in these facilities to strengthen preventive measures and screen out potentially infected workers. Also, infection disease guidelines were introduced and the institutions were required to comply with the guidelines. Thirdly, though the community-based care centers were closed, care services like meal delivery are still maintained for older adults (Kim 2020).

There are, at present, other measures for all age-groups to effectively control the number of cases in Korea. Those measures are therefore highlighted. They include massive testing by using drive-thru and walk-thru model, effective tracing with information technology and low-cost treatment due to coverage provided by the National Health Insurance Service (Kim 2020; Kwon 2020; Ministry of Health and Welfare 2020).

Since the measures and policies in both countries are acknowledged to be effective, the following paragraphs will explore factors contributing to the effectiveness of these measures and policies.

5 Factors that Determine the Effectiveness to Control the Pandemic

Firstly, the major factor should be the high level of compliance of the public in both countries. When the government of Korea encouraged citizens to maintain social distance and adopt hygiene behaviors such as washing hand and wearing masks, citizens are generally willing to comply with these recommendations. The compliance is demonstrated by the more than 90% of residents including older adults who avoid crowded places and gathering. Also, over 50% of residents have begun to wear masks and to wash hands after the COVID-19 outbreak in Korea (Statista 2020b). Similar situation has been observed in Japan. The public have, thus, complied with the recommendations of avoiding "3Cs" and staying at home. Yamada et al. (2020) found that older adults in continuing care retirement community spend less time in common areas and decrease their daily walking distance.

There are two interrelated factors contributing to the compliance in both countries: Trust in government and culture. Travaglino and Moon (2021) found that compliance is associated with trust in government. The governments released accurate and updated information for the public during the pandemic, which increases trust of citizens in government. This transparent communication between the government and the public is essential, which builds the trust to the government (Kwon 2020). If insufficient information about the virus is given by the government, the public will reduce their trust in the government, thereby, lowering the extent of compliance to the healthcare measures. For example, lacking of governmental supervision on the pandemic during the early stage of MERS outbreak, the Korean government fail to provide sufficient information to the public. Therefore, a widespread distrust occurred (Lee and You 2020; Travaglino and Moon 2021).

Cultural values can also be a significant determinant in compliance. The values of a society or community can be divided into two categories: individualism and collectivism. Individualistic cultures emphasize independence, so individual goals are prioritized while collectivism focuses on interdependence, in which group-level goals are valued (Travaglino and Moon 2021). Frey et al. (2020) found that people in countries with collectivist culture tend to follow the restriction to mobility, revealing the relationship between collectivist culture and compliance. As Japan and Korea are two countries that emphasize collectivist culture, residents would be more willing to follow instructions from the government like wearing masks (Tashiro and Shaw 2020). Furthermore, collectivist culture and trust in government is interrelated. Trust in government is not only related to the performance of government but also is associated with a culture valuing cohesive relationships. Therefore, people in a culture of collectivism are more likely to have faith in governmental actions (Travaglino and Moon 2021). It should be noted that there are other reasons to trust in government, apart from culture (Bouckaert and Van de Walle 2001). Also, compliance is only one type of conformity; another type of conformity is internalization. Internalization is related to accepting information about reality and thus having accurate conception of reality and behaving properly. Study showed that no cross-cultural difference (individualism vs collectivism) in internalization was found (Oh 2013). Therefore, citizens in individualist culture could still accept the accurate information about pandemic released by the government and change their behaviors.

Apart from collectivist culture, the customs and greeting styles in both countries quite correlate with the policies emphasizing wearing masks and maintaining social distance. As a result, it may appear natural for the citizens of these two countries to comply with those epidemic prevention measures. It is found that people in East Asia have a custom to wear masks for various reasons, not just for sickness (Li et al. 2020). For example, in Japan, citizens would normally use masks to prevent respiratory infections. Therefore, during the outbreak of COVID-19, this custom protects the infection of virus to some extent (Iwasaki and Grubaugh 2020). Regarding greeting style, unlike some western cultures where kissing and hugging are the acceptable forms of greeting, citizens in Japan and Korea prefer to bow for greeting people. This act avoids close contacts among citizens (Iwasaki and Grubaugh 2020). Hence, the Japanese and Korean population not unexpectedly comply, in general, with the policy of maintaining social distance.

Secondly, previous experiences of dealing with other epidemics also contribute to the effectiveness of controlling number of cases. Japan and Korea experienced other infectious diseases before, so lessons learned may strengthen the capacity of the governments; thus, older adults have already equipped some knowledge on controlling infections. In Japan, the influenza epidemic in 2009 raised awareness of prevention measures of citizens, especially older adults (Takahashi et al. 2017). Therefore, older adults will draw on a historical memory to adopt preventive measures during COVID-19, such as wearing masks (Lim et al. 2020). Also, in Korea, a previous outbreak of MERS enriched the knowledge and practice of hand-washing among the older adults (Song and Yang 2016), which may increase compliance of hygiene behaviors recommended by the government in the COVID-19 pandemic. In addition, the experience in MERS enabled the government to improve their pandemic response. For example, more comprehensive testing for COVID-19 has been implemented. (Frey et al., 2020).

Thirdly, ongoing preparedness for infectious control in healthcare facilities in both countries may be helpful to address COVID-19. In Japan, before the outbreak of COVID-19, Kariya et al. (2018) found that long-term care facilities for older adults have already equipped infection control manuals and related professionals. Almost all long-term care facilities followed the guidelines of the Society for Healthcare Epidemiology of America-a worldwide recognized protocol. While in Korea, before this pandemic, the hospitals had run simulations of different outbreak conditions to enhance their readiness and capacity for controlling epidemics (Our World in Data 2020).

6 Lessons Learned in These Two Countries

After examining the countries' measures and policies to control the infections in older adults, and those factors influencing the effectiveness of related measures and policies, the following experiences can be learned from Japan and Korea.

Firstly, the cautious attitude, which is rooted in the Eastern Asian culture and history, towards COVID-19 for taking prompt response to prevent outbreak is a key to epidemic control. From aforementioned timeline, it can be seen that after the first confirmed case occurred, the governments in both countries rapidly reacted to control the pandemic. However, when the first case was observed in the U.K., the government did not take the needed consistent action. Not until the first death occurred in the county did the government start to carry out relevant measures (Mafham et al. 2020). Therefore, the number of infected cases, especially at the beginning stage, in both Japan and Korea were significantly lower than that in the Western countries like the U.K.

Secondly, it is essential to enhance the public compliance by providing sufficient and accurate information to build trust in the government. In particular, it is important that the information is made accessible to the older adults. Also, the information enabled the public to take the appropriate measures to guard against infection (Lee and You 2020). According to an online survey on COVID-19 (Geldsetzer 2020), it is found that the citizens in the U.K. and the U.S. held misconceptions pertaining to effective preventive measures. Some of these misconceptions resulted from inaccurate information disseminating via social media. Therefore, it is crucial for health authorities to work with social media to provide accurate information and also to identify misinformation.

Thirdly, as the pandemic may last for a significant period—possibly into 2022, a new lifestyle needs to be promoted such as changing the greeting style and promoting the habit of washing hands through health promotion programs. Older adults, in particular, may reduce physical activities under the pandemic. How to maintain the physical and mental health of the population group should be paid attention by the social service agencies. The agencies may need to help older adults to adapt to new lifestyle. More importantly, older adults living alone or having low income may need additional care. Because they may face more issues under the pandemic; relevant policies and measures should be provided to support this age group. For example, the government in Korea is formulating plans to provide financial support and voucher programs for vulnerable populations such as the older adults living alone (Kwon 2020).

Lastly, other countries of the world should continuously improve the measures to control infections. The experiences of Korea and Japan show that the effectiveness of controlling the pandemic depends on ongoing preparedness of healthcare facilities. Therefore, governments should enhance the capacities of healthcare facilities to control infections through gaining experience in this pandemic, and provide training for healthcare professionals. Moreover, the vulnerability of long-term care facilities is revealed during the pandemic, so the infection control measures taken and the knowledge level of staff should be further examined so as to improve their effectiveness in controlling infections.

7 Conclusion

The book chapter introduced the situations of coronavirus prevention in Japan and Korea, as well as their measures/policies to reduce risks of infection on older adults. This chapter also identified several factors that led to the effectiveness of these measures and policies, including high level of compliance of the citizens (which was influenced by the culture and customs, and trust in government), previous experiences in dealing with other epidemics, and ongoing preparedness of healthcare facilities. Through these examinations, other countries can draw a few notable lessons from these two countries: firstly, to provide supports on older adults, which represent a vulnerable population during the pandemic. Though the individualist culture in some countries may influence the compliance of citizens, the governments in these countries may still increase trust of citizens in government by providing accurate and sufficient information about the pandemic and counter-infection measures. As the pandemic may last for a significant period, the governments need to support older adults to adapt their lifestyle under the new normal.

References

Bouckaert, G. & Van de Walle, S. (2001) Government performance and trust in government. Available at: https://www.researchgate.net/profile/Steven_Van_de_Walle/publication/228767477_Government_Performance_and_Trust_in_Government/links/02e7e521e026c60989000000.pdf. (Accessed 28 January 2020).

Frey, CB. Chen, C. & Presidente, G. (2020) Democracy, culture, and contagion: Political regimes and countries responsiveness to COVID-19. *COVID Economics* 18: 1–20. https://www.oxfordmartin.ox.ac.uk/downloads/academic/Democracy-Culture-and-Contagion_May13.pdf.

Gai, R. Tobe, M. (2020) Managing healthcare delivery system to fight the COVID-19 epidemic: experience in Japan. *Glo Health Res Policy* 5: 23. https://doi.org/10.1186/s41256-020-00149-0.

Geldsetzer, P. (2020) Use of rapid online surveys to assess people's perceptions during infectious disease outbreaks: a cross-sectional survey on COVID-19. *J Med Internet Res* 22: e18790.

Iwasaki, A. & Grubaugh, ND. (2020) Why does Japan have so few cases of COVID-19? *EMBO Mol Med* 12: e12481.

Jijitsushin New Online. (2020) Heart consultation, surge in April New Corona impact, more than 4900-Ministry of Health, Labour and Welfare. Available at: https://www.jiji.com/sp/article?k=2020052900799&g=cov. (Accessed 9 September 2020).

Kariya, N., Sakon, N. & Komano, J. et al. (2018) Current prevention and control of health care-associated infections in long-term care facilities for the elderly in Japan. *J infection and chemotherapy* 24: 347–352.

Kim, HS. (2020) The impact of COVID-19 on long-term care in South Korea and measures to address it. LTccovid.org. https://ltccovid.org/wp-content/uploads/2020/05/The-Long-Term-Care-COVID19-situation-in-South-Korea-7-May-2020.pdf. (Accessed 26 August 2020).

Korea Centers for Disease Control & Prevention. (2020) Press release. Available at: http://www.kdca.go.kr/board/board.es?mid=a30402000000&bid=0030.

Korean Society of Infectious Disease, Korean Society of Pediatric Infectious Disease, Korean Society of Epidemiology et al. (2020) Report on the epidemiological features of Coronavirus Disease 2019 (COVID-19) outbreak in the Republic of Korea from January 19 to March 2, 2020. *J Korean Med Sci*, 35: e112. https://doi.org/10.3346/jkms.2020.35.e112.

Kwon, S. (2020) COVID-19: Lessons from South Korea. *Health System Global*. https://healthsystemsglobal.org/news/covid-19-lessons-from-south-korea/. (Accessed 26 August 2020).

Lee, M. & You, M. (2020) Psychological and behavioral responses in South Korea During the Early Stages of Coronavirus Disease 2019 (COVID-19). *Int J Environ Res Public Health* 17: 1–14. https://doi.org/10.3390/ijerph17092977.

Li, T., Liu, Y. & Li, M. et al. (2020) Mask or no mask for COVID-19: A public health and market study. *PloS one* 15: e0237691.

Lim, WS., Liang, CK. & Assantachai, P. et al. (2020) COVID-19 and older people in Asia: Asian Working Group for Sarcopenia calls to actions. Geriatr Geron Int 20: 547–558. https://doi.org/10.1111/ggi.13939.

Mafham, MM. Spata, E. & Goldacre, R. et al. (2020). COVID-19 pandemic and admission rates for and management of acute coronary syndromes in England. *The Lancet* 396: 381–389. https://doi.org/10.1016/s0140-6736(20)31356-8.

Ministry of Health, Labour and Welfare. (2020) Basic policies for Novel Coronavirus disease control by the government of Japan. Available at: https://www.mhlw.go.jp/stf/seisakunitsuite/bunya/newpage_00032.html. (Accessed 9 September 2020).

Ministry of Science and ICT. (2020) How we fought COVID-19: A perspective from Science & ICT. Available at: http://www.mofa.go.kr/eng/brd/m_22591/view.do?seq=28&srchFr=&srchTo=&srchWord=&srchTp=&multi_itm_seq=0&itm_seq_1=0&itm_seq_2=0&company_cd=&company_nm=&page=1&titleNm=. (Accessed 9 September 2020).

Ministry of Health and Welfare. (2020) Korean government's response system. Available at: http://ncov.mohw.go.kr/en/baroView.do?brdId=11&brdGubun=111&dataGubun=&ncvContSeq=&contSeq=&board_id=. (Accessed 9 September 2020).

Oh, SH. (2013) Do collectivists conform more than individualists? Cross-cultural differences in compliance and internalization. *Social Behavior and Personality: An International Journal* 41: 981–994.

Oshitani, H. (2020) The new phase of COVID-19 response in Japan (2020/7/13). Ministry of Health, Labour and Welfare. Available at: https://www.mhlw.go.jp/content/10900000/000648616.pdf. (Accessed 9 September 2020).

Our World in Data. (2020) Emerging COVID-19 success story: South Korea learned the lessons of MERS. Available at: https://ourworldindata.org/covid-exemplar-south-korea. (Accessed 9 September 2020).

Park, H. & Yu, S. (2020) Mental healthcare policies in South Korea during the COVID-19 epidemic. *Health Policy Technol* 10. https://doi.org/10.1016/j.hlpt.2020.06.006.

Shahid, Z. Kalayanamitra, R. & McClafferty, B. et al. (2020) COVID-19 and older adults: What We Know. *J Am Geriatr Soc* 68: 926–929. https://doi.org/10.1111/jgs.16472.

Song, M. & Yang, N. (2016) A Study on hand hygiene for infectious disease control in elderly. *Adv Sci Technol Lett* 132: 130–135.

Statista. (2020a) Coronavirus (COVID-19) in Japan. Available at: https://www.statista.com/statistics/1105162/japan-patients-detail-novel-coronavirus-covid-19-cases-by-age-and-gender/. (Accessed 9 September 2020).

Statista, (2020b). Coronavirus (COVID-19) in South Korea-Statistics & facts. Available at: https://www.statista.com/topics/6082/coronavirus-covid-19-in-south-korea/. (Accessed 9 September 2020).

Takahashi, S., Sato, K. & Kusaka, Y. et al. (2017) Public preventive awareness and preventive behaviors during a major influenza epidemic in Fukui, Japan. *J Infect Public Health* 10: 637–643. https://doi.org/10.1016/j.jiph.2017.04.002.

Tashiro, A. Shaw, R. (2020) COVID-19 pandemic response in Japan: What is behind the initial flattening of the curve? *Sustainability* 12:5250.

The Government of the Republic of Korea. (2020) COVID-19, testing time for resilience: In recovering from COVID-19: Korean. Available at: https://www.preventionweb.net/publications/view/71638. (Accessed 9 September 2020).

Travaglino, AG. & Moon, C. (2021) Explaining compliance with social distancing during the COVID-19 pandemic: A cross-cultural study of trust and self-conscious emotions in the United States, Italy, and South Korea. *Frontiers in Psychology* 16. https://doi.org/10.3389/fpsyg.2021.565845.

Wake, J., Ohwa, M. & Matsuo, K. et al. (2020) Japan. In: COVID-19 and social work: A collection of country reports. IASSW. Available at: https://www.iassw-aiets.org/wp-content/uploads/2020/07/IASSW-COVID-19-and-Social-Work-Country-Reports-Final-1.pdf. (Accessed 9 September 2020).

World Health Organization. (2020a) WHO Coronavirus Disease (COVID-19) Dashboard. Available at: https://covid19.who.int/. (Accessed 9 September 2020).

World Health Organization. (2020b) WHO Coronavirus Disease (COVID-19) Dashboard. Available at: https://covid19.who.int/table. (Accessed 9 September 2020).

Yamada, Y., Uchida, T. & Ognio, M. et al. (2020) Changes in older people's activities during the COVID-19 pandemic in Japan. *J Am Med Dir Assoc* 21: 1387–1388. https://doi.org/10.1016/j.jamda.2020.07.039.

Where Everyone Plays a Part: Singapore's Health EDRM Responses in Face of the COVID-19 Crisis

Ghee W. Ho

Abstract Singapore faced the impact of the COVID-19 first as an imported disease and later having a relatively less severe community outbreak, and a more severe sub-community outbreak among migrant workers. Singapore named its lockdown as the Circuit Breaker, and lobbied community support for containing the disease. High quality health services help to provide a sense of security and confidence to the effectiveness of the government among residents of Singapore. Systematic communications of the disease characteristics and situations to the public also play an important role to enhance community resilience. Being a city state, Singapore's unique approach to control the spread of the disease may not be applicable to other countries; however by sharing its experience, it might help other countries to develop their idiosyncratic plans to combat COVID-19 within their own borders.

Keywords COVID-19 · Health EDRM · Public-health crisis · Whole-community approach

1 Introduction

On New Year's Eve 2020, China reported to the World Health Organization, W.H.O., regarding a cluster of cases of pneumonia in Wuhan, Hubei Province, which we now know as the novel Coronavirus SARS-CoV-2. Within three days into the New Year, Singapore's Ministry of Health, MOH, began screening travelers from Wuhan. By the third week of January 2020, Singapore set up a Multi-Ministry Task Force, MTF, to deal with the novel Coronavirus outbreak, and began to identify, quarantine and treat traveler with pneumonia symptoms and a 14-day travel history to China (Yong 2020).

The MTF is backed up by the Homeland Crisis Executive Group (HCEG), which was originally set up to coordinate responses across ministries during the national crisis. Singapore being a state contributor to W.H.O.'s Health Emergency

G. W. Ho (✉)
Beijing Normal University Hong Kong Baptist University United International College, Zhuhai, China
e-mail: gheeho@uic.edu.cn

S.X.B. Zhao et al. (eds.), *COVID-19 Pandemic, Crisis Responses and the Changing World*, https://doi.org/10.1007/978-981-16-2430-8_9

and Disaster Risk Management, EDRM Framework, has set up the HCEG to facilitate the government to take proper actions in the processes Disaster Preparedness, Prevention, Response, and Recovery (World Health Organization 2019). Health EDRM is based on the following set of core principles and approaches that define policies and practices:

1. Recognizing the importance of risk assessment and reduction;
2. Comprehensive emergency management, encompassing the cycle of preparedness, prevention, response and recovery;
3. Covering all kinds of hazards;
4. Community and people centered practices;
5. Multi-sectoral and multidisciplinary collaboration; involving all levels of health care particularly primary health, and
6. Health as a basic human right ethics (WHO 2019).

With the Prime Minister as the Advisor, the MTF is co-led by the Minister of Health and the Minister of National Development, and MTF members are Ministers from the various ministries. The mandate given to the MTF is to manage the national response to the novel Coronavirus outbreak, and to oversee the community response against the spread of the disease as well as to work with the international community in following up on developments relating to the outbreak (gov.sg 2020). This paper aims to describe and discuss the responses of the Singapore government as well as the other stakeholders in combating the COVID-19.

2 Initial Impact of COVID-19 in Singapore

On 23 January 2020, a traveler from Wuhan was identified as the first confirmed case of the Coronavirus in Singapore. The MTF continued to monitor for new confirmed cases. The Singapore government developed the Disease Outbreak Response System Condition (DORSCON) to reflect the severity of a disease outbreak situation. The system is color-coded, starting from Green indicating "mild, severe but noncontagious", to Yellow indicating "severe, contagious spreading outside Singapore", to Orange indicating "severe, but contained", to Red indicating "severe and spreading widely". On 7 February, the DORSCON level was raised from Yellow to Orange (Ng 2020). Some citizens responded by involving themselves in panic hoarding of toilet paper and food; spreading of rumors; and blaming particular group of people: for example: foreign visitors, travelers in transit and migrants, for the outbreak. One possible source of the increase in fear and anxiety as well as an overwhelming sense of helplessness may have been an initial lack of information and the apparent uncertainty of the circumstance.

As such the MTF initiated daily briefing on the developments of the outbreak. The public were provided details of the viral spread such as to whom, the locality and the numbers involved. Daily information on new cases and clusters as well as the number of deceased and those recovered were also published by the media. The MTF also deployed infectious disease and medical specialists to engage the public on public health measures, such as wearing masks, maintaining personal hygiene, keeping hands clean, participating in contract tracing initiatives through mobile devices and observing social distancing of 1 m apart. These measures were designed to protect them from contracting and/or limiting the spread of the virus.

On 11 February 2020, WHO renamed the disease Corona Virus disease 2019 (COVID-19). By then, the outbreak in Singapore seemed under control. In early March 2020, during the initial phases of the COVID-19 outbreak across Singapore, the island state was hailed as the gold standard by WHO for the handling of the crises. This would include Singapore's consolidated approach in contact tracing, quarantine, social and health-care measures in limiting and controlling the spread of COVID-19. Singapore seems to have successfully contained the outbreak of the virus within its borders. However, in less than a month, the situation took a downturn. Confirmed cases in the community, and in particular, within the migrant workers' dormitories sub-community increased drastically. Meantime increasing numbers of Singaporeans and permanent residents who continued to return globally too, were found to be infected. Singapore subsequently, took the unprecedented step to close its borders to tourists and short-term visitors with effect from 23:59 on 23 March 2020 culminating eventually in a nation-wide lockdown on 7 April 2020. At that point, the number of confirmed infected cases had increased to 1000 with 4 succumbing to the disease.

Five days before the "Circuit Breaker", as the nation-wide lockdown was then renamed as the Prime Minister announced the impending lock-down on a nationally televised broadcast, urging Singaporeans and residents to stay calm and united to face the upcoming adversity together with courage. He also advised people to take sensible precautions, help each other stay calm and carry on with life. The Prime Minister also cautioned the public about the negative social and economic impact the COVID-19 pandemic will have. He explained the reason for, and the process of the "Circuit Breaker" while assuring that the government is prepared to handle the crises and able to lead the public through the difficult times ahead.

3 The "Circuit-Breaker"

Originally, the "Circuit-Breaker" or lockdown period was designed to last from 7 April 2020 to 4 May 2020, and later extended to 1 June 2020. During the "Circuit-Breaker" period, non-essential services, workplaces and schools were being shut down. The general public were to stay in their homes and only go out, if absolutely necessary, such as getting groceries, food and seeking medical attention. Take away and food delivery services were allowed, and groceries stores could remain open. The public was obligated to observe social distancing and contact tracing measures, as well as wearing masks when outside (Ministry of Health 2020).

By late April, the situation within the migrant workers dormitories worsened. Daily, large numbers of confirmed cases (initially ranging from thousands and later falling to hundreds) of these migrant workers were discovered, as the virus spread among these dormitories. In contrast, in the local community, the outbreak seemed to be under control, with less than 100 daily number of confirmed cases being detected. Daily new cases peaked at 596 cases on 19 April 2020, and began on a downward trend. With the local community daily confirmed cases also decreasing, the MTF on 28 May 2020 announced the three-phased plan to restart social and economic activities in a safe, orderly and progressive manner at the end of the "Circuit Breaker". Eventually, on 2 June 2020 "Circuit-Breaker" ushering the phase 1 of reopening, with 408 daily new cases in the migrant dormitories and no local community cases. In all, there were confirmed cases of COVID-19 infection, of which 33,027 were from the migrants' dormitories, and 1619 from local community, of which 22,466 fully recovered and were discharged from hospitals, and 24 deaths.

4 Phases 1 and 2 for Reopening

During the 17 days Phase 1 period of reopening of the lockdown, residents by and large were allowed to go back to work, starting with businesses that operate in settings with lower risks of transmission. Some non-essential services were allowed to reopen, which include air-conditioner servicing, hairdressing and vehicle servicing. However, retail-outlets remained closed and dining-in at restaurants was still not allowed. Moreover, limited to one visit per day, households could receive up to 2 visitors per day, who must be children and/or grandchildren from the same household. Graduating primary, secondary school and junior college students were to attend school, while others alternated weekly between online home-based learning and attending lessons at school. And, as the confirmed cases figures continued to decline, Phase Two of reopening began on 19 June 2020 (gov.sg 2020).

In Phase Two, social distance rule of keeping individuals 1 m apart, was extended to be enforced between groups, with no more than five persons per group, and with no mixing between groups. Furthermore, businesses may re-open their physical retail outlets, as well restaurants and food stalls dine-in were allowed to resume. However, live music and video screenings were not allowed in all food and beverage outlets. Larger public venues with high human traffic, such as shopping malls were subjected to capacity limits, in order to prevent crowds or long queues from building up. Personal wellness, and home-based services were also allowed to resume, and public facilities were reopened. As for returning to work, the safety management measures for workplaces during phase 1 will continue to be in effect. Kindergarten, primary, secondary and junior college students returned to school daily from 29 June 2020, however, Institutes of Higher Learning continued to conduct most lessons online, except for practical and laboratory-based lessons, and gradually increased the number of students back on campus.

While the vast majority of activities were allowed to resume at the beginning of Phase Two, activities or settings where large numbers of people were likely to come into close contact in enclosed spaces, and for prolonged periods of time, remained prohibited. These include religious congregations and large cultural venues, such as concerts, conferences and trade fairs. Persistently the MTF reminded the public to continue to maintain a high level of hygiene, and social responsibility. And further urged Singaporean and residents to maintain disciplined and vigilant, and to find the strength and will to collectively achieve a COVID-safe Singapore (gov.sg 2020).

As of 14 September 2020, Phase 2 of the reopening was still in effect, and there were 48 new confirmed cases of COVID-19 infection, with 5 imported cases and no new community and death cases. In all, there were 57,454 confirmed cases of COVID-19 infection of which 54,220 were migrant dormitory cases and the rest were local community and imported cases. The number of death toll at 27, and 56,802 persons infected by the COVID-19 virus fully recovered, with 625 persons still under hospital care in Singapore at that point in time.

5 Treatment Needs and Recovery from the Disease

According to the MOH, about 99% of the people infected will fully recover from the disease, of which about 80% will recover from the disease without needing special treatment; in particular, children and young adults. In other words, around 20% of the people who are infected will have difficulty in breathing and require hospital care. COVID patients who are over 60 years-old, or with underlying chronic medical conditions such as diabetes, hypertension or cardiovascular diseaseare at greater risk of developing serious complications. Overall, the MOH concluded that illness due to COVID-19 is minor in general (MOH 2020).

The economic impact of the COVID-19 pandemic on Singapore has been significant, primarily due to the "Circuit Breaker" lockdown restricting international travel, and trade. The labor market second quarter report indicated relative to the first quarter the number of retrenchments increased by more than doubled, from 3720 to 8130. And approximately 11,350 people lost their jobs in Singapore during the first 9 months of the year 2020. The most affected sectors of the economy include tourism-related industries including air transport and accommodation; consumer-facing sectors, such as retail; and outward-oriented sectors, including manufacturing and trade; domestically-oriented sectors such as construction and real estate; and the food & beverage services sector, such as restaurants, and bars. However, the economy did observe a significant positive rise in demand for online sales and services. Nevertheless, the 2020 Gross Domestic Product (GDP) growth forecast for the Singapore economy shrunk by 3 per cent, from "-4.0 per cent to -1.0 per cent" to "-7.0 per cent to -4.0 per cent" (Saw et al. 2020),

6 Contributing Factors to Controlling COVID-19 for Singapore

It is not by accident that the Singapore has been successful in containing the COVID-19 outbreak with a low death rate (about 1%). Its accomplishment can be attributed to a variety of factors.

1. Previous Severe Acute Respiratory Syndrome (SARS) experience and world class health care system

In Singapore, there were 238 cases and 33 deaths from the 2003 SARS outbreak; ever since, the Homeland Crisis Executive Group (HCEG) began to progressively prepare for the next Public Health Crisis. A system of Public Health Preparedness Clinic was setup throughout Singapore, and the National Centre for Infectious Diseases was established. These advanced medical care facilities are equipped with negative pressure rooms, ventilators and more, to provide testing and medical care services during future infectious diseases outbreak. (Ministry of Health 2014)

Singapore's health care is ranked by W.H.O., as No. 6 in the world. With a population of close to 5.6 million, there is one medical doctor for every 520 citizens and residents, and one nurse for every 150 citizens and residents. Moreover, the public hospitals in Singapore, 10 in total, offer affordable and high-quality public health care, through government subsidized public health care system, as well as national insurance, and community health assist scheme.

Together, Singapore's post-SARS preparedness combined with a strong health care infrastructure have provided a strong foundation required to combat the COVID-19 outbreak.

2. Government's strong leadership and adoption of a crisis management strategy

The MTF's prompt and effective action has won public approval. The transparency and the integrity of information of the Taskforce accentuated via the strategic use of the media has built trust with the citizens. This trust in turn enables and facilitates effective crisis management efforts (WHO 2019). Information from trustworthy sources reduces the anxiety of the public and increases the sense of hope as well as control over the situation. Moreover, not only the government's consistent and joint actions reflect the seriousness of the crisis, but the confidence of the public was also enhanced by the government's strong arm enforcement of those placed under the 14 days quarantine order.

3. Info-communications infrastructure and development of innovative digital applications

For the past six years Singapore has invested heavily in info-communications infrastructure and innovative apps. This infrastructure enables learning outside the classroom by enabling students and teachers to have access to interactive digital teaching and learning resources from home. In addition, the e-resources facilitated teachers' delivery of interactive online classes to their students at home, especially during the "Circuit Breaker" lockdown period. Furthermore, through similar technologies daily business activities can continue with employees working in and away from the offices: thereby, minimizing the negative impact of schools and office closures on education and business, respectively. Moreover, it is such high levels of preparedness and investment in info-communication infrastructures and digital applications development that allow Singapore to quickly launch its contact tracing apps, "Trace Together" and "Safe Entry," during the early stages of the COVID-19 outbreak. As well, the use of digital video communication and social apps have helped to maintain social and emotional connectedness among family members and friends during the extended lockdown period,

4. Awareness of the psychological and economic impact

When individuals are confined to their homes for relatively long time, psychological responses including anxiety, loneliness, difficulty in concentrating, low motivation, a state of distraction, stress, negativity, desperation, financial strain, and apprehension about future are not uncommon (Rogowska et al. 2020). The government understands the importance of addressing the psychological needs of its citizens, thereby establishing community outreach programs and psychological distress hotlines with NGOs and government agencies such as MOH, in order to provide psychological help and care services. Moreover, to help ease financial strain, the government has consecutively announced four stimulus budgets promising to pour in fund, amounting to 100 billion SGD, to attempt to counter the negative economic impact of the COVID-19 pandemic (Chan 2020).

The government is also cognizant about the psychological impact of the preventive COVID-19 measures even as they were being implemented. For instance, at the beginning of the ordeal, the public were advised to wear a mask only when they are sick and not hoard masks from the front-line medical workers. A possible reason was to prevent a panic due to the limited supply of masks available to the public in the retail market. Nevertheless, every household was given five single use masks free of charge and the seniors were encouraged to use them when necessary. Later, reusable masks were distributed to every citizen, and on April 14 the wearing of masks in public became mandatory after which the government continued to distribute upgraded masks to every citizen even as the supply of masks in the open market has become ample. This intervention had further enhanced the perception that there is an abundant supply of masks available to the public, so that they feel secure and safe.

5. Culture of high trust in the government

However, regardless of the government's level of preparedness and health care infrastructure, the successful managing of the crisis would not be possible without the support, trust and concurrence from the population. The consenting behaviors of the population could be attributed to the high level of trust earned by the founding government, which has been in power ever since 1965. Singapore's undeniable progress from a third world to a first world nation in the past 65 years has won the government much support and praise from its people.

Government community building activities through the mass media coupled with education promoting multicultural integration has also instilled a strong sense of patriotism and national identity among its citizens. Furthermore, since 1968, the compulsory enlistment of every 18-year-old male citizen to a 2–2.5 years term of national service with the Armed Forces or Civil Defence (ENLISTMENT ACT 1970) And after they had completed their national service, enlistees are still liable to periodic call ups thereafter, for operationally ready or reservists training up to the age of 45. The unique military experience has not only contributed to a sense of brotherhood and unity among its citizens; it has also imputed a sense of obligation towards the well-being of the country and instilled the social capital that the government can call upon when the support of the population is needed.

6. Where everyone plays a part

The Government supports community enhancing activities to promote social harmony and unity. SG United NGOs conducted unite Singapore campaigns such as, getting people to openly express their gratitude to front line personnel, and to participate in the whole nation singalong event, so as to boost the morale of its people. Moreover, people were urged to practice social responsibility to uphold good personal hygiene, to observe safe distancing measures, to wash hands regularly, to wear masks and to seek medical help immediately when feeling sick. In addition, the public is also reminded to participate in using contact tracing mobile apps, such as Safe Entry and TraceTogether. Individually, these are things people can do to protect themselves and others. Collectively, these actions will keep COVID-19 from spreading uncontrollably within the community. Everyone has a part to play in maintaining societal cohesion and resilience in the fight against COVID-19 (The Straits Times's post 2020).

7 Conclusion

As mentioned earlier Singapore is unique in many aspects as a city state. Its multicultural population also necessitates its government to be very effective in public communication. In addressing COVID-19, Singapore can be regarded as one of the few successful examples of demonstrating a "whole community" collaboration in disaster management (Low 2020). Singapore has vast economic and social resources, together with well-prepared infrastructure, manpower and experience in dealing with SARS, therefore enabling its government and its people to work effectively together to form a united front against the COVID-19 outbreak in the community, with the exception of migrant workers' dormitories sub-community outbreak, which relatively took a longer time, but was eventually contained and came under control. Singapore's experience may not be relevant to less developed countries with larger and more diverse populations and vast areas; however, Singapore's "where everyone plays a part" approach could be shared with other nations.

References

Chan, D. (2020) Combating a crisis: the psychology of Singapore's response to COVID-19. *World Scientific.*

ENLISTMENT ACT. (1970) Available at: https://sso.agc.gov.sg/Act/EA1970.

Gov.sg. (2020) Post-circuit breaker—when can we move on to phases 2 and 3? Available at: https://www.gov.sg/article/post-circuit-breaker-when-can-we-move-on-to-phases-2-and-3.

Low, J. (2020) COVID-19 crisis management: an early look. Available at: https://www.csc.gov.sg/articles/covid-19-crisis-management-an-early-look.

Ministry of Health. (2014) MOH pandemic readiness and response plan for influenza and other acute respiratory diseases. Available at: https://www.moh.gov.sg/docs/librariesprovider5/diseases-updates/interim-pandemic-plan-public-ver-_april-2014.PDF.

Ministry of Health. (2020) Circuit breaker to minimize further spread of COVID-19. Available at: https://www.moh.gov.sg/news-highlights/details/circuit-breaker-to-minimise-further-spread-of-covid-19.

Ng, J.S. (2020) Novel coronavirus: S'pore moves to Dorscon Orange, as 3 new cases confirmed with no apparent link to previous cases or recent travel to China. Available at: https://www.todayonline.com/singapore/wuhan-novel-coronavirus-spore-moves-dorscon-orange-3-new-cases-confirmed-no-apparent-links-previous-cases.

Rogowska, A.M., Kuśnierz, C. & Bokszczanin, A. (2020) Examining anxiety, life satisfaction, general health, stress and coping styles during COVID-19. Pandemic in polish sample of university students. *Psychology Research and Behavior Management*. 13, 797–811.

Saw, C., Lin, J., & Wong, Y. J. (2020) *Impact of the COVID-19 pandemic on the Singapore economy*. Second Quarter Report, Economics Division, Ministry of Trade and Industry.

The Straits Times's post. (2020) Community spirit despite restrictions. Available at: https://www.sgunited.gov.sg/stories/community-initiatives/community-spirit.

World Health Organization. (2019) *Health emergency and disaster risk management framework*. Licence: CC BY-NC-SA 3.0 IGO. Available at: https://www.who.int/hac/techguidance/preparedness/health-emergency-and-disasterrisk-management-framework-eng.pdf.

Yong, M. (2020) Timeline: How the COVID-19 outbreak has evolved in Singapore so far. Available at: https://www.channelnewsasia.com/news/singapore/singapore-covid-19-outbreak-evolved-coronavirus-deaths-timeline-12639444.

COVID-19 Outbreak in India: Country Features and Social Impact

Md. Nazrul Islam

Abstract India-one of the world's most densely populated countries is severely affected by the COVID-19 pandemic and has the second largest number of confirmed cases followed by the USA as on September 15, 2020. This chapter analyzes the overall features of the outbreak within the country as well as the micro social impacts caused by the coronavirus in India. Based on thematic content of various newspapers, magazines, and other media reports qualitative analyses, it is possible to understand the country features and social impact of the novel coronavirus pandemic. The first part of the chapter gives a general overview of the outbreak and government responses, and the second section scrutinizes the social impact in relation to micro level socio-economic consequences and epidemiological concerns. In mainstream reports, the impact of COVID-19 outbreak in India has been presented through the macro-economic indicators and emphasis on the negative economic impacts such as decline of growth rate, shrinking Gross Domestic Product (GDP), etc. However, the micro level socio-economic impacts of the outbreak, which are largely caused by the government interventions i.e., lock down, social distancing, etc., persist beyond the statistical number and have spread to every corner of the society. Although statistics revealed that the case fatality rate and death per hundred thousand is relatively low in India compared to other severely affected countries there are reasons beyond the standard epidemiological claims for this trend, reasons which are not properly addressed. This chapter concludes that while, from an epidemiological point of view, India has, thus far, been successful in handing the crisis brought by the global outbreak; however, the social consequences are much larger and need to be taken in consideration before claiming any success.

Keywords COVID-19 · Coronavirus · India · Inequality · Epidemiology · Socio-economic · Social impact

Md. N. Islam (✉)
BNU-HKBU United International College, Zhuhai, China
e-mail: nazrul@uic.edu.cn

S.X.B. Zhao et al. (eds.), *COVID-19 Pandemic, Crisis Responses and the Changing World*, https://doi.org/10.1007/978-981-16-2430-8_10

1 Introduction

The first case of coronavirus infection in India was reported on 30 January 2020-more than a month later than China where the coronavirus outbreak originated. However, the first case of coronavirus death in India was reported nearly a month and half later on March 12, 2020 in the state of Karnataka. The victim was a 76-year old man who returned from Saudi Arabia with a history of hypertension, diabetes, and asthma and tested positive (*The Economic Times* 2020). With her 1.3 billion people India is currently having the second highest number of confirmed COVID-19 cases followed by United States of America, and the total number of confirmed cases rose to 4,930,236 as of September 15, 2020 when the death tools reached to 80,776 (Statista.com 2020a). The objective of this chapter is twofold: firstly, to provide a brief overview of the COVID-19 outbreak in India and analyze the governments' responses to tackling the crisis; and secondly, to explore the social impact of the pandemic in relation to micro level socio-economic consequences and epidemiological significance. The first part of the chapter discusses the general situation of the COVID-19 outbreak in India and provides statistical information from different states. This section also analyses the government responses to the crisis, particularly various advisory responses, lockdowns, social distancing measures, travel restriction, and quarantine measures taken by the government. The second section of the chapter scrutinizes the social impact in particular and argues that the novel coronavirus has different impact on diverse social-economic groups in India, impacts which are encoded to social stratification and inequality. This section also includes an analysis on the epidemiological success claims by the Indian government in global arena and its' potential discrepancies.

2 COVID-19 Outbreak in India: An Overview

The Republic of India is a diverse yet unified country in terms of her history, language, and religion. The pluralistic nature of India is found in the geographical location of the various states, the varying levels of socio-economic development, and rates of urbanization. Social segregation and inequality is a common feature in India and is caused by a variety of factors. India is divided into a total of 28 states[1] and 9[2] union territories and administered by various state governments and the central government. States are administered by their legislatures and elected chief ministers as heads of the state government, while the union territories are administered directly by the

[1] The 28 states in India are: Andhra Pradesh, Arunachal Pradesh, Assam, Bihar, Chhattisgarh, Goa, Gujarat, Haryana, Himachal Pradesh, Jharkhand, Karnataka, Kerala, Madhya Pradesh, Maharashtra, Manipur, Meghalaya, Mizoram, Nagaland, Odisha, Punjab, Rajasthan, Sikkim, Tamil Nadu, Telangana, Tripura, Uttar Pradesh, Uttarakhand, and West Bengal.

[2] The 9 Union Territories in India are Delhi, Jammu & Kashmir, Ladakh, Dadra and Nagar Haveli, Daman and Diu, Puducherry, Chandigarh, Andaman and Nicobar Islands, and Lakshadweep.

Table 1 Top five Indian states for COVID-19 positive case and related death

State	Number of cases	Number of death
Maharashtra	967,349	27,787
Andhra Pradesh	527,512	4634
Tamil Nadu	480,524	8090
Karnataka	421,730	6808
Uttar Pradesh	285,041	4112

Source This table is prepared by the author and based on the data available in the Indian Government statistics. Available at: http://www.vidyagyaan.com/general-knowledge/india/list-of-28-states-9-union-territories-and-their-capitals-in-india/ (Accessed September 10, 2020)

central government or union government. The land size and population density, nature of rural-urban segregation, degree of socio-economic development, and political philosophy of individual state government varies greatly from state to state in India.

The impact of COVID-19 outbreak also varies from state to state while some states are more severely affected than others. Because of the uneven development, access to health care, test facilities, affordability, etc. some states witnessed much larger number of cases. According to the Indian government statistics, the highest number of positive cases have been identified in the state of Maharashtra, which reached to 967,349 out of India's total 4,470,166 (Government of India 2020a) confirmed cases as on September 10, 2020. The fatality in Maharashtra is also the highest among Indian states and accounted for 27,787 deaths out of India's total 75,062 (ibid.) death victims on the same date. Among the union territories Delhi encountered the highest number of COVID-19 positive cases and stands at 201,174 as on September 10, 2020. The death toll in Delhi also reached to 4638 (ibid.) as on September 10, 2020. The following Table 1 shows the top five states in India, which experienced the highest number of COVID-19 positive cases and causalities.

3 Government Responses

The Indian constitution recognizes a division of legislative responsibilities between the union government and the state, and both the union government and the state governments are authorized by the constitution to legislate on matters related to public health. The union law is usually enforced by the central government and deals with epidemic disease at ports of entry and exit and port and interstate quarantine. At the union level, The Epidemic Diseases Act 1897, which was enacted during the British colonial era, provides the legislative framework for the prevention of epidemics (Ahmad 2020). State legislatures oversee matters relating to public health and sanitation, hospitals, dispensaries, etc. within their own state jurisdiction and are empowered to adopt all measures to prevent the outbreak of epidemic diseases. The

COVID-19 outbreak began in India on January 30, 2020 when an Indian student at China's Wuhan University returned to Indian state of Kerala and tested coronavirus positive. Since then, both the Indian central government and different state governments have taken measures to stop the spread of the virus and protect its citizens. These includes declarations of emergency, closure of institutions and public meeting places, mandatory quarantine, lock down, restriction on traveling and issuing visas, and other restrictions intended to limit the spread of the virus. The government responses and actions may be broadly categorized into three areas: responses related to advisory, lockdown and social distancing, and travel restriction and quarantine.

4 Responses Related to Advisory

The Indian central government set up a 'group of ministers' under the direction of Prime Minister Narendra Modi to review, monitor and evaluate regional preparedness and measures taken (Ahmad 2020). The group of ministers on March 11, 2020 suggested that the Indian Ministry of Health and Family Welfare should advise all state and union territories to invoke section 2 of the Epidemic Disease Act, 1897, which "gives power to the States and Union Territories to take special measures and formulate regulations to contain the spread of the grave disease" (Saikia 2020). The Act further stipulates that

> when a state government is satisfied that any part of the state is visited by or threatened with an outbreak of any dangerous epidemic disease and if they find that the ordinary provisions of the law for the time being in force are insufficient for the purpose, may take strict measures and temporary regulations can be observed by the public which shall deem necessary to prevent the outbreak of such disease. The government is given the power to inspect persons traveling by railways and other means of transportation. The State Government is allowed to set up hospitals with temporary accommodation for the people who are suspected by the inspecting officer of being infected with any such disease which is seen as being grave. (ibid.)

The central government on the same day also invoked section 69 of The Disaster Management Act, 2005, which explains the "Delegation of powers" and noted "The National Executive Committee, State Executive Committee, as the case may be, by general or special order in writing, may delegate to the Chairperson or any other member or to any officer, subject to such conditions and limitations, if any, as may be specified in the order, such of its powers and functions under this Act as it may deem necessary" (The Indian Parliament 2005: 27). The central government of India also declared COVID-19 a 'notified disaster' on March 14, 2020 and offer assistance under the State Disaster Fund, which was set up under the above Act (Ahmad 2020).

5 Lockdown and Social Distancing

Lockdown was one of the major strategies adopted by India in order to prevent the further spread of the COVID-19 outbreak. The nationwide lockdown came into force with the announcement of Prime Minister Narendra Modi on March 24, 2020 on behalf of the union government for a period of three weeks. This time frame was extended subsequently for four occasions and was in place until June 30, 2020 with some relaxations. Transport services, schools, factories, various business, and services were closed during this period and nearly 1.3 billion Indian people were asked to stay at their homes. Different Indian state governments also adopted various lockdown measures and restrictions depending on their local circumstances.

In addition to lockdown related to social distancing the Indian union government proposed various interventions through the Ministry of Health and Family Welfare and these includes closure of all educational establishments including schools, universities, gyms, museums, cultural and social centres, swimming pools and theatres. Students were advised to stay at home, and online education was promoted if practicable. The government proposed to explore the possibility of postponing exams although ongoing exams could be conducted after ensuring physical distance of one meter amongst students. The government encouraged private sector organizations/employers to allow employees to work from home whenever feasible; meeting were encouraged through video conferences as well as the minimization or rescheduling of meetings involving large number of people unless necessary. Restaurants were encouraged to ensure various measures such as handwashing, proper cleanliness of frequently touched surfaces, physical distancing (minimum1metre) between tables, and the use of open air seating, where practical, with adequate distancing. The government proposal suggested that already planned weddings be of limited size and discouraged all non-essential social and cultural gatherings. The government also suggested that local authorities have a dialogue with organizers of sporting events and competitions involving large gatherings and advised them to postpone such events. They were further encouraged to have a dialogue with opinion leaders, religious leaders, traders associations, and other stakeholders to regulate mass gatherings, working hours, etc. One meter distance between customers during commercial activities was suggested and measures to reduce peak hour crowding in markers were advised. The government advised avoidance of any non-essential travel and the maximization of social distancing in public transport as well as regular and proper disinfection of surfaces. Hospitals were asked to follow the necessary protocol related to COVID-19 management and prescribed and restrict family/friends/children visiting patients in hospitals. There were few proposed interventions related to hygiene and physical distancing, avoiding shaking hands and hugging, special protective measures for delivery men/women working in online ordering services, and keeping communities informed consistently and constantly (Government of India 2020b).

6 Travel Restriction and Quarantine

Since January, 2020 The Indian Union Government consistently issued various travel advisories from and to India as well as guidelines for domestic travel and guidelines for international arrivals with quarantine requirements. As on March 11, 2020 the Ministry of Health and Family Welfare issued Consolidated Travel Advisory for Novel Coronavirus Disease (COVID-19). The consolidated advisory contained a total twelve directives and the following issues were at the forefront: Firstly, all existing visas (except diplomatic, official, UN/International Organizations, employment, project visas) stood suspended till 15th April 2020. This came into effect from 1200 GMT on 13th March 2020 at the port of departure. Visas of all foreigners already in India were to remain valid, and they may contact the nearest relevant offices for extensions/conversions etc. of their visas or any consular service, if they choose to do so. Any foreign national who intended to travel to India for compelling reasons were advised to contact the nearest Indian Mission. Secondly, visa free travel facility granted to Overseas Citizens of India (OCI) card holders was kept in abeyance till 15th April, 2020. This measure came into effect from 1200 GMT on 13th March 2020 at the port of departure. OCI card holders already in India could stay in India as long as they wanted. Thirdly, there were also special restrictions related to some severely affected countries such as Italy, the Republic of Korea, China, Iran, France, Spain and Germany. Passengers traveling from and or having visited these countries and desirous of entering India needed a certificate of having tested negative for COVID-19 from the designated laboratories authorized by the health authorities of these countries. This measure came into effect on 10th March, 2020 and would remain in place till cases of COVID-19 subsided. All incoming travelers, including Indian nationals, arriving from China, Italy, Iran, Republic of Korea, France, Spain and Germany after 15th February, 2020 were advised to go under quarantined for a minimum period of 14 days. This came into effect on 13th March, 2020 at the port of departure. And fourthly, incoming travelers, including Indian nationals, are advised to avoid non-essential travel and were advised to quarantine for a minimum of 14 days on their arrival in India. Indian nationals were further strongly advised to refrain from travelling to China, Italy, Iran, the Republic of Korea, France, Spain and Germany (Government of India, Ministry of Health and Family Welfare 2020c: 1–2).

The Ministry of Health and Family Welfare, Government of India also issued two more guidelines on domestic travel and international arrivals in India as of May 24 which were subsequently revised. The guideline for domestic travel (air/train/inter-sate bus) includes items, such as precautionary measures to be followed in the airports/railway station/bus terminals and in public transportations, terminal screening to all passengers, personal and environmental hygiene, social distancing, sanitization, self-isolation, etc. (Government of India 2020d: 1).

The guideline also stipulated that States can develop their own protocol with regard to quarantine and isolation as per their assessment (ibid.). Another guideline was issued for international arrivals by the Ministry of Health and Family Welfare on

May 24, 2020 as a precautionary measure to restart a good percentage of international passenger flight to and from India before August, 2020 (Aiyappa 2020). The guideline included a total of sixteen points related to mandatory quarantine and exemption of quarantine in exceptional circumstances and other issues already mentioned in the guideline for domestic travel (ibid.: 1–2).

All these above mentioned measures taken by the Indian union government and state governments to prevent the spread of COVID-19 outbreak and control public health have severe social impacts in different arena of peoples' lives. In the following section the social impact of COVID-19 outbreak in India and the impact of government measures have been scrutinized.

7 Social Impact

On September 26, 2020, the *Times of India* published a report on how India's *Dangal* wrestlers forced to take odd jobs for a living because of the COVID-19 outbreak. The report shared several stories of the wrestlers. Sangram, a champion from Haryana state was featured in one anecdote. The 26-year old wrestler had earned, previous to the pandemic several hundred thousand Indian rupee (1 USD = 73 INR app.) a year by means of mud wrestling, popularly often known as *Dangal* in India. Sangram was at the time of the report working as a porter at a state's authorities warehouse in Haryana state and making only 5000 Indian rupee a month and struggling to feed his five members household, the report added (*Times of India* 2020). Another report was published on August 22, 2020 in *The Hindu* under the title *Differential impact of COVID-19 and lockdown* stressed that lockdown in India caused sharp rise in unemployment. The report used statistical evidences and suggested that the sudden rise of unemployment was not caste neutral. Through using the data from the Centre for Monitoring Indian Economy (CMIE)'s Consumer Pyramids Household Survey, the report asserted that while the proportion of employed upper castes dropped only 7% between December 2019 and April 2020 the fall among the scheduled castes (lower caste) was 20% during the same period, nearly three times higher (Deshpande and Ramachandran 2020). The anecdotal evidence suggests the wide-ranging impacts of COVID-19 outbreak and adoption of the lockdown approach. Thus, the social impact of COVID-19 outbreak is primarily related to existing inequality in Indian society and is fostered by the various policies and measures taken by both the union government and state governments. The inequality in socio-economic conditions, access to health care, geographical location related to urban-rural divide, gender, and so on prevails all over India. In the following sections, the social impact of COVID-19 outbreak in India has been scrutinized from socio-economic and epidemiological aspects.

8 Economic Impact

COVID-19 pandemic has catastrophic consequences for the global economy in both developed and developing countries. Since the pandemic began in January 2020, various global industries such as hotel and tourism, aviation, entertainment, etc. have collapsed. Other businesses are hard hit because of the lockdown interventions of governments in various countries. Traditional service sectors such as education, government services were also severely impacted although some services were resumed online thanks the assistance of or the support of the Information and Communication Technologies (ICT).

The economic impact of COVID-19 outbreak in India is related to socio-economic inequality and is exacerbated by the preventive measures imposed by the government such as social distancing and quarantine, lockdown, widespread suspension of normal mobility, travel restriction, and the general shutdown the economic activity. Although the macro economic impact often shown in indicators such as growth rate, GDP, etc. the micro social impacts are largely unreported in mainstream media outlets. These micro social impacts are caused by the existing social hierarchy and inequality in India. An International Labor Organization (ILO) Report suggested that the two billion people working in the informal sector (mostly in emerging and developing economies) worldwide are particularly at risk because of the COVID-19 pandemic (Press Trust of India 2020a). The UN'S labor body further reported that about 400 million workers in India working in the informal economy are at risk of falling deeper into poverty during the COVID-19 outbreak. Many of these workers lost their job and were forced to return to their hometown and villages in the rural areas during the pandemic (ibid.). Returning to a countryside home without any savings in hand these workers became victims of starvation, indebtedness, and extreme stress, which are often unseen in various reports (Ray and Subramanian 2020). The long and stringently enforced lockdown in India also seriously disrupted the massive supply chain in both agriculture in the rural areas and economic activity in urban centers. Millions of migrant workers from the urban city centers have been forced to return to their rural homes without cash, food, or the prospect of re-employment (ibid.). The lengthy period of enforced co-habitation between intimate partners of these migrant workers during the lockdown period caused the increase of domestic violence (ibid.).

Along with the rurally based migrant workers who worked in the urban areas, coronavirus posed a similar threat to urban low end socio-economic groups in India. A London School of Economics report suggested that the COVID-19 outbreak has "exacerbated the pre-existing inequities in urban India" and has left the "lockdown generation" with lower employment rates (Press Trust of India 2020b). The report, titled *City of dreams no more: The impact of COVID-19 on urban workers in India*, further noted that "workers in the bottom half of pre-COVID labor income group suffered bigger income losses than the top half following the coronavirus-induced lockdown" (ibid.). By decimating livelihoods in urban areas, the outbreak created a new underclass of workers in India who lost jobs and are being pushed into poverty;

many of them, the report concluded, are low paid young informal workers from lower socio-economic groups (ibid.).

The coronavirus outbreak in India and the lockdown measures to prevent the spread of the virus caused a rural-urban digital divide. The divide is evident in education, telemedicine, banking, e-commerce, e-governance, etc. Education provides an example of this trend, as many students from rural household were unable to participate in their online classes' simply because their family didn't have a mobile phone or access to information and communication technology, the internet in particular. Even if some rural household purchases a mobile phone to facilitate their children's study there is no power supply with which to charge the phone (Pandey 2020). According to the survey on Key Indicators of Household Social Consumption on Education in India conducted by the National Statistical Office, Ministry of Statistics and Program Implementation from July 2017 to June 2018 (NSS 75TH Round), only 4.4% rural households have a computer, and 14.9% rural households have internet facilities compared to 23.4 and 42.0% of urban households respectively (Government of India 2019: 47). A similar rural-urban divide exists with the ability to operate a computer and use internet among persons. While 32.4% urban persons (37.5% male and 26. 9% female) of age 5 years and above have the ability to operate computers the percentage among rural persons is 9.9 (male 12.6% and female 7.0%). Further, 37.1% of persons (43.5% male and 30.1% female) from the same age group in the urban area have the ability to use internet where only 13.0% rural persons (17.1% male and 8.5% female) have the same ability (ibid.: 48). India is a country which has a clear division of access to resources between its social groups. This division is visible between the urban and rural population as well as between the male and female population, and in all spheres of the society. Such disparities in access to basic needs occur with regard to education, health care, food, shelter, communication technology, etc. These inequitable disparities are key factors in producing the devastating socio-economic consequences proceeding from the coronavirus pandemic. Many of these impacts contributed negatively towards the disadvantageous group while the advantageous segment of the society might suffer less. When people's mobility was restricted because of the lock down and some of the essential services went to online systems—for instance the updating of health information, e-commerce, e-education, e-banking, e-government, etc.–only those having ability to use internet got access to resources. It is presumed that the vast majority of the Indian rural and urban population stayed out of the e-government services related to essential health care during the COVID-19 outbreak.

The protective measures implemented, such as social distancing, economic lockdown, suspension of mobility, quarantine, etc. were primarily based on practices first exercised in the developed economies where substantial economic support from the government for each citizen or households in-need was available. In order to attend to the global trend of responding to the COVID-19 pandemic the Indian government followed the same path and received international praise. However, as an emerging economy with nearly 1.3 billion people and great sectoral and occupational vulnerability, following the global trend in responding to the COVID-19 outbreak caused a social disaster. Recent research shows that lockdown and limiting economic activities by the government "must be accompanied by an extensive and careful system of compensatory transfers to provide sustained and effective protection against this danger" (Ray and Subramanian 2020). This, however, did not happen in India, and critics suggest that there are more lives lost in India from the severe economic and social dislocations than COVID-19.

9 Epidemiological Question and Government Success

The public health impact of COVID-19 outbreak in India is perceived in governmental organizations from an epidemiological approach. Various statistics related to the virus infection, such as number of total confirmed case, number of total death caused by the virus, case fatality rate, the number of confirmed positive case per one hundred thousand in the country, etc. have become important determinants to evaluate the severity of the outbreak. This epidemiological approach also assesses the success and failure of individual countries' governments based the number of deaths. Mortality is the most important factor in assessing the severity of the pandemic, and countries around the world adopted such approach. India was not an exception, and the Indian government gave the highest emphasis on reducing the case fatality rate from the COVID-19 outbreak. Medical professionals were on the forefront to advise the government on taking measure to control the outbreak and prevent the spread of the virus. Ministry of Health and Family Welfare was selected to monitor the situation, take necessary steps, and save lives. According to the World Health Organization (WHO) Coronavirus Disease (COVID-19) Dashboard as on September 15, 2020 India had the world's second largest number of confirmed cases, followed by USA, and stands at 4,930,236 cases with 80,776 deaths (World Health Organization 2020a) (see Table 2).

One of the noteworthy features in Table 2 is that India has the lowest case fatality rate and lowest number of confirmed cases out of one hundred thousand in population, yet it was among the top twelve countries according to the number of infection as on September 15, 2020. These countries represent diverse continents–including Europe, North American, South American, and Asia–and belong to developed, emerging and developing economies. Spain–a western European country with a developed economy had a case fatality rate of 5.0% and the number of infection per hundred thousand populations was 63.88 as on September 15, 2020. Another Latin American developing country–Peru had a case fatality rate of 4.2%, with the infection of 96.0 person per hundred thousand population on the same date. However, the case fatality rate in India is only 1.6%, and the number of confirmed cases per one hundred thousand peoples is 5.89–much lower than that of the both previously mentioned developed and developing countries. The number of deaths in India from the COVID-19 is 34 per million populations, which is far lower than many European and North American countries (Biswas 2020). The Indian government did make obvious efforts to take

Table 2 Case fatality features from COVID-19 in India

No	Country	No. of confirmed cases	No. of confirmed death	Case fatality rate (%)	No of death per 100 K
1	USA	6,462,135	193,119	3.0	59.45
2	India	4,930,236	80,776	1.6	5.89
3	Brazil	4,330,455	131,625	3.0	63.02
4	Russian Federation	1,068,320	18,635	1.7	12.86
5	Peru	729,619	30,710	4.2	96.00
6	Colombia	716,319	22,924	3.2	46.57
7	Mexico	668,381	70,821	10.6	56.30
8	South Africa	649,793	15,447	2.4	26.82
9	Spain	566,326	29,747	5.0	63.88
10	Argentina	555,537	11,412	2.1	26.22
11	Chile	436,433	12,012	2.8	64.14
12	Iran	404,648 (World Health Organization 2020b)	23,313 (ibid.)	5.8 (Johns Hopkins University 2020)	28.50 (ibid.)

Source This table is prepared by the author and based on the data available in the World Health Organization (WHO) Coronavirus Disease (COVID-19) Dashboard and Coronavirus Resource Center, Johns Hopkins University as on September 15, 2020

credit through presenting impressive data and through publicizing its responsibility for the success at home and abroad in handling the pandemic.

However, many epidemiologists ignored the fact that the relatively low case fatality rate in India is not only caused by the efficient handling of the outbreak by the government and her allied agencies. There are other factors that played a role, such as the nature of Indian demography. India is one of the world's youngest countries. According to Statista.com, the median age of Indian population is 28.4 in 2020 (Statista 2020b), which could be considered a "demographic dividend" for the country (Basu 2007). Experience having demonstrated that the elderly population is more vulnerable to infection and causality of the COVID-19 outbreak in various countries, particularly in the west, India was able to minimize the case fatality rate because of the large number of young people, critics argue.

10 Conclusion

Up until the time of writing, the Indian government handled the COVID-19 outbreak using an epidemiological approach and initiated all the measures implemented globally for tackling the pandemic. Apparently the interventions brought success for the government, since the case fatality rate was relatively low. However, India is a country of social inequality based on caste, gender, socio-economic segregation, and rural-urban location. The novel coronavirus outbreak and government responses have different impacts on diverse social groups. For example, one study shows that the case fatality rate among females is more than that among males, and Indian women may face higher risk of death from coronavirus infection than men. While the global case fatality statistics revealed that there is more causality among male than female, Indian statistics have gone in the opposite direction. Studies suggest that, in India, although males shared a higher burden (66%) of COVID-19 infections than females (34%), the case fatality rate among males is 2.9%, while that for females it is 3.3% (*India Times* 2020). Even in some of India's neighboring countries such as Bangladesh which has similar socio-economic conditions, the case fatality among males is much higher than that of females. The Ministry of Health and Family Welfare, Government of Bangladesh official said on July 8, 2020 that the death rate for men in Bangladesh from COVID-19 infection was 79.24%, while it was 20.76% for women (Sakib 2020). Thus, gender inequality is an issue that needs to be taken into consideration in India when adopting measures to respond the COVID-19 outbreak for the government. Most of the measures taken up to now to tackle the situation were focused on to reduce fatality and minimize economic cost. These measures might have economic and epidemiological merits. However, the government should initiate new programs for severely affected disadvantaged groups to minimize the social cost.

References

Ahmad, T. (2020) FALQs: India's government response to COVID-19 (Novel Coronavirus). Available at: https://blogs.loc.gov/law/2020/03/falqs-indias-government-response-to-covid-19-novel-coronavirus/?__cf_chl_jschl_tk__=f879e6761f16d5fc89b1b150755d429af7980b51-1599927504-0-Aa8Z-hWMF-yl32_6V4cj_qaTgp7zSKK4iXWiZCa0zBrPb7SMO-Q7cR4yemPLcDnB-6WhLAXWsHXG0X0r5IjXpRX9OeGz6RbqriXy8izdqz6UxF4xy6uq6216tZ5HCKFjHvLZP7SZro9Brbc-GeLjIQY1qtcJ2vfCLnKzZNp2ML8TrQDRm-sCPDZHr7Yj2xo0TfdKPu-IM1YarKxrtPGbKisqp8lxh05WmEIphmO4jGrfxYqS8zMu7CPO2ZDmKs4mvRws7MjtP8gD1BnzD79qTjX-DcmjUuZg_jz9cpFyrAvf13Ta-0lAJ3ss1A03DhGOtRmWI80VSSnoocy_-a6lyBdvNJ9qAZlk6JI4s_MpHALRxsqVkIBkgxhH88yDX0YAyg (Accessed 12 September 2020).

Aiyappa, V. (2020) 14 day quarantine mandatory for international travelers. Available at: https://www.oneindia.com/india/14-day-quarantine-mandatory-for-international-travellers-3094007.html (Accessed 14 September 2020).

Basu, K. (2007) India's demographic dividend. *BBC News*, July 25, 2007. Available at: http://news.bbc.co.uk/2/hi/south_asia/6911544.stm (Accessed 16 September 2020).

Biswas, S. (2020) Coronavirus: How many COVID-19 deaths is India missing? *BBC News*, August 17, 2020. Available at: https://www.fr24news.com/a/2020/08/coronavirus-how-many-covid-19-deaths-is-india-missing.html (Accessed 14 September 2020).

Deshpande, A., & Ramachandran, R. (2020) Differential impact of COVID-19 and the lockdown. *The Hindu*, August 22 (Accessed 13 October 2020).

Government of India. (2019) *Key indicators of household social consumption on education in India, National Statistical Office, Ministry of Statistics and Program Implementation.* New Delhi:

National Statistical Office. Available at: http://www.mospi.gov.in/sites/default/files/publication_reports/KI_Education_75th_Final.pdf (Accessed 15 September 2020).
Government of India. (2020a) COVID-19 state wise statistics. Available at: https://www.mygov.in/corona-data/covid19-statewise-status (Accessed 10 September 2020).
Government of India. (2020b) Advisory on social distancing measure in view of spread of COVID-19 disease. Available from: https://www.mohfw.gov.in/pdf/SocialDistancingAdvisorybyMOHFW.pdf (Accessed 14 September 2020).
Government of India. (2020c) Ministry of Health and Family Welfare, consolidated travel advisory for novel coronavirus disease (COVID-19). Available at: https://www.mohfw.gov.in/pdf/ConsolidatedTraveladvisoryUpdated11032020.pdf (Accessed 14 September 2020).
Government of India. (2020d) Ministry of Health and Family Welfare, guidelines for domestic travel (air/train/inter-state bus travel), P1. Available at: https://www.mohfw.gov.in/pdf/Guidelinesfordomestictravel(airortrainorinter-statebustravel).pdf (Accessed 14 September 2020).
India Times. (2020) Females in India may have higher COVID-19 death risk than males, study says. Available at: https://www.indiatimes.com/news/india/females-in-india-may-have-higher-covid-19-death-risk-than-males-study-516126.html (Accessed 22 September 2020).
Johns Hopkins University. (2020) Coronavirus Resource Center. Available at: https://coronavirus.jhu.edu/) (Accessed 15 September 2020).
Pandey, K. (2020) COVID-19 lockdown highlights India's great digital divide. Available at: https://www.downtoearth.org.in/news/governance/covid-19-lockdown-highlights-india-s-great-digital-divide-72514 (Accessed 14 September 2020).
Press Trust of India. (2020a) COVID-19 impact: 400 million workers in India may sick into poverty. Available at: https://www.oneindia.com/international/covid-19-impact-400-million-workers-in-india-may-sink-into-poverty-3067621.html (Accessed 15 September 2020).
Press Trust of India. (2020b) COVID-19 exacerbated pre-existing inequities in urban India: Report. Available at: https://economictimes.indiatimes.com/news/economy/indicators/covid-19-exacerbated-pre-existing-inequities-in-urban-india-report/articleshow/77871809.cms (Accessed 15 September 2020).
Ray, D., & Subramanian, S. (2020) India's response to COVID-19 is a humanitarian disaster. *Boston Review*, July 16. Available at:http://bostonreview.net/global-justice/debraj-ray-s-subramanian-indias-response-covid-19-humanitarian-disaster (Accessed 13 September 2020).
Saikia, B. (2020) *The Epidemic Diseases Act, 1897*. Available at: https://www.thelawbug.com/epidemic-act-1897/ (Accessed 14 September 2020).
Sakib, SM Najmus. (2020) *Bangladesh: Nearly 80% of coronavirus deaths are in men*. Available at:https://www.aa.com.tr/en/asia-pacific/bangladesh-nearly-80-of-coronavirus-deaths-are-in-men/1903694 (Accessed 22 September 2020).
Statista. (2020a) *Coronavirus (COVID-19) deaths worldwide per one million population as of September 10 by country*. Retrieved from the https://www.statista.com/statistics/1104709/coronavirus-deaths-worldwide-per-million-inhabitants/ (Accessed 10 September 2020).
Statista. (2020b) India: Average age of the population from 1950 to 2050. Available at:https://www.statista.com/statistics/254469/median-age-of-the-population-in-india/ (Accessed 16 September 2020).
The Economic Times. (2020) Karnataka announces India's first coronavirus death, March 13, 2020. Available at:https://health.economictimes.indiatimes.com/news/industry/state-minister-announces-indias-first-coronavirus-death/74604253 (Accessed 9 September 2020).
The Indian Parliament. (2005), The Disaster Management Act, 2005, p. 27. Available at:https://www.ndmindia.nic.in/images/The%20Disaster%20Management%20Act,%202005.pdf (Accessed 14 September 2020).
Times of India. (2020) India's Dangal wrestlers forced to take odd jobs for a living, September 26. Available at:https://newsindia.ictv.in/indias-dangal-wrestlers-forced-to-take-odd-jobs-for-a-living-more-sports-news/ (Accessed 13 October 2020).
World Health Organization. (2020a) WHO corona virus disease (COVID-19) Dashboard. Available at: https://covid19.who.int/table (Accessed 15 September 2020).

World Health Organization. (2020b) Coronavirus disease (COVID-19) dashboard. Available at: https://covid19.who.int/?ftag=MSF0951a18 (Accessed 15 September 2020).

Fighting the Invisible Enemy—COVID-19: How Ghana Fared

Gabriel Owusu

Abstract All countries, just as Ghana, have been affected by the global pandemic caused by the novel coronavirus, COVID-19. The unique nature of individual countries—culture, political system, economy and philosophy—has resulted in varied patterns of solutions, strategies, approaches and results. Ghana's social, economic and cultural background cannot be overestimated in analyzing the COVID-19 situation in the country. This paper seeks to give a concise country report on the COVID-19 in Ghana in reference to the country's background (social, economic and political), response strategies, and the trends in the country. Ghana has various characteristics that set it apart from other countries, yet some common underlying factors among countries cannot be ignored as well. In view of these characteristics, the paper analyzes and expounds on the peculiar factors, situations and strategies realized in Ghana's COVID-19 battle. It makes observations from the trends of events, offering recommendations based on the analyses.

Keywords Ghana · COVID-19 · Pandemic · Directives · Health

1 Introduction

In the wake of the COVID-19 pandemic, how would a country such as Ghana fare in the face of already existing conditions, systems and economy? To gain a comprehensive understanding of Ghana's response to the COVID-19 pandemic, an overview of the country's background is necessary. Ghana is a lower middle-income country with a Gross Domestic Product (GDP) currently estimated at $69.76 billion USD (2020),[1] with per capita of $1807.10 in 2018 (yet, one of the highest in West Africa).[2] As an emerging economy, Ghana's economy continued to expand in 2019 as the first quarter Gross Domestic Product (GDP) growth was estimated at 6.7%, compared

[1] Source: World Bank (https://www.worldbank.org/en/country/ghana/overview).

[2] See Appendix 1.

G. Owusu (✉)
Belt and Road School, Beijing Normal University, Zhuhai, China

S.X.B. Zhao et al. (eds.), *COVID-19 Pandemic, Crisis Responses and the Changing World*, https://doi.org/10.1007/978-981-16-2430-8_11

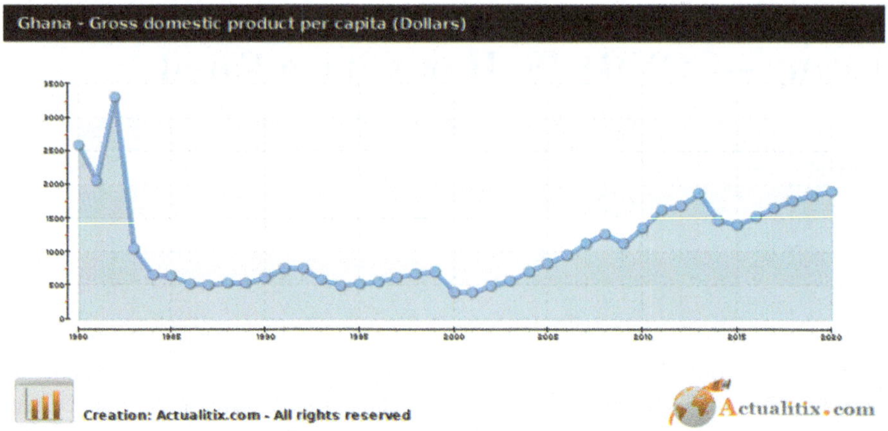

Fig. 1 Pattern of Economic Growth in Ghana [*Source* IMF, 2015; Ghana Health Service (https://www.ghanahealthservice.org/COVID19/latest.php#)]

with 5.4% in the same period of the previous year, 2018. Also, its growth in the non-oil sector was significantly improved at an estimated annual rate of 6.0%. Apparently, the relatively high quarterly growth was driven by a strong recovery in the services sector, which grew by 7.2% compared with 1.2% in 2018.[3] Ghana's GDP per capita is currently estimated at 1807.10 US dollars in 2018—representing only 14% of the world's average.[4] The diagram below shows the GDP growth over the past three decades (Fig. 1).

Undeniably, the demographic features of any country are a key to understanding its approach to the pandemic. How do the country's demographics contribute to the degree of infection and death amongst its general population, and how do the trends in population growth inform the response of the government to the global pandemic? Accordingly, Accra, the capital, is the most densely populated city in Ghana, having over 2.2 million inhabitants. Overall, the population of the country appears youthful: 65% between the ages of zero and 45 years.[5] The youthful attributes of the population presents both hope and challenge for Ghana. Whereas it offers a potential for an increase in the quantity and the quality of the labour force, it also presents the problem: how to provide education, training and employment to the teeming population. Failing to meet the needs of this youthful population could spell doom for the future of Ghana as well as to Africa at large, which faces similar issues in demographics.

Again, the pre-pandemic state of human development is worth noting. How would COVID-19 affect the quality of living in Ghana? It is necessary, therefore, to assess the pre-pandemic situation in the country. According to the United Nations Development

[3] https://www.worldbank.org/en/country/ghana/overview.

[4] See https://tradingeconomics.com/ghana/gdp-per-capita.

[5] See Appendix 2.

Program (UNDP), Ghana has been classified in the Human Development category, with an HDI value of 0.596, achieving an 142nd rank out of 189 countries and territories listed. It observes that Ghana's HDI value has increased by only 31.1% between 1990 and 2018.[6] The high deficit in physical and social infrastructure has left Ghanaians, by and large, with relatively low standards of living compared with those of the Western countries. The lack of access to health facilities, for example, has led to the high maternal mortality and a rise in diseases such as measles and tuberculosis. There is low life expectancy, low literacy rate, high maternal mortality, and amongst a substantial portion of the population, there is a minimal access to potable water and sanitation. According to the Ghana Statistical Service report of 2017, 6.8 million Ghanaians, representing 23.4% of the population, could not afford to spend more than GH 4.82 cedis (approximately US$1—a day in 2016/17.[7]

Even though Ghana has achieved relatively positive development, attaining a lower middle-income status in 2010, Ayelazuno (2013) has observed the paradox between these economic indicators and the actual wellbeing of most Ghanaians—noting that the people "still suffer grinding poverty." Indeed, there remain areas in Ghana with low levels of education, inadequate health facilities, lack of potable drinking water, no access to good roads and the existence of outmoded cultural practices. Cases of insecurity, poverty, corruption, gender inequality among others continue to be prevalent in some parts of Ghana today. Nzeribe G. et al. (2019) argue that African countries, not only Ghana, remain plagued by infrastructural deficits, corruption, insecurity and inequalities.How does the COVID-19 pandemic pose significant challenges for the present and in the future? It was in this situation that the COVID-19 pandemic greeted the nation of Ghana, and the battle goes on of at the time this paper is written.

2 The Advent of COVID-19

Shortly after the novel coronavirus had been recorded in China, various countries around the world inevitably were obliged to welcome the '*unwanted visitor,*' compelling the World Health Organization (WHO) to declare a global pandemic. Ghana was definitely no exception. On March 12, 2020, two cases of the COVID-19 were confirmed in Ghana—the first time since the disease broke out in December 2019 and spread across the world.

Speaking at a press conference on March 12, 2020 the Minister of Health, Mr. Kwaku Agyeman-Manu, who eventually tested positive for the virus,[8] said the 'Noguchi Memorial Institute for Medical Research' in Accra confirmed the two

[6] UNDP report, 2018.

[7] Ghana Living Standards Survey Round 7, Ghana Statistical Service (2017).

[8] The President, in one of his COVID-19 national broadcasts, revealed that the Minister of Health had tested positive for the virus. See https://africa.cgtn.com/2020/06/15/ghanas-health-minister-tests-positive-for-covid-19-president-says/#.

cases after tests on March 12, 2020. According to the minister, the two foreigners arrived in the country from Norway and Turkey and had been kept in isolation. The minister then admonished Ghanaians on the protocols recognized to prevent the spread of the Novel Coronavirus.

The Ghanaian president, President Nana Akufo-Addo, on March 15, 2020, in his first address to the nation on COVID-19, restricted all public gatherings including church activities, conferences, workshops, funerals, festivals, political rallies, schools among others from holding. This was in attempt to reduce the spread of COVID-19. These measures were not adequate to prevent the initial increase in cases in March from 2 to 153, forcing the government to adopt a more restrictive set of measures. Thus, President Akufo-Addo in his fourth COVID-19 address announced a partial lockdown in the country involving Accra, Tema, Kumasi and Kasoa. The lockdown measures were to take effect from Monday, March 30, 2020, until the following 15 days.

A key precautionary measure after recording a few cases of the virus was the disinfection of all open spaces, markets and bus stations across the country. This exercise was to begin from Accra, Metropolis on March 23, 2020.[9] It was conducted under the supervision of the Minister of Local Government and Regional Development.

As of September 30, 2020, Ghana has recorded 46,482 cases of the novel coronavirus, 45,651 recoveries, including 301 deaths.[10] The country has since been stricken with great shock, which continues to exert notable psychological and emotional stress on its citizens. The opening of basic schools and high schools alike has been postponed to the following year (2021). Loss of jobs, sense of insecurity and restrictions on movement have shaped the lives of Ghanaians in the time of COVID-19. What have been the trends of events, strategies and notable changes in the Ghanaian society after the advent of COVID-19? How effective have the country's efforts in fighting this pandemic been?

The strategies adopted by the Ghanaian government were not so different from what we have witnessed in many other countries. However, the unique situations in each country contributes to the varying expectations and outcomes as well as changes in the dynamics of the situation. This paper considers the dimensions of government's preparedness and the response strategies in combating COVID-19.

3 Ghana's COVID-19 Preparedness Strategies

According to Murphy, B. (2012), preparedness takes place in advance of any risk event such as pandemics, flood and other natural disasters. Even though no country had the luxury to prepare adequately as to prevent COVID-19 from spreading to its boarders, time allowed Ghana to implement basic preparedness measures. The

[9] Source: Daily Guide (https://dailyguidenetwork.com/ghana-disinfects-markets-in-fight-against-covid-19/).

[10] See https://www.ghanahealthservice.org/covid19/.

main source of public awareness and its increased sensitization has been the mass media. In this regard, the country had already been encouraging and promoting the observance of personal hygiene and the use of hand sanitizers. Thus, in the wake of the COVID-19, these practices had become the norm in most public institutions in the country. The President of Ghana added his voice to the general guidelines in the media, emphasizing the need for observing personal hygiene through regular handwashing (with soap), avoiding or reducing physical contacts and the regular use of hand sanitizers. As a means of further sensitizing the Ghanaian people to the necessary health protocols, the president refrained from 'customary' handshakes with dignitaries during the 63rd Independence Day celebration in Kumasi, on March 6, 2020.

The government of Ghana has set up isolation and treatment centres in all the administrative regions in the country as part of the preparedness measures of the country. Currently, the country boasts of two fully equipped centres of research. They are the Noguchi Memorial Institute of Medical Research (NMIMR)—initially, the sole centre for testing—in Accra and the Kumasi Centre for Collaborative Research (KCCR) in Kumasi responsible for testing samples from the Southern and Northern Sectors respectively.

Another key measure of preparedness is the inauguration of the National COVID-19 Team. The key members of the National COVID 19 team include:

Dr. Nsiah Asare, the Presidential adviser on health, an experienced medic and former Director of Health Services.
Dr. Anarfi Asamoa- Baah a former Deputy Director General of World Health Orgnization (WHO), directly appointed to coordinate issues of COVID 19 at the Presidential level.
Dr. Okoe-Boye, the Deputy Minister of Health who is an expert in Medicine and Public Health.

Thus, before the country registered the first two cases, relevant effective measures had been implemented. Such policies included regular testing of persons arriving from abroad and those showing symptoms, public education to create awareness on the available information about the pandemic. The public education campaigns have advocated regular washing of hands, the use of hand sanitizer and nose masks as well as the need to avoid overcrowded areas.

4 Ghana's Response Measures

The response phase of crisis management has been viewed by scholars such as Statoil (2013) as the act of putting 'preparedness' into action. Following the advent of COVID-19 and the eventual escalation in the number of cases, the government came up with preventative measure to mitigate the spread of the virus within the borders of the country. With the help of the Telecommunication Companies in Ghana, the Ghana Health Service (GHS) has acquired the data sufficient for effective contact tracing across the length and breadth of the country. Thus, Ghana Health Service (GHS) is able to conduct a real time online monitoring system for COVID-19 in the country. This initiative is key in the government's efforts to prevent the spread of the virus within the borders of the country. Ghana has taken a multi-faceted approach to addressing the pandemic as discussed below:

5 Directives on Restricted Movements and Public Gatherings

In view of the need to avoid overcrowding, the President of the Republic granted amnesty to eight hundred and eight (808) prisoners on March 26, 2020.[11] The measure was done upon the recommendation of the Prison Service Council and in consultation with the Counsel of State in as provided by the Constitution of Ghana. The directive would reduce the overcrowded conditions in the prison and thereby minimize the risk of COVID-19 spread.

More to that, schools, conferences, social gatherings, sporting activities and political rallies were all put on hold as enhanced measures against the spread of COVID-19.[12] As of now, with the exception of school-re-opening, other social gatherings are permitted but under the condition of strict adherence to COVID-19 protocols.

In a public address by the Ghanaian president, on March 27, 2020, the cities of Accra and Kumasi, a densely populated city, were put under a total lockdown. As a consequence, economic activities as well as free movements were to be halted in these cities starting from March 30, 2020. These restrictions also came with a new transport policy, which reduced the number of passengers permitted within a commercial vehicle. The measure was undertaken in concomitant with the already-imposed restriction on the closure of churches activities, mosques, schools, and a ban on all public gatherings, which had previously been announced on March 15, 2020.

As was to be expected, these measures soon heightened the vulnerability of many individuals and social groups, especially those within the areas under lockdown.[13] The aged, the physically challenged, women and low-income earners were generally faced with severe challenges of affording basic necessities. In response to the hardships suffered as a result of the directives, the National Disaster Management Organization (NADMO), together with the Ministry of Gender and Social Protection, launched a programme, which would help supply relief items including food and other necessities to those disadvantaged populations. This initiative received support from private philanthropists, Non-Governmental Organizations

---

[11] See https://desertherald.com/covid-19-ghana-grants-amnesty-to-808-prisoners/.

[12] Source: Ghana Web (https://www.ghanaweb.com/GhanaHomePage/NewsArchive/Coronavirus-Ban-on-public-gathering-includes-nightclubs-Akufo-Addo-898660).

[13] Source: https://www.cnbcafrica.com/news/2020/04/20/ghana-lifts-lockdown-on-key-regions-as-covid-19-cases-reach-1042/.

(NGOs), Faith-based Organizations and Metropolitan, Municipal and District Chief Executives (MMDCEs).

The closure of the land, air and sea borders of the country was announced on March 21, 2020[14] with a mandatory fourteen-day quarantine and testing for all travelers from countries with more than 200 COVID-19 cases. Although the Kotoka International Airport reopened for regular international passenger travel on Tuesday, September 1, 2020, the country's land and sea borders remain closed until September 30, 2020.[15] In accordance with these directives, the Ghana Tourism Authority (GTA), in a press release on March 23, 2020, announced the closure of all beaches and tourist sites in the country.

6 Communication/Public Education and Stakeholder Engagement

To ensure the effective implementation of COVID-19 protocols, the government of Ghana has engaged periodically with key stakeholders since the inception of COVID 19 in the country. Such stakeholders include trade unions, leadership of political parties, religious leaders, chiefs, representatives of key public institutions, Civil Society Organizations (CSOs) and Non-Governmental Organizations (NGOs). This initiative has helped to ensure the utmost cooperation of all segments of the Ghanaian society in the fight against the "invisible enemy."

Deliberate efforts have been made to educate the public on the need to abide by various protocols initiated by the government. Ghanaians are also becoming educated on the appropriate use of Personal Protection Equipment (PPEs). Public education campaigns have been organized mainly through the media in various indigenous languages. The National Commission on Civic Education (NCCE) has been at the core of these campaigns conducted in partnership with various public and private agencies.

Another important source of information and public education has been the regular 'presidential addresses.' The first came on March 12, 2020,[16] the day following the announcement by the World Health Organization (WHO), declaring COVID-19 a pandemic. President Nana Addo-Danquah Akuffo-Addo's maiden official address focused on the government's line of action in the COVID-19 fight. The President informed the public of the government's readiness and preparedness to combat the novel coronavirus and gave the assurance that all points of entry including land borders and airports were ready to screen all travelers entering the country and

[14] Source: https://alternativeafrica.com/2020/03/22/ghana-begins-complete-lockdown-closes-land-sea-borders-over-covid-19/.

[15] See more at: https://www.travelandtourworld.com/news/article/ghana-reopens-air-borders-for-international-tourism/.

[16] https://www.moh.gov.gh/president-akufo-addo-addresses-nation-on-measures-taken-by-govt-to-combat-the-coronavirus-pandemic/.

subject the visitors to a formal set of protocols. He further declared the commitment of his government to spend at least $100 Million on interventions such as expansion of infrastructure, procurement of materials and equipment, and public education among others. His advice to the nation was that residents should minimize, if not avoid foreign travel as much as possible.[17]

In addition, the Minister of Information has been conducting periodic press briefings. The briefings continue to provide as a channel for information exchange between Government and the general public. The role of the media is indispensable as it has provided and continues to avoid officials with the medium for public education on COVID 19 and its protocols.

7 Legal Instruments/Legislation on the COVID-19 Pandemic

Laws, in conformity with the national constitution, must back actions of democratic governments. Thus, the Ghanaian government, a democracy, operated in accordance with constitutional legislative/executive instruments. In view of this institutional framework, the President of Ghana provided a legal backing to the COVID-19 response directives by passing various Executive Instruments (E.Is). So far, three of such instruments, all passed and published in the Gazette on March 23, 2020 have provide the legal basis for the actions undertaken by the government in response to the epidemic:

"Establishment of Emergency Communications System Instrument, 2020" (E.I.63).

"Imposition of Restrictions (Coronavirus Disease (COVID-19) Pandemic) Instrument, 2020" (E.I. 64).

"Imposition of Restrictions (Coronavirus Disease (COVID-19) Pandemic) (No. 2) Instrument, 2020" (E.I. 65).

The fourth, "Imposition of Restrictions (Coronavirus Disease (COVID-19) Pandemic) (No. 3) Instrument, 2020" (E.I. 65) has been passed more recently. It was published in the Gazette on April 3, 2020.

8 Fiscal Policies to Support Local Businesses/General Intervention Policies

As part of the response to COVID-19 crisis, the government has employed various fiscal measures including the ease of transactions, scrapping/reduction of electronic transaction charges and the reduction of monetary policy rate. The central bank, Bank of Ghana (BoG), as part of its response measures, has reduced the monetary policy

[17] Access the president's speeches on http://www.presidency.gov.gh/.

rate by 150 basis points to 14.5% in addition to a 2% reduction in interest rates; all as forms of stimulants, which would help reduce the level of shock and vulnerability the pandemic has inflicted on businesses.[18] The measure was intended to encourage businesses to access loan facilities as a means to avoid collapse. The central bank has also collaborated with the 'Ghana Interbank Payment and Settlement Systems (GHIPSS)' to reduce the electronic transaction, notably Mobile Money charges, thereby encouraging online as opposed to in-person transactions.

Another fiscal response policy comes in the form of relaxing the country's tax system. The Ghana Revenue Authority (GRA) has come up with flexible terms such as a two-month extension of annual tax returns and field auditing and a scraping of penalties for taxpayers who redeem their outstanding debts by the end of June, 2021. The measure would offer a breathing space for businesses and private individuals in the midst of the pandemic. Importers also had their share of the "national cake" when the President announced that the government would waive off rent charges and demurrages for the months of March and April 2020 with the view of easing the financial loss due to COVID-19.

More so, the Ghanaian government has instituted a soft-loan scheme that would aid and stabilize middle and small-scale businesses. The government is collaborating with the National Board for Small Scale Industries (NBSSI), Trade Unions (TUs), as well as some Commercial and Rural Banks, to implement this important initiative. According to the President, the scheme would provide a loan facility up to a total of 600 Million cedis, with will a one-year moratorium and two-year repayment period for micro, small and medium scale businesses.

9 The Role of Academia, Research, Science and Technology

Academic and research institutions across the country have played a crucial role in the fight against COVID-19. University of Ghana (UG), Kwame Nkrumah University of Science and Technology (KNUST), the Centre for Plant Medicine Research (CPMR), Noguchi Research Institute of Medical (NMIMR), among others have served as the base for research for the country during the pandemic. For instance, the Kwame Nkrumah University of Science and Technology (KNUST) collaborated with Incas Diagnostics to a Rapid Diagnostic Test (RDT) kits.

These research and academic institutions provided invaluable guidance in launching the Ghana COVID 19 Tracker App, a technological means to trace contact of patients infected with COVID-19.[19] More so, under the guidance of these institutions, Ghana continues to encourage the local production of facemasks, surgical

[18] News by YEN: https://yen.com.gh/150795-monetary-policy-committee-bank-ghana-reduces-policy-rate.html.

[19] Read more at https://newsghana.com.gh/ghana-launches-covid-19-tracking-app/.

gloves, scrubs and other PPEs, with the assistance of academic and research institutions. Such locally-made products are required to undergo the normal process of authentication from the Ghana Standards Authority (GSA).

10 Health Infrastructure and Facility Expansion

As the background information shows, the country lacks crucial infrastructure and social amenities. Thus in the wake of COVID-19, the government announced the allocation of $100 million to fund the expansion of infrastructure, purchase of materials and equipment, and public education on COVID-19.[20] The Majority Leader of Ghana's Parliament believes that the pandemic presents the country with the opportunity to expand its health infrastructure.[21]

Seven more testing faculties have been added to the initial two centres—the Noguchi institute of Medical Research and the Kumasi Center for Collaborative Research—to enhance quick testing and delivery of test results.[22] To aid those living in remote villages and communities, the country has enlisted the use of medical drones. Such smart use of technology ensures that test samples and results are transported to and from such places in time without difficulties.

In addition, there is an on-going construction of a hundred-bed isolation and treatment facilities in Ga East Municipal Assembly, as part of the infrastructural expansion. Such measures only partially described the many proposed infrastructural projects nationwide.

11 Private Initiatives

The crucial role of private individuals and organizations cannot be overemphasized. The Ghana COVID-19 Relief Support (GCRS) is a typical example of private initiatives in the combat of COVID-19. It is a "private sector-led initiative to complement efforts of government and other institutions in Ghana in combatting the novel Coronavirus (COVID-19)."

Again, as Bhatt, M., and Reynolds, T. (2012) argue, that the local communities play a critical role in the Disaster Management (DM) cycle. Local authorities, especially those whose areas suffered from the lockdown have come up with support funds targeting the vulnerable and less privileged in those localities. For instance, His

[20] Source: China Daily (https://www.chinadaily.com.cn/a/202003/12/WS5e69aa86a31012821727e7fc.html).

[21] See https://www.ghanaweb.com/GhanaHomePage/NewsArchive/Coronavirus-has-given-us-an-opportunity-to-expand-health-infrastructure-Majority-Leader-946903.

[22] Source: President's 18th speech (https://www.ghanaweb.com/GhanaHomePage/NewsArchive/FULL-TEXT-Akufo-Addo-s-ninth-address-on-Ghana-s-enhanced-response-to-COVID-19-947872).

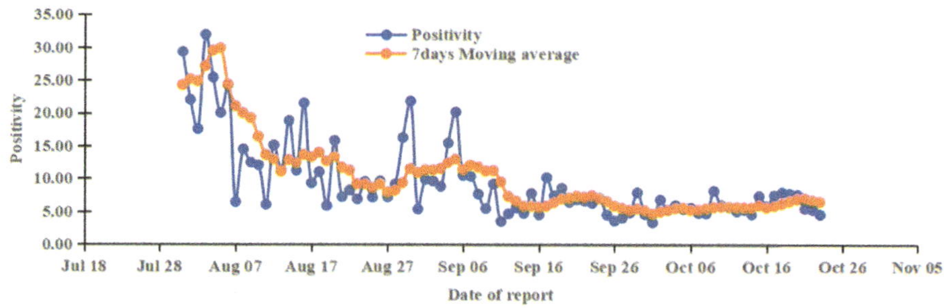

Fig. 2 COVID-19 positivity rate in Ghana between July 29 and October 23, 2020 [*Source* Ghana Health Service (https://www.ghanahealthservice.org/COVID19/latest.php#)]

Royal Majesty Otumfuo Osei Tutu II, whose city (Kumasi) was affected by the lockdown has set up a 1 million Ghana cedis fund to assist the vulnerable in his locality and beyond. Ghanaian communities in the diaspora have also contributed to the efforts of battling the pandemic in Ghana. For instance, Ghanaians in Denmark and Sweden have supported government's effort with a cheque for 8272 cedis through the Ministry of Foreign Affairs.[23]

12 Observations and Analysis from GHANA'S COVID-19 Battle

A careful observation reveals some notable trends. To begin with, Ghanaians have begun to depend more on indigenous resources for self-development. This is not to suggest that Ghana has independently fought the pandemic; many countries and international organizations supported the country with PPEs, Experts, and funds. However, the nature of the crises has provided an impetus for the national leaders to look within their borders to harness resources for their people's survival. The local manufacture of PPEs and various research collaborations adequately attest to the claim. As Mr. Alhassan Andani remarked, the pandemic has been a "wake-up call" on the country to be self-reliant.[24]

Again, taking into account the background information and the trend of events in the country, the actions of the Ghanaian government have been generally commendable, especially given the limited resources available to the nation. The fatality rate has been relatively low. The active cases have substantially reduced. The data below shows the rate of positivity in the samples in Ghana in recent months (Fig. 2).

---

[23] Source: GhanaWeb (https://www.ghanaweb.com/GhanaHomePage/diaspora/Ghanaians-in-Denmark-and-Sweden-donate-towards-coronavirus-fight-1096801).

[24] Source: Joy News (https://www.myjoyonline.com/business/economy/covid-19-is-a-wakeup-call-for-ghana-to-be-self-reliant-alhassan-andani/).

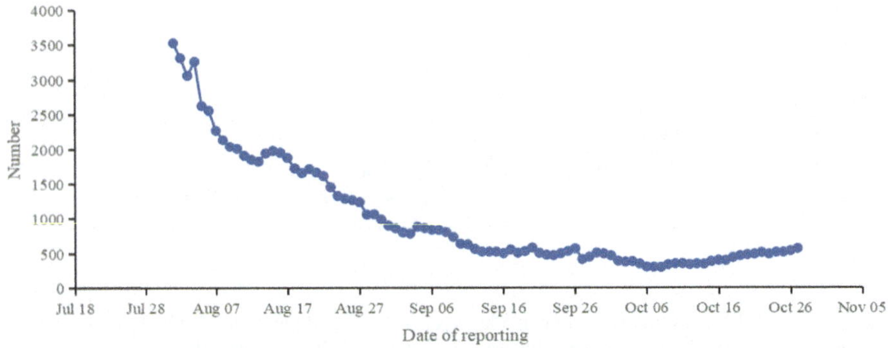

Fig. 3 Pattern of active COVID-19 cases in Ghana from August to October, 2020 [*Source* Ghana Health Service (https://www.ghanahealthservice.org/COVID19/latest.php#)]

As of October 26, the COVID-19 positivity rate has notably fallen as compared with earlier figures in June and July this year.

The number of active COVID-19 cases have been on a steady decline following the peak in July. This remarkable drop in the cases, as shown in the data below, confirms that government's efforts have yielded results (Fig. 3).

More so, the advent of COVID-19 has caused government's attention to focus more on the Health Sector. The increased attention suggests that the nation may benefit from an upturn in the quality of healthcare facilities. Government's immense resource-allocation to the health sector will not only serve the fight against the pandemic, but also promote the general standard of health services in the country. On April 26, 2020, the President disclosed the intention of the government to construct eighty-eight (88) new district hospitals within the space of a year, and an additional the six (6) regional hospitals; one in each of the newly created regions.[25]

However, the nature of the Ghanaian economy, coupled with the resource constraints contributed to the shortfalls and common lapses in the process. For example, the lockdown directed was impeded by the immense hardship it brought on low-income earners and the unemployed. As *Daily Post* reports, market women flouted the directive at certain times as a means of sustaining their families. According to the report, some of the women lamented the immense hardship the lockdown directive had brought to their families. "…It's better, I leave this world," a frustrated woman cried out in tears.[26] The situation further revealed the vulnerability of the Ghanaian society—where there are huge disparities between classes. This level of disparity calls for both long-term and short-term restructuring of the economy, which could make the society more resilient in unforeseen crisis that, may arise in the future.

[25] See https://www.modernghana.com/news/998184/covid-19-govt-to-construct-88-district-hospitals.html.

[26] Source: DailyPost (https://dailypost.ng/2020/04/25/covid-19-lockdown-kaduna-residents-storm-mini-markets-flout-social-distancing-order/).

Again, the economic impact of COVID-19 has been notable. The Minister for Finance speaking on "Economic Impact of the COVID-19 pandemic on the Economy of Ghana" on March 30, 2020, outlined the government's expectation of the pandemic's impact on the Ghanaian economy. He also mentioned the fiscal and monetary measures taken by the Government of Ghana to mitigate those impacts.[27] As it stands, many private workers, especially those in the informal sector, have hardly recovered from the financial crisis resulting from the COVID-19 pandemic. In a survey conducted by the Ghana Statistical Service (GSS) in collaboration with the United Nations Development Programme (UNDP), it was observed that about 770,000 workers, representing 25.7% of the total workforce, have experienced a reduction in their wages and/ or salaries. Also, approximately 42,000 employees were laid off during the country's COVID-19 partial lockdown.[28] Ghana National Council of Private Schools (GNACOPS), has lamented that about 94,000 private school teachers are likely to lose their jobs due to COVID-19. Mr. Enoch Kwasi Gyetuah, the Director of GNACOPS, explained that the suspension of schools left private school owners with no choice than to release their teachers. Indeed, the government acknowledged the loss of employment due to the pandemic. The Ghana Statistical Service (GSS) has noted that at least 72,087 workers, representing 2.3% has lost their jobs due to the pandemic.[29] Government must, therefore, initiate additional social intervention programs, create jobs and encourage entrepreneurship in order to minimize the hardship the pandemic poses.

Socially, the advent of COVID-19 has heightened social isolation in the country, especially for the aged. People-to-people interactions, which used to characterize the Ghanaian society has almost been eliminated by the pandemic. As Professor Charles Mate-Kole, the Director for the Centre for Ageing Studies, University of Ghana, observes, "The outbreak of COVID-19 in Ghana has worsened the social isolation of older adults and threatened their health status."[30] It is recommended that religious groups and various social agencies take on an active role of educating and sensitizing the public to ameliorate the situation.

13 Conclusion

To draw the curtains down, Ghana's COVID-19 battle has been multifaceted. Government's directives have been warmly received; the few who flouted these directives largely did so out of economic hardships. It seems feasible to view the various plans,

[27] https://taxnews.ey.com/news/2020-0838-ghana-announces-plans-to-provide-relief-to-taxpayers-in-response-to-covid-19?uAlertID=Sd%2fG8rua1oj6%2fl58EZ2AiA%3d%3d.

[28] Source: Ghana Statistical Service (GSS), 2020. Also, UNDP, Ghana (www.gh.undp.org).

[29] See https://www.undp.org/content/dam/rba/docs/COVID-19-CO-Response/UNDP-rba-COVID-assessment-Ghana-business-tracker.pdf.

[30] See https://www.ghanabusinessnews.com/2020/10/02/covid-19-has-worsened-self-isolation-of-older-persons/.

strategies and policies as worth emulating especially, in low-income countries in Africa and other parts of the world. As an instance of a notable success, the local production of PPEs and the research by indigenous institutions has saved the country lots of costs and accorded international honor to the country. The *battle* as it stands requires cooperation and extensive research. All countries must collaborate in finding a lasting solution to this global crisis.

A holistic approach to general health and its related issues is crucial in these times. Losing sight on any area to focus only on COVID-19 may pose an existential threat to national survival. The pandemic must be vigorously fought, but not to neglect the likes of malaria and HIV/AIDS, which continues to cost thousands of lives around the globe. This is to say that countries with limited resources ought to ensure considerable attention is paid to other health concerns, which could equally pose serious threats as COVID-19.

Appendices

Appendix 1

See Fig. 4.

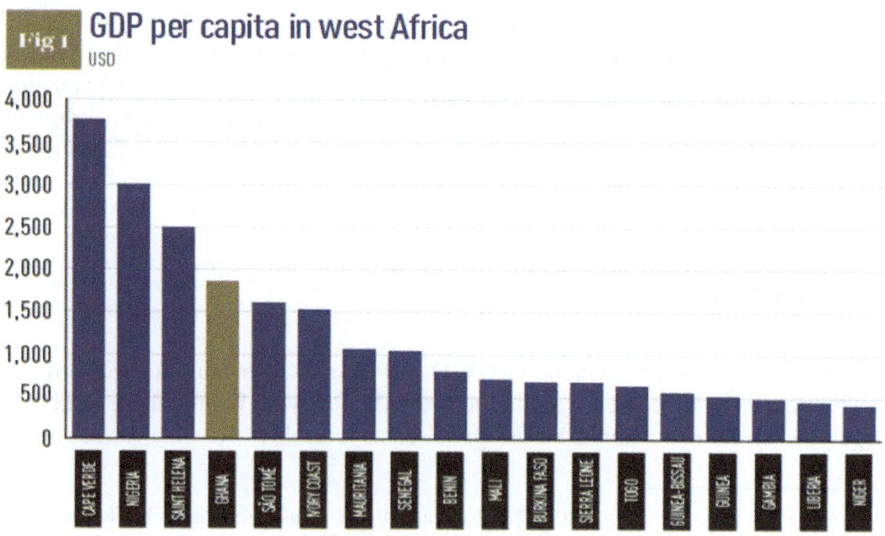

Fig. 4 GDP per capita ranking in West Africa (*Source* The World Bank)

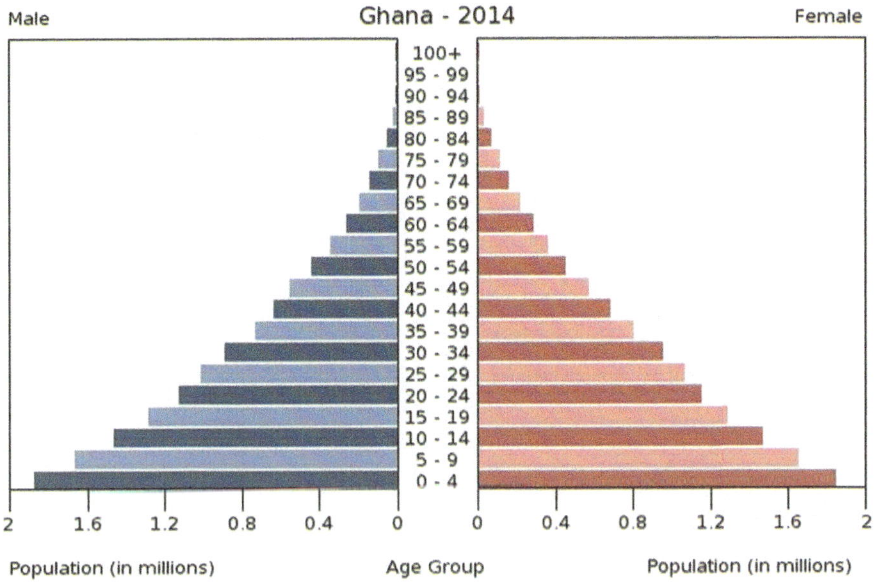

Fig. 5 Ghana's population structure

Appendix 2

See Fig. 5.

References

Ayelazuno, J.A. (2013) Neoliberalism and growth without development in Ghana: A case for state-led industrialization. *Journal of Asian and African Studies*, 80–99.

Bhatt, M.R. and Reynolds, T. (2012) Community-based disaster risk reduction: Realizing the primacy of community. *Disaster, Risk and Vulnerability: Mitigation Through Mobilizing Communities and Partnerships*. Montreal: McGill-Queen's University Press, pp. 71–90.

Murphy, B.L. (2012) Community-level emergency management: Placing social capital.

Nzeribe, G., et al. (2019) Developmental challenges of African developing economics. 10 (2019): 53–80.

Statoil, A.S.A. (2013) The In Amenas Attack: Report of the Investigation into the Terrorist Attack on In Amenas. *Prepared for Statoil ASA's board of directors*. Google Scholar. Available at: http://www.statoil.com/no/NewsAndMedia/News/2013/Downloads/In%20Amenas%20report.pdf (Accessed 5 December 2014).

The "Perfect Storm": A Failed Response to the Pandemic in the United States

Charles Lowe and Benjamin Barber

1 Context and Introduction

During an interview that aired on *Axios* on *HBO* on Monday, August 3rd, 2020, President Trump claimed that the numbers, despite their appearance, indicated that the US response had been relatively effective worldwide—the assertion was based on a low death rate vis-à-vis other countries and the high number of tests conducted. The report from Center of Disease Control (CDC) present a starkly difference picture of the progress of the pandemics in the United States. As of August 6, 2020, there have been 4,802,491 total cases, 157,631 total deaths, and 1465 cases per 100,000 in the United States (cited in CDC COVID Data Tracker). And while it is true that US ranks 24th in case-fatality ratios, Jessica Craig (2020, para. 15) notes that the statistic is driven by the age of the victim and is, therefore, highly misleading. In countries such as Belgium and the United Kingdom, where the median age is relatively high, 41.9 and 40 years, respectively, the death rate is much higher. In sharp contrast, in Uganda, where the median age is 15.9, the per capita death rate is extremely low, 0.01. In either case, the statistic does not speak to the effectiveness of the country-wide response to the pandemic. A more revealing statistic is the death rate per 100,000. Here, the US ranks 8th worldwide, higher than Brazil and France and lower than Belgium and the United Kingdom. And although there has been an increase in the number of tests, when considering population size, the U.S., as Craig (para. 20) observes, "comes [in] ninth place, having conducted 174 tests per 1,000 people"—a per capita rate significantly below the rates, for instance, in Luxembourg at 691 per 1,000 people, the United Arab Emirates at 525 and Denmark at 268.

Further, although numbers of tests given have risen from 640,000 per day in early July to 755,000 per day in early August and are far more than in April and May

C. Lowe (✉) · B. Barber
Division of Humanities and Social Sciences, Beijing Normal University-Hong Kong Baptist University United International College (BNU-HKBU UIC), Zhuhai, China
e-mail: charleslowe@uic.edu.cn

S.X.B. Zhao et al. (eds.), *COVID-19 Pandemic, Crisis Responses and the Changing World*, https://doi.org/10.1007/978-981-16-2430-8_12

according to the COVID Tracking Project, Sarah Mervosh and Manny Fernandez (2020, para. 4) report in *The New York Times* that

> With testing chemicals and other equipment in short supply, and a surge in coronavirus cases nationwide leading to skyrocketing demands, many Americans are still having to wait many days for results, effectively rendering those tests useless.

According to an online survey representing 19,000 people from 50 states and Washington, DC, by researchers from Harvard University, Northeastern University, Northwestern University, and Rutgers University, as of August 3, 2020, individuals tested in July 2020 waited, on average, approximately 4 days, the same wait time for those who reported taking a test in April. Overall, approximately 10% of those surveyed waited 10 days or more. The recommended return time, according to the CDC, is 24–48 hours.

A closer examination of the picture reveals strong differences in the rate of return amongst race groups. African Americans "surveyed reported an average wait time for results of five days, and Hispanic respondents reported an average wait time of 4.6 days, compared with 3.9 days for white people" (Sarah Mervosh and Manny Fernandez 2020, para. 7). The reasons behind the delay is traceable to "critical shortage of certain equipment and supplies, including reagents, the chemical ingredients needed to detect whether the coronavirus is present in a sample" (Sarah Mervosh and Manny Fernandez 2020, para. 9).

Hence, a substantial body of evidence indicates that the national and state authorities have failed in the months since the first stay-at-home order on March 19th in California to develop an adequate testing strategy to address the emergency. The use of masks, even though it is widely accepted that usage will reduce both the user's chances of infection and the spread itself, reveals a similarly troubling failure. Anastasia Moloney (2020, para. 6) reports that, according to a survey of 169,000 people in over 100 countries by U.S.-based data company Premise, the United States has a low level of mask usage even compared to countries in Latin America:

> Nearly one in five Americans said they never wear a mask when leaving the house, while 37 percent of the 7,649 people in the United States surveyed said they sometimes wear one." That is despite 73 percent of Americans saying they are "concerned" or "very concerned" about the spread of COVID-19 in their community.

The degree of mask usage, we have observed anecdotally, varies significantly regionally as does adherence to social distancing guidelines. However, overall, what is apparent even from a superficial reading of the data is that the United States on federal and state levels, as well as individually, has failed to address the crisis in a manner close to adequate, considering the scale of the growing pandemic. That failure has had tragic results economically, socially, and of course regarding loss of life as well as the long-term impact on public health.

Here, we offer a disclaimer. Neither of us are public health professionals and, therefore, cannot speak authoritatively on the nuances of medical solutions to the pandemic. Further, the knowledge base appears to be changing radically as epidemiologists determine more about the virus. However, as noted above, the evidence, uncovered thus far, indicates that neither government nor its citizens are acting on the knowledge available: e.g. the government is failing to provide sufficient resources for testing, and its citizen have failed to wear mask in adequate percentages. Hence, as the US has the resources and expertise to address the crisis, the question becomes, what factors sociologically, culturally, and ideologically have contributed to the overall failure? And will these factors continue to determine a failure on the part of US citizens and their federal and state governments to address the crisis, and will such failures continue to inform the US responses to the virus and especially Americans willingness to participate in a government vaccine programme for COVID-19?

Obviously, this subject is incredibly broad as are the answers to the questions, which have extraordinarily far-reaching consequences. Our consideration will have much more narrow direction, starting from an observation by Richard Horton that traces the failure to frame an adequate response to COVID-19 in the United States to a belief of Americans generally in their impregnability, a belief that "informs not just a response to a pandemic, but attitudes to climate change and other threats" (cited in Booth 2020).

This paper, in support of the contention, will draw attention to how a perception of American exceptionalism has informed the failed response, thus far, to the pandemic—a failed response, that, as we have seen, has informed the failure on the part of the US government to provide adequate resources and the failure of a significant portion of its citizens to take adequate public safety measures, such as wearing a mask. There are, we will argue, other elements at play, including a profound distrust of central authority prevalent in the post-Watergate era and a President with a constituency expressing a strain of anti-intellectualism that, Richard Hofstadter famously observes, has its roots in colonial European and an Evangelical Protestant heritage. All these factors, accelerated by an engine of the mass media, came together to produce, so to speak, the "perfect storm."

2 Discourse in a Crisis

Implicit in this statement, however, is the notion that—absent any one of these elements—the response to the pandemic may have been very different. Hence, the failure, thus far, to meet the present emergency, the paper will also argue, may not be predictive of responses to the future challenges, including other possible pandemics and large scale issues such as global warming. Indeed, the differences in responses to the pandemic regionally shows the difficulty of determining whether the failure bespeaks a flaw in the American character or merely represents an unfortunate convergence of certain discursive strains to produce an inadequate response to a potential existential threat. Discourse, as characterized in the OED, represents "a spoken or written treatment of a subject in which it is handled or discussed at length; a dissertation, treatise, homily, sermon, or the like" (cited in *The Chicago School of Media Theory* 2020). Discourse constitutes in its most reductive terms a sort of unit of language organized around a particular subject matter and meaning.

The non-specific definition is certainly relevant to our consideration, drawing attention to the connotations of the language used to describe the virus as well as on the adverse impact of the language in contemporary use in promoting an adequate policy to address the pandemic. Our analysis will, further, draw focus to the power relations underlying the discursive frames which all share a subversion of traditional notions of medical authority in a "position of power" (cited in Nimmon and Stenfors-Hayes 2016) informing public health policy.

As a prominent example of how medical discourse has become an area for contestation, even the name ascribed to the virus has acquired politically charged connotations. The use of the term, COVID-19, foreshadows a communicator wishing to imbue the disease with a non-geographic and time-specific character in conformance with the WHO's original rationale for the change in name (cited in Forster 2020, para. 2).

However, in the U.S., various politicians have, as shall be discussed, applied the terms, "China virus" and "Wuhan virus", specifically to counter the intentions of the WHO. One object in President Trump's use of these terms has apparently been to shift attention away from the management of the pandemic and accentuate, instead, its perceived genealogy.

According to Marietta Vazquez in *Yale School of Medicine* (2020), renaming COVID-19 the "Wuhan Virus" or "China Virus," has the profoundly negative consequence of highly politicizing language surrounding the disease. Vazquez goes on to note that "we can better prevent the spread of COVID-19 and protect those who may have it when we speak about it with empathy, and care." By suggesting the creation of an etiquette for speaking of the virus, she implies that many in the public need such a code. As an example, Dr. Vazquez offers the following prescription: "**DO**: Talk about people "acquiring" or "contracting" COVID-19. **DO NOT:** Talk about "transmitting COVID-19," "infecting others," or "spreading the virus" as it implies intentional transmission and assigns blame." The concern is that the victim-laden language will link the disease with weakness and criminality, thus discouraging the public from seeking out testing and/ or submitting to a quarantine. Hence, the language used to describe the disease, the patients, the transmission, etc. has, in Dr. Vazquez and our views, the "power" to encourage or dissuade the public from seeking testing and treatment and thereby, either to flattening the curve or to creating the conditions behind what is at present an exponential rise in cases.

Our study will examine a few, by no means all, factors behind a linguistic environment wherein a code becomes necessary in order for a general public to perceive the straightforward fact that, as Dr. Vazquez puts it, "pathogens do not discriminate." The challenge in effecting such a public-health friendly discourse points to a resistance on the part of the general public. One source of this resistance, we will argue, is the embeddedness of American exceptionalism as a part of political discourse.

3 Discourses of American Exceptionalism, Anti-Intellectualism, and Loss of Trust in Government

There is a combination of factors that have shaped the discourse that has propelled the failed response to the pandemic in the United States. In this section, we will enumerate and define some major factors informing the direction of the discourse and ultimately reflect on how these factors work together to disseminate a false sense of American immunity to the threat of COVID-19. We will define the nature of American exceptionalism, recount the widespread loss of faith in the trustworthiness and efficacy of the governmental authority, consider the American predilection towards anti-intellectualism, and the American tendency to collective amnesia after historical health catastrophes, specifically the influenza pandemic of 1918. By defining and discussing each factor and how they work together, we will prepare the way to showing how they impede the development of a national discourse that would help to curb and control the predations of COVID-19 in the United States.

Distrust of a central government authority appears widespread in the United States in the in later part of the twentieth and early part of the twenty first century, a distrust which has spurred the fractious racial, economic, and social divisions. During the COVID-19 pandemic, the profound skepticism towards national governmental authority is on full display. However, the anxiety about the potential misuse of federal power has been a constant refrain in America's continued interpretation, elaboration, and interrogation of the constitution.

3.1 Loss of Trust in Government

The widespread dissent against the human cost of the war in Vietnam combined with the Watergate scandal that would lead to Richard Nixon's resignation of the presidency in 1974 was a crucial inflection point in the general public's faith its federal government. When Nixon came to office in 1969, opposition to the federal government's continued fight against the Vietnamese people was widespread. In his *People's History of the United States*, Howard Zinn notes that in the 1970s "middle-class and professional people unaccustomed to activism began to speak up. In May 1970, the *New York Times* reported from Washington: '1000 "ESTABLISHMENT" LAWYERS JOIN WAR PROTEST'" (Zinn 1980, p. 478). The *Wall Street Journal* is an important sounding board where the financial elites within the country expressed anxieties about the strategies and tactics pertaining to the war and where the political establishment in Washington began to break ranks with the administration's insistence on the use of American forces in a limited war in Vietnam (1980, p. 478). The dissent against the war contributed to a diminishment of faith in government:

> As early as 1970, according to the University of Michigan's Survey Research Center, "trust in government" was low in every section of the population. And there was a significant difference by class. Of professional people, 40 percent had "low" political trust in the government; of unskilled blue-collar workers, 66 percent had "low" trust. (1980, p. 529)

Across American society, individuals both on the left and right were beginning to question the moral capacity of their government to protect their values and represent their voices on national and international issues: "An article in the *American Political Science Review* by Arthur H. Miller, reporting on the extensive polling done by the Survey Research Center, said that the polls showed 'widespread, basic discontent and political alienation'" (Zinn 1980, p. 532). This general disaffection was confirmed and intensified by Watergate—the revelation of the Nixon administration's activities in election sabotage, information theft, and lying to American's about the war in Vietnam. The House of Representatives forwarded eight resolutions calling for Nixon's impeachment. When, in August 1974, it became clear that the majority of the Senate would vote in impeach, Nixon resigned (1980, p. 532). Although his Republican successor, Gerald Ford, would pardon Nixon for the crimes he had been convicted of in the Senate, the act was not generally viewed positively, contributing to Ford's eventual defeat in 1976. Though the political establishment and mainline media sources hailed Nixon's impeachment as a victory for the American democratic system of checks and balances (Zinn 1980, p. 533), the trust placed in the federal government by average citizen remained severely shaken.

Lynn Vavreck (2015) has forwarded the hypothesis that increased transparency in the workings of government has made citizens more suspicious of the central government in the United States and elsewhere, suggesting that the scepticism conforms to a tradition of the patriotic critique of British rule prior to the American Revolution. She asserts that most Americans agree on the importance of "peace, security and economic growth. But they disagree on the steps to get there" (Vavreck, para. 4). Vavreck notes that a poll taken by the American National Election Study in 1958 showed that 73% of Americans put faith in the federal government, while—in a study conducted by the Pew Research Centre in 2014—"roughly 24 percent of the adult population in the United States trusted the federal government to do what was right most or some of the time" (2015, para. 6). Noting the historical events that track along with this decline, she writes:

> The drop in trust over the decades has not been completely steady; the farthest fall came in the period starting with the Vietnam War, and continuing with the Watergate Hotel break-in, Richard Nixon's resignation, Gerald Ford's pardon of Mr. Nixon, the energy crisis and stagflation. (2015, para. 7)

Falloffs in economic development, natural disasters, and the threats of war and terrorism have since been the driving forces in the continually declining confidence of Americans in their central government (Vavreck 2015, para. 10). However, trust in the central government also varies depending on party allegiances. Vavreck points out that confidence in the central government, though declining overall, is lower among those polled whose party does not currently hold power: "gaps of 15 points or more during the presidencies of Mr. Nixon, Mr. Reagan, Bill Clinton, George W. Bush and

Barack Obama" register large differences in partisans' confidence in the government. She goes on to observe that "[t]he data also show that the average partisan gap over an administration is getting bigger, suggesting that something other than disagreeing about the steps to achieve common goals may be driving declining faith in Washington" (2015, para. 12). This decline in trust in governments is not unique to the United States, however. Citing *The Economist*'s, Justin Wolfers, Vavreck notes that "[t]here is increasing transparency across all types of institutions today relative to the 1940s and 1950s.… That very transparency might be the root of declining trust" (2015, para. 14).

3.2 Discourses of American Exceptionalism

Though Americans may have a declining faith in their federal government's capacity to do the right thing nationally and internationally, many Americans, nevertheless, share a belief in the unique role of United States as a beacon of freedom and justice among the nations of the world, an understanding which has been termed: American exceptionalism, a term coined ironically by Stalin as a rationalization for his excommunicating the American communist, Jay Lovestone and his acolytes from the Communist International (2015, para. 7). Stalin was asserting the incompatibility of American market capitalist values with the communist future he imagined for the world.

Writing within the context of the 2012 presidential election, Uri Friedman recalls the biblical image of a nascent New England colony—proffered to his fellow colonists by Puritan lawyer John Winthrop—"as a city upon a hill" (Friedman 2012, para. 2). In a 1630 speech aboard the *Arabella* designed to exhort the colonists he was leading to the New World, Winthrop borrowed his image from Christ's Sermon on the Mount: "Ye are the light of the world. A city that is set on a hill cannot be hid" (Matt. 5:14). The idea that America uniquely manifests—or at least aspires to manifest—Christianity's highest moral ideals persist in its rhetorical championing of freedom, justice, and equality. Married to this idea of America's unique spiritual mission is the notion that it will receive providential help in achieving its goal of becoming the city on the hill, providential help which will take the form of its political, technological, intellectual, and economic dominance in the world (Bell 1975, p. 197). In the early 1970s, sociologist Daniel Bell declared the death of American exceptionalism and global ascendency in a 1975 essay titled, "The End of American Exceptionalism." Bell writes: "Today, the belief in American exceptionalism has vanished with the end of empire, the weakening of power, the loss of faith in the nation's future. There are clear signs that America is being displaced as the paramount country" (1975, p. 197). Commenting on the corruption of American institutions and internal division, Bell calls for an end to the myth of American exceptionalism.

Bell's rejection of American exceptionalism represents, however, a minority view at least in the popular discourse. Americans, by and large, did not give up on their unique national status, and in fact, the challenge by Bell and other critics of the

War might have reinforced the desire to claim national pre-eminence. Illustrating the predominance of American exceptionalism in public life, Reagan's successful campaign against Carter in 1980 centered on slogans such as "Making America Great Again" and "It's Morning in America." The outcome of slogans based on a belief in American exceptionalism was a landslide victory, Reagan winning 489 out of a possible 538 electoral votes.

Conversely, the perception of Carter as challenging American exceptionalism became a cautionary tale to American political leaders, both Democrats and Republicans, even for those who might, otherwise, question the sustainability of the U.S.'s leading position as a consumer of non-renewable resources. Further, as the U.S. increasingly faces challenges such as global warming, which suggest the country unexceptionally faces issues similar to other countries around the globe, American reaction has been to double down on the optimistic belief in American impregnability (cited in Booth 2020, para. 29).

However, it should also be noted that exceptionalism represents one of many competing discourses in U.S. public life from liberal internationalism, dating back at least to the Wilsonian period in the early twentieth century to environmentalism, a discourse reaching back at least to the nineteenth century with the writings of Henry Thoreau and John Muir. Friedman incisively observes that the Trump-Reagan campaign slogan "Make American Great Again," and the Trump slogan, "Keep America Great Again," may define a singular moment. Nevertheless, it cannot be overemphasized that, regardless of who wins the upcoming election, American exceptionalism will, most likely, remain a powerful component of the national conversation and identity. Even Biden's slogan, "Build Back Better," contains Reaganesque optimism, although with Biden, there is also a recognition of a paradoxical need for multilateralism, wherein the U.S. is one of many co-equal partners in a global community.

3.3 Discourses of Anti-Intellectualism

Since the early colonial period in the seventeenth and eighteenth centuries, the faith in America's providentially afforded moral goodness has combined with a related tendency to subordinate rigorous intellectualism to a popular anti-intellectualism. In his 1963 *Anti-intellectualism in American Life*, Richard Hofstadter defines anti-intellectualism as a set of interrelated attitudes and ideas that manifest "a resentment and suspicion of the life of the mind and of those who are considered to represent it; and a disposition constantly to minimize the value of that life" (1963, Sect. 1.2). Hofstadter's book looks back to instances of anti-intellectualism he observed in political and public life during the Eisenhower administration, especially as it manifested in the McCarthyism of the 1950s. After giving a number of examples of how anti-intellectualism is expressed in public life, Hofstadter sums up the attitude: "Intellectuals, it may be held, are pretentious, conceited, effeminate, and snobbish; and very likely immoral, dangerous, and subversive. The plain sense of the common man… is an altogether adequate substitute for… formal knowledge and expertise acquired in the schools" (1963, Sect. 1.3). Hofstadter goes on to qualify, with rigor, those who may hold anti-intellectualist attitudes, noting that they may come from the realms of politics, religion, business, or the arts. Further, he concedes that the individual may be deeply engaged in a life of the mind themselves—often concerned with forwarding the ideas of influential intellectuals of the past over those of contemporary thinkers (1963, Sect. 1.4). He asserts that he does not see anti-intellectualism as a "positive creed," but an attitude that sometimes accompanies "justifiable intention[s]" (1963, Sect. 1.4), such as the valuation of egalitarianism (1963, Sect. 2.5). Ultimately, he argues that anti-intellectualism

> first got its strong grip on [American] ways of thinking because it was fostered by an evangelical religion that also purveyed many humane and democratic sentiments. It made its way into our politics because it became associated with our passion for equality. It has become formidable in our education partly because our educational beliefs are evangelically egalitarian. (1963, Sect. 1.4)

Hofstadter readily acknowledges that within the Christian tradition there has been a long struggle about whether the intellect or emotional impulse should take pride of place (1963, Sect. 3.1). However, anti-intellectualism in America is born of a preference for the affective experiences afforded by the Protestant faith rather than the intellectual rigour of its ethics and theology. Hofstadter does acknowledge that the Protestant evangelicalism, present at America's founding, contained a strong pro-intellectual element, as historically evidenced by Protestants' commitment to building many of the nation's most prestigious seats of higher education.

Nevertheless, Hofstadter asserts that, early in American life, Protestant "forces of enthusiasm and revivalism won their most impressive victories" over the Protestant intellectual forces, who were only able to find refuge in the select churches institutions they created (1963, Sect. 3.1). The tendency in popular Protestant religion, he claims, is towards a religiosity of emotions that elevates emotion and impulse over the mind and takes offence if its movements are impugned by an intellectualist argument. This propensity has broadly inflected American intellectual, social, and political life in ways that ensure sophisticated, articulate, and highly informed arguments are routinely sidelined for the emotional sensation of vague, yet morally plausible appeals.

All of these factors—the tendency to have a near-religious faith in America's special status, a lack of faith in the centralized authority of the federal government, the affinity with anti-intellectualism in pursuit of ethically justifiable goals, and the predilection to collective amnesia in the aftermath of previous health catastrophes—have led many Americans to believe, write about, and speak of their immunity to apparently foreign threats such as a virus, the name of which, as we have stated, has become a contested rhetorical space.

4 Medical Discourse on Pandemics in the Media, Past and Present

A recent article in *The New York Times* entitled, "The Mask Slackers of 1918," notes that the resistance to governmental authority, characteristic of the U.S. failure to adequately address the present pandemic, is not, in fact, a new phenomenon. Christine Hauser (2020, para. 3) observes further, "[i]n 1918 and 1919, as bars, saloons, restaurants, theaters and schools were closed, masks became a scapegoat, a symbol of government overreach, inspiring protests, petitions and defiant bare-face gatherings. All the while, thousands of Americans were dying in a deadly pandemic." Likewise, the mask acquired a negative meaning in the discourse of the period, called muzzles, germ shields, and dirt traps. They gave people a "pig-like snout" (para. 1). The resultant rejection of commonsensical public health measure by many no doubt heavily contributed to the eventual high death toll, estimated by the CDC to be 675,000 Americans out of 50 million worldwide.

However, one significant difference between now and then was the role played by social media. With the Spanish flu, there appeared to a collective amnesia regarding the virus. As Segal (2020, para. 6) notes, "[w]ith rare exceptions, it didn't crop up in novels, paintings, plays, or movies. Even scholars overlooked the subject. The first major account of the flu, "Epidemic and Peace"—later reissued as "America's Forgotten Pandemic"—was published in 1976 by Alfred Crosby, who was baffled by the absence of any impression left by the disaster."

It is doubtful that such will be the case with the pandemic occurring a hundred years later. Instead, social media will play a pivotal role in publicizing the threat of the virus, intensifying the anxieties of the general public, as well as in fragmenting the responses to the pandemic and, in some notable cases, spreading misinformation. Recently, in an article entitled, "Building trust while influencing online COVID-19 content in the social media world," digital social networks were described as a "viral entity," spreading "misinformation" (Limaye 2020, para. 3) The authors (Limaye 2020, para. 2) identify an important effect of social media in altering collective notions of "legitimacy":

> The idea of legitimacy has changed in the context of social media platforms. Users increasingly see trusted individuals within their peer networks who support production and exchange of valued information as authoritative sources of information. As that information is further disseminated, it often increases in its perceived legitimacy. This method of sharing and validating information contrasts with methods more directly controlled by intermediaries (e.g. traditional media), who have specialised knowledge and special responsibilities related to information verification and sharing.

Social media has had the effect of reinforcing the tendency with the U.S. to question the "legitimacy" of the medical specialists and traditional media. These entities are often perceived as a threat to the user's virtual community which becomes a sole source for "information." Such a shifting of "legitimacy" can have tragic effects when proper information is needed to address an emergency. As a prominent illustration, the slickly produced documentary *Plandemic* gained millions of hits, far more than the daily readership of a traditional media source, arguing that masks cause the virus and claiming that the virus was a direct descendent of SARS and that it would take "800 years" for a virus to evolve so quickly—despite the extensive evidence that viruses can change radically as entities within a two-week period (Neuman 2020, para. 40). The video also promoted conspiracy theories undermining the reputation of a leading epidemiologist, Dr. Anthony Fauci, and suggesting, again without evidence, that hospitals receive an extra payment of 13,000 USD if a death can be ascribed to COVID-19 (Fichera 2020, para. 5). The viral nature of "misinformation" has rendered attempts to remove the faux documentary as meaningless.

Social media has, thus far, played a significantly adverse role, impeding the efforts by U.S. medical experts, including Fauci and some political officials, to implement the necessary public measures to fight the virus. However, the role of social media may already be changing, indicated anecdotally by the number of public health messages, encouraging the use of masks, on *YouTube* and other social media vehicles.

5 Anti-Vaccination Discourse

Many experts, including Dr. Anthony Fauci, have predicted that a vaccine will become available either by the close of 2020 or the start of 2021 (Weise 2020, para. 3). One significant question in the near future then will be whether the mistrust of experts and central authority, anti-intellectualism as well as possibly American exceptionalism will, likewise, deter Americans in sufficient numbers from taking the vaccine. This is not an idle speculation. A recent poll conducted by Gallup has found that 65% stated that "if a vaccine were FDA-approved and available to them at no cost," they would take such a vaccine (O'Keefe 2020, para. 2). However, 35% stated they would not. Further, "a poll in May by The Associated Press-NORC Center for Public Affairs Research offered an even bleaker picture. It found that only about half of Americans said they would be willing to get a coronavirus vaccine. One in five said they would refuse and 31 percent were uncertain" (Hoffman 2020, para. 15).

That even a significant minority would choose not to take a vaccine under such favorable circumstance will at the very least impede heavily efforts to flatten the curve. Therefore, it is our view that addressing the pandemic in the U.S. is not merely a matter of achieving a scientific remedy but of altering long-standing attitudes infused with an anti-intellectual and distrust of government discourse that has affected America's failed response to the pandemic.

As Philip Ball (2020, para. 1) noted, there is a "small but fervent anti-vaccination movement." This movement has deep roots in American history and, fueled by Facebook and other social media, had achieved a significant following even before the pandemic. Neil Johnson, a physicist at George Washington University led a wide-ranging pre-pandemic study where they found that over 1,300 pages on Facebook expressed views consistent with the Anti-Vaccine Movement "followed by about 85 million individuals" (cited in Ball 2020, para. 3). The tendency to oppose government's promotion and mandates regarding vaccine use has become further exacerbated during the present pandemic by the President's long running championing of the anti-malarial drug, hydroxychloroquine, as a viable treatment for COVID-19.

The President's rhetoric surrounding the efficacy and safety of this drug began in March of 2020 and continued—despite multiple science-based sources disavowals of its beneficial effects against coronavirus—into August. On March 19, the President declared the "drug a 'game changer'" and announced "the FDA [would] fast-track approval of unproven coronavirus treatments including chloroquine and hydroxychloroquine" (Cathey 2020, para. 6). In late March, the FDA approved the use of hydroxycholoroquine as an emergency measure and—in early April after the death of a man who ingested "a form of cholorquine used to clean fish tanks," apparently trying to self-medicate against coronavirus (2020, para. 11)—the President repeated his endorsement of the drug, asking "What really do we have to lose?" (2020, paras. 14, 16). In April, the NIH undertook studies to examine the safety and effectiveness of the drug, as a trial study in Brazil indicated that it was linked to fatal heart problems (2020, para. 19, 20). In mid-April, the President continued to hail the drug's effectiveness and fired Dr. Rick Bright the head of the government agency "overseeing the rapid production of a coronavirus vaccine" in apparent retaliation for his request for funding of scientifically proven and safe treatment of the virus (2020, para. 24). May saw the *Journal of the American Medical Association* publish a study stating that hydroxycholoroquine "is not effective against COVID-19 and is associated with cardiac arrest" (2020, para. 31). Through the spring and into the summer, independent and government physicians continued to state that the drug was not effective. However, by early August the president was holding firm to his claim that the drug could be effective (2020, para. 56). It is plausible that the politicized clash between the president's rhetoric on hydroxycholoroquine and the dissemination of scientific evidence dismissing the drug's usefulness has stoked public anxiety about accepting medical advice from government sources on what coronavirus drugs are effective. Such conflicting discourse may ultimately hamper future efforts to widely vaccinate against the virus.

Added to this is suspicion of government medical advice, especially around vaccination, in social media-based anti-vaccination communities (made up mostly of parents of young children) and the African-American community, who have historically been subject to unethical government testing programmes that have undermined their community's health. Beginning in the late 1990s an online movement that linked autism to measles and mumps vaccinations began to circulate. The theory, with the study it was based upon, has now been discredited, but many online organizations, notably a group called Crazy Mothers, have continued to promote this and other theories about the long-term negative health effects of childhood vaccinations (cited in Reich 2020). Anti-vaccination groups have been outspoken and influential online and may well undermine public confidence in any vaccine that the government puts forward during the pandemic (Ball 2020). As Jan Hoffman noted in a *New York Times* piece the government's notorious Tuskegee syphilis experiment—in which "from 1932 to 1972, doctors intentionally did not treat Black men for the disease, so they could study the progress of symptoms" (2020, para. 12)—has made African-Americans suspicious of government-funded drugs and treatments for disease.

As has been stated, the suspicion is not only confined to the African-American community, but is shared by the general public. Hoffman (2020, para. 15) further cites interviews with Americans who would, prior to the current pandemic, accept medical advice and treatment from the government, but are now less likely to because of skepticism over its competence (2020). This doubt has been largely directed at the government's programme to rapidly create a vaccine—a Whitehouse initiative dubbed Operation Warp Speed, which is made up of both private and government researchers (*Fact sheet: explaining operation warp speed*, 2020). The name of the programme suggests that research will likely be rushed, which has led to broad-based concern that the drug it produces will prove unsafe and ineffective (Hoffman 2020, para. 25). Many are also concerned companies in the pharmaceutical industry will benefit at the expense of average and, especially, disadvantaged Americans (Hoffman 2020, para. 13). Citing broad-based online reaction to the programme, University of Colorado sociologist Jennifer Reich wrote:

> distrust [of pharmaceutical companies] goes hand in hand with anti-vaccine sentiment. Prior to Covid-19, I often heard complaints from those critical of vaccines about the revolving door between Big Pharma and government. Many of these concerns seem confirmed by the creation of Operation Warp Speed … this May. (2020, para. 12)

Public health researchers have echoed these concerns about government initiatives to produce and roll out a vaccine that, Americans will feel, may be safely taken. Medical researchers from the Johns Hopkins Centre for Health Security and the anthropology department at Texas State University have published a report titled "The Public's Role in COVID-19 Vaccination," which states:

> Baseline vaccine hesitancy and uneven access to vaccines, coupled with the country's currently charged political environment and fragmented pandemic response, call for effective planning and implementation of a COVID-19 vaccine program. If poorly designed and executed, a COVID-19 vaccination campaign in the United States could undermine the increasingly tenuous belief in vaccines and the public health authorities that recommend them—especially among people most at risk of COVID-19 impacts. (Schoch-Spana et al. 2020, p. 1)

Based on the observations of these researchers, it seems clear that the strains of discourse surrounding the issue of the efficacy and safety of creating and effectively disseminating a vaccine for COVID-19 are fraught and confused, a circumstance which may well ensure that—even if an effective vaccine is created in the near or distant future—many Americans may not choose not to be inoculated, inclined to believe the rhetoric that the vaccine will compromise their own health and, thereby, the health of the nation as a whole.

6 A Pro-Vaccine Alternative

However, such a dire outcome is only one possible scenario. It assumes that the government under the present leadership will continue to propagate unproven cures such as hydroxycholoroquine and use unfortunate terminology, such as "warp speed," suggesting the vaccine has not been fully vetted. However, the government has historically been successful in overcoming the efforts of a vociferous minority to impede inoculation efforts. By 1952, small pox was, according to the CDC, eradicated in North America, including the U.S ("History of Small Pox" 2016, para. 16). Similarly, the efforts to eradicate polio through the widespread use of a vaccine were highly effective. Throughout the entire region of the Americas, North and South America was judged polio-free by the World Health Organization in 1994. Interestingly, Alissa Greenberg (2020) observes the remarkable similarities between the socio-political environments in the US in 1946 and in 2020 before the discovery of a vaccine, where, in both cases, Americans adopted a pessimistic outlook, assuming the necessity to live with the outbreak, or as President Trump put matters, "it is what is." Historically, the US has, in fact, ignored, in actual practice, the nightmarish scenarios propagated by an extensive conspiracy network—and accepted the advice of experts.

According to a CDC analysis of a national 2017 immunization survey "of children born in 2015, 1.3 percent had not received any of the recommended vaccinations." The story is not entirely positive. That percentage compares adversely "with 0.9 percent in 2011 and with 0.3 percent of 19- to 35-month olds who had not received any immunizations when surveyed in 2001. As is noted further, "even though that figure is a tiny fraction of the estimated 8 million children born in the past two years who are getting vaccinated, the trend has officials worried" (cited in Sun 2018, para. 4).

7 Conclusions, Implications, and Lessons for Other Countries

Then, what can one conclude about the historical practices of Americans regarding actual vaccine use? How does such a practice play into the widespread belief in American exceptionalism, and what, if any, lessons are there for other nations? First, the widespread acceptance of guidelines and mandates set by public health experts may, in part, be a product of a faith in the ability of authorities, as exemplified in the post-World War II period, to solve what had previously been unsolvable challenges such as the reoccurrence of small pox and polio epidemics. Such an optimistic outlook contributed to the popular support for extensive government programmes fueling the development of an interstate highway system and a space program in the 50s and 60s, climaxing famously with the landing of a man on the moon in the late 60s. However, the faith in the government and expert authority to solve a public health emergency was not entirely limited to the greatest generation. In the late twentieth and early twenty-first centuries after overcoming societal prejudices and widespread doubt, the government was able to craft public health policies that addressed the AIDs epidemics. Most recently, the U.S., under an Obama-Biden presidency, managed, as part of a multilateral effort, to meet the challenges posed by an Ebola outbreak.

While there may be, then, a reason for optimism in regard to a substantial portion of Americans eventually choosing to become inoculated, such a positive outcome will be dependent on the ability of the government and experts to find the appropriate discursive note. In the meantime, we believe the U.S. government must also modulate its discourse so as to promote widely accepted measures such as testing, tracing, and social distancing. In addition, Americans may need to accept, at least within some hotspots, the necessity of reinstituting a lockdown. It may also be necessary to consider whether more aggressive measures are needed to counteract the misinformation spread on Facebook and other social media against the use of face masks and on the lack of efficacy of vaccines. While Facebook and Twitter have taken measures, including removal of such posts and labeling such posts as inaccurate, their implementation has been on a very limited scale.

A policy advocating limited action is, however, not an option. According to a recent “projection from researchers at the University of Washington’s Institute for Health Metrics and Evaluation – one of the more prominent teams modeling the pandemic”—by December 1, 2020, the U.S. death from COVID-19 could reach nearly 300,000”—an increase of nearly 80 percent over the next 5 months (cited in Aizenman 2020, para. 1). The long-term consequences, both in human and economic suffering, of a large-scale failure to participate in a vaccine program would be catastrophic—not only for the US but for the world.

What, if any lesson then, may other countries derive from the U.S. experience? First, as our analysis suggests, the reasons for the failure are rooted within a particular discursive strain embodied by the present President and his constituency that embraces American exceptionalism as well as a distrust of the federal government, scientists, and other intellectual policymakers—thereby, creating a ‘perfect storm.’ Nevertheless, a general lesson can be deduced: In countries around the world, the discourse that informs and designs policy for controlling future health crises must be modulated to address each particular nation’s historical and cultural discourse. Like the U.S., every country has its own set of prevailing discourses that could undermine its efforts to control a virus’s spread. Ultimately, attention to the best epidemiological advice must be combined with careful analysis of the ways we think and speak about ourselves as nations if future messaging is to be effective in controlling the virus in the U.S. and around the globe.

References

Aizenman, N. (2020) 300,000 deaths by December? 9 takeaways from the newest COVID-19 projections. *NPR*, 6 Aug. Available at: https://www.npr.org/sections/health-shots/2020/08/06/900000671/300-000-deaths-by-december-9-takeaways-of-the-newest-covid-19-projections (Accessed 15 August 2020).

Ball, P. (2020) Anti-vaccine movement could undermine efforts to end coronavirus pandemic, researchers warn. *Nature*, 13 Mar [online]. Available at: https://www.nature.com/articles/d41586-020-01423-4 (Accessed 12 August 2020).

Bell, D. (1975) (2020) The End of American Exceptionalism. *National Affairs*, 44, 193–224 [online]. Available at: https://www.nationalaffairs.com/public_interest/detail/the-end-of-american-exceptionalism (Accessed 7 August 2020).

Booth, W. (2020) Lancet editor Richard Horton has harsh words for Trump, hope for science. *Washington Post*, Jul 29. Available at: https://www.washingtonpost.com/world/europe/lancet-richard-horton-trump-vaccines/2020/07/29/1209b610-d048-11ea-826b-cc394d824e35_story.html (Accessed 30 July 2020).

Cathey, L. (2020) Timeline: Tracking Trump alongside scientific developments on Hydroxychloroquine. *ABC News*, 8 Aug [online]. Available at: https://abcnews.go.com/Health/timeline-tracking-trump-alongside-scientific-developments-hydroxychloroquine/story?id=72170553 (Accessed 12 August 2020).

CDC COVID Data Tracker. CDC, 8 Aug 2020. Available at: https://www.cdc.gov/covid-data-tracker/#cases (Accessed 8 August 2020).

Craig, J. (2020) Charts: How the U.S. ranks on COVID-19 deaths per capita—And by case count. *NPR*, 5 Aug [online]. Available at: https://www.npr.org/sections/goatsandsoda/2020/08/05/899365887/charts-how-the-u-s-ranks-on-covid-19-deaths-per-capita-and-by-case-count (Accessed 8 August 2020).

Fishera, A., Spencer, S. H., Gore, D., Robertson, L. & Kiely, E. (2020) The Falsehoods of the 'Plandemic' Video. FactCheck.Org. A Project of The Annenberg Public Policy Center, 8 May [online]. Available at: https://www.factcheck.org/2020/05/the-falsehoods-of-the-plandemic-video/ (Accessed 7 August 2020).

Forster, V. (2020) Coronavirus gets a new name: COVID-19. Here's why that is important. *Forbes*, 11 Feb [online] Available at: https://www.forbes.com/sites/victoriaforster/2020/02/11/coronavirus-gets-a-new-name-covid-19-heres-why-renaming-it-is-important/#a8cee57548ed (Accessed 7 August 2020).

Friedman, U. (2012) 'American Exceptionalism': A short history. *Foreign Policy*, 18 Jun [online]. Available at: https://foreignpolicy.com/2012/06/18/american-exceptionalism-a-short-history/ (Accessed 7 August 2020).

Greenberg, A. (2020) What polio in post-WWII America can teach us about living in a pandemic. *NOVA*, 29 Jul. Available at: https://www.pbs.org/wgbh/nova/article/polio-pandemic-coronavirus-vaccine/ (Accessed 15 August 2020).

Hauser, C. (2020) The mask slackers of 1918. *The New York Times*, 3 Aug [online]. Available at: https://www.nytimes.com/2020/08/03/us/mask-protests-1918.html (Accessed 7 August 2020).

'History of Anti-Vaccination Movements.' The College of Physicians of Philadelphia. Available at: https://www.historyofvaccines.org/content/articles/history-anti-vaccination-movements (Accessed 15 August 2020).

'History of Small Pox.' CDC 30 Aug 2016. Available at: https://www.cdc.gov/smallpox/history/history.html (Accessed 15 August 2020).

Hoffman, J. (2020) Mistrust of a coronavirus vaccine could imperil widespread immunity. *The New York Times*, 18 Jul [online]. Available at: https://www.nytimes.com/2020/07/18/health/coronavirus-anti-vaccine.html (Accessed 12 August 2020).

Hofstadter, R. (1963) *Anti-intellectualism in American Life*. New York: Alfred A. Knopf.

Limaye, R. J. et al. (2020) Building trust while influencing online COVID-19 content in the social media world. *The Lancet* [online]. Available at: https://www.thelancet.com/journals/landig/article/PIIS2589-7500(20)30084-4/fulltext (Accessed 7 August 2020).

Moloney, A. (2020) Wear a face mask? Many in the U.S. say no, while in Latin America most say yes. Reuters, 6 Aug. Available at: https://news.trust.org/item/20200806161041-83qji/ (Accessed 8 August 2020).

Mervosh, S and Fernandez, M. (2020) 'It's Like Having No Testing': Coronavirus test results are still delayed. *The New York Times*, 7 Aug. Available at: https://www.nytimes.com/2020/08/04/us/virus-testing-delays.html (Accessed 8 August 2020).

Neuman, S. (2020) Seen 'Plandemic' We take a close look at the viral conspiracy video's claims. *NPR,* 8 May. Available at: https://www.npr.org/2020/05/08/852451652/seen-plandemic-we-take-a-close-look-at-the-viral-conspiracy-video-s-claims (Accessed 17 August 2020).

Nimmon, L and Stenfors-Hayes, T. (2016) The "Handling" of power in the physician-patient encounter: perceptions from experienced physicians. *BMC Med Educ.* 2016; 16: 114. Available at: https://www.ncbi.nlm.nih.gov/pmc/articles/PMC4835893/ (Accessed 6 August 2020).

O'Keefe, S. M. (2020) One in three Americans would not get COVID-19 vaccine. GALLUP 7 Aug. Available at: https://news.gallup.com/poll/317018/one-three-americans-not-covid-vaccine.aspx (Accessed 15 August 2020).

Reich, J. (2020) How anti-vaxxers are thinking about a Covid-19 vaccine. *Vox*, 28 Jul [online]. Available at: https://www.vox.com/first-person/2020/7/28/21337621/coronavirus-covid-19-vaccine-anti-vaxxer (Accessed 12 August 2020).

Schoch-Spana, M., Brunson, E., Long, R., Ravi, S., Ruth, A., Trotochaud, M. on behalf of the Working Group on Readying Populations for COVID-19 Vaccine. (2020) COVID-19 *Vaccination: Planning Recommendations Informed by Design Thinking and the Social, Behavioral, and Communication Sciences*, July [online], Baltimore: Johns Hopkins Center for Health Security. Available at: https://www.centerforhealthsecurity.org/our-work/pubs_archive/pubs-pdfs/2020/200709-The-Publics-Role-in-COVID-19-Vaccination.pdf (Accessed 12 August 2020).

Segal, D. (2020) Why are there almost no memorials to the flu of 1918? *The New York Times*, 14 May [Online]. Available at: https://www.nytimes.com/2020/05/14/business/1918-flu-memorials.html (Accessed 14 May 2020).

Sun, L. (2018) Percentage of young U.S. children who don't receive any vaccines has quadrupled since 2001. *Washington Post*, 11 Oct [Online]. Available at: https://www.washingtonpost.com/national/health-science/percentage-of-young-us-children-who-dont-receive-any-vaccines-has-quadrupled-since-2001/2018/10/11/4a9cca98-cd0d-11e8-920f-dd52e1ae4570_story.html (Accessed 15 August 2020).

The Chicago School of Media Theory [Online] Available at: https://lucian.uchicago.edu/blogs/mediatheory/keywords/discourse/ (Accessed 6 August 2020).

Vasquez, M. (2020) Calling COVID-19 the "Wuhan Virus" or "China Virus" is inaccurate and xenophobic. Yale School of Medicine. [Online] Available at: https://medicine.yale.edu/news-article/23074/ (Accessed 6 August 2020).

Vavreck, L. (2015) The long decline of trust in government, and why that can be patriotic. *The New York Times*, 3 Jul [online]. Available at: https://www.nytimes.com/2015/07/04/upshot/the-long-decline-of-trust-in-government-and-why-that-can-be-patriotic.html (Accessed 7 August 2020).

Weise, E. and Weintraub, K. (2020) We're one-third of the way to a widely available coronavirus vaccine, experts say. *USA TODAY,* 30 Jun [online]. Available at: https://www.usatoday.com/in-depth/news/health/2020/06/30/covid-vaccine-progress-widely-available-coronavirus-expert-panel/3242395001/ (Accessed 15 August 2020).

Zinn, H. (1980) *A People's History of the United States*. London: Longman.

'A Mild Dose of the Flu': The Discourse of the COVID-19 Crisis in Brazil and the Impact of the Pandemic on the Internationalization of Brazilian Higher Education

John Corbett

Abstract On 24th March 2020, in a televised interview, Brazilian President Jaír Bolsonaro notoriously dismissed the symptoms of the COVID-19 virus as a 'gripezinha', which can be translated into English as a 'mild dose of the flu.' While his characterization of the illness was consistent with the Brazilian leader's other pronouncements about the virus and with his claims that he and his compatriots would be relatively immune to its impact, it was this expression, repeated endlessly, that came to symbolize the *laissez-faire* attitude of the leadership to the crisis. By November 2020, COVID-19 had resulted in over 150,000 deaths in the country, and Brazil was third only to the USA and India in virus-related fatalities. The pandemic also arrived in Brazil at a time of defunding of public universities generally, and governmental hostility towards the humanities and social sciences in particular. This chapter considers ways in which the humanities and social sciences in Brazil might respond to the constraints imposed by the pandemic by drawing on the tradition of critical discourse analysis and the more recent innovations of the digital and medical humanities. The chapter also considers the likely impact of the economic and health crisis on Brazilian public universities' plans for internationalization.

Keywords COVID-19 · Brazil · Gripezinha · Internationalization of higher education

1 Introduction

While Brazil is no stranger to epidemics, the COVID-19 pandemic of 2020 has emerged as a distinctive force in the national public debate. In the five years before the COVID-19 pandemic in 2020, the country's healthcare system had faced successive waves of mosquito-borne diseases, in particular chikungunya, dengue and zika. While these epidemics caught the public imagination to a greater or lesser extent, it is the COVID-19 pandemic, the first global health crisis in the age of social media, that has

J. Corbett (✉)
Division of Humanities and Social Sciences, Beijing Normal University-Hong Kong Baptist University United International College (BNU-HKBU UIC), Zhuhai, China
e-mail: johnbcorbett@uic.edu.cn

S.X.B. Zhao et al. (eds.), *COVID-19 Pandemic, Crisis Responses and the Changing World*, https://doi.org/10.1007/978-981-16-2430-8_13

dramatically affirmed the polarization in Brazilian political beliefs and exposed the decline in national affluence after the optimistic years of economic growth. Despite the impact of the recent economic downturn on Brazil's public finances, the relatively affluent years for the Brazil-Russia-India-China-South Africa (BRICS) nations at the start of the millennium had left a tangible legacy of research labs, facilities, agencies and trained staff, all primed to deal with recurring medical crises. And yet, at the time of writing, in the middle of November 2020, Brazil has suffered one of the worst rates of infection and mortality in the world, third in the world, behind the USA and India. The Microsoft News website that tracks infections and deaths in Brazil relates that there have been 5,783,647 confirmed cases, and that there have been 164,332 fatalities so far (2020).

The advent of the virus coincided with recent cuts in federal funding for public universities, particularly in the areas of the humanities and social sciences, whose practitioners have generally been voices raised in opposition to the current federal government (Borges 2019). The COVID-19 pandemic also presents a challenge to public universities that are trying to respond to globalizing impulses in higher education by attempting to internationalize, since student and staff exchanges have been suspended. The most obvious manifestation of internationalization in Brazil had been, until the outbreak of the pandemic, physical movement of faculty and students to overseas institutions on funded or subsidized exchanges. This kind of mobility came to an abrupt halt.

It would hardly be an exaggeration, therefore, to state that the position of the humanities and social sciences in Brazilian public universities in the wake of the COVID-19 pandemic appears to be weak. However, the present chapter argues that there is still a range of active and powerful roles that the arts and social sciences can play in Brazilian public life during and after the pandemic. First of all, we can draw on the established tradition of critical discourse analysis to highlight contradictions in the responses to the crisis from the federal government and the scientific community. Secondly, new developments in the digital humanities and social sciences can complement the work of healthcare providers in addressing the impact of the virus and monitoring public understanding of the health response. Universities can also extend recent trends towards 'internationalization at home' to continue fostering global relationships even when faculty and student travel has been curtailed. And, finally, we can draw on the medical humanities to complement overly medicalized responses to the pandemic, by bearing witness to the stories that people tell, and will continue to tell, about their own and others' experiences of COVID-19.

To illustrate these possibilities, the chapter first gives a brief account of the Brazilian context and argues that the *laissez-faire* attitude of the government to the health crisis is in part ideological, and in part a consequence of the fragmented nature of Brazilian political institutions. This is followed by a critical analysis of the federal government's discursive construction of the COVID-19 virus, and in particular its characterization of the disease as 'a mild dose of the flu' that could be treated by remedies such as wormicides—characterizations that contradicted those of the scientific community. The chapter then focuses on ways in which the humanities and social sciences can go beyond a critical exposure of governmental rhetoric, justifiable though that might be. The analysis of social media texts about the pandemic illustrates how the digital humanities might complement healthcare responses to the crisis; the nascent Brazilian approach to university internationalization is presented as a possible model for others to follow; and the medical humanities are offered as one means by which the value of the arts and social sciences can be affirmed during and after the health crisis. These various exemplars demonstrate that there is a viable future for the humanities and social sciences in Brazil even as these disciplines are threatened by a hostile government, a reduction in federal funding, and the consequences of a global health crisis.

2 The Brazilian Context

Its ethnically diverse population of 212,784,888 makes Brazil the sixth most populated country in the world (Worldometer 2020). The distribution of Brazilian citizens across the 3,286,488 square miles of its terrain is uneven, with the majority of Brazilians having been described, since colonial times, as being like 'crabs, clinging to the coast' (Skidmore 1999, p. 79). Since the end of a military dictatorship that lasted from 1964–1985, Brazil has been an elective democracy, with executive and legislative branches at federal level, and an independent judiciary. The federal legislature is characterized by a large number of separate political parties (currently 30 parties hold seats in Congress) that enter into mutually beneficial but often uneasy and temporary alliances.

Since the president must command over 50 percent of the public vote, the process of election usually whittles a number of candidates down to two final players. The current president, Jair Bolsonaro, was elected in 2018, as the then leader of the relatively minor Social Liberal Party (PSL) which, after the election, held 52 of the 513 seats in Congress. A former army captain, President Bolsonaro built his platform on a right-wing, populist agenda and nostalgia for the perceived discipline of military rule, which played to widespread disenchantment with corruption scandals that had tainted successive democratic governments. A substantial part of his support derives from the evangelical Christian churches, whose number of adherents has rapidly grown amongst the Brazilian working classes, giving them considerable political power (Hunter and Power 2019). His liking for blunt, inflammatory public statements predictably earned him the nickname 'the Tropical Trump' (e.g. Financial Times Editorial Board 2020). Since the 2018 election, President Bolsonaro has cut his ties with his former party, which is now led by one of his sons, and he governs as an independent. His Vice-President, Hamilton Moura, leads the Brazilian Labor Renewal Party (PRTB), while the largest party in Congress remains the Labor Party (PT) with 56 seats. Commenting on the early years of Brazilian democracy after the military dictatorship, Skidmore (1999, p. 192) observes:

> Such fragmentation, accompanied by weak party discipline, encouraged individual wheeling and dealing by congressmen and made consensus on policy action, especially with regard to the economy, virtually impossible.

The "fragmentation," "wheeling and dealing," and lack of "consensus" that Skidmore describes as being part of the earlier phase of Brazilian democracy continue to characterize the current Brazilian government, playing their part in the federal response to the COVID-19 crisis.

A coordinated response to the COVID-19 crisis would have required not only a much higher degree of consensus and common purpose at the federal level but also at the state and municipal levels of government. There are 26 states in Brazil, each with its own elected governor, as well as a number of autonomous municipalities, effectively larger towns and cities that elect a mayor. Municipalities vary in size; the largest, the city of Sao Paulo, has over 9 million inhabitants, almost twice the population of Ireland. The federal Health Minister oversees national healthcare strategy, but implementation of medical provision is through the *Sistema Único de Saúde* (SUS), or Unified Health System, which is administered at municipal level. Basic healthcare is a right of all Brazilian citizens and permanent residents, but, for those who can afford it, there is an extensive private health system, which funds clinics and hospitals, the most famous of which is the Albert Einstein Hospital in São Paulo, where the first Brazilian case of COVID-19 was admitted at the end of Carnival, on 25th February 2020, and confirmed on the following day.

Politics at municipal, state and federal level are interlinked and they are also characterized by short-term alliances and individual careerism. To take one example, the former mayor of São Paulo, João Doria, resigned in 2018, after only a year in office, to stand, successfully, for the post of state governor. A member of the Brazilian Social Democracy Party (PSDB), he supported Bolsonaro in the final run-off stage of the presidential election in 2018, but he has since distanced himself from the president, almost certainly because he intends to make a bid for the post himself in 2022 (Bonin 2020). The impact of the fragmented and antagonistic politics of Brazil on the health crisis is evident in heated public arguments between Doria and Bolsonaro on the desirability of testing a vaccine that had been developed in China, in the state of São Paulo, and on whether, if a vaccine were to be proved safe and effective, there should be state legislation on compulsory vaccination.[1]

The public discourse around COVID-19 in Brazil, and the public health response to the crisis, then, must be understood in the context of a nation where centralized control is limited, political relations at all levels, federal to municipal, are fractious, and public trust in politicians and governmental institutions is low. The country remains a site of severe inequality, where millions live in slums, parts of which are no-go zones run largely by drug gangs, while a small proportion of wealthy urbanites

[1] See, for example, https://veja.abril.com.br/blog/thomas-traumann/a-nova-guerra-da-vacina/ ('The New Vaccine War;' Traumann, 2020) and https://www.correiobraziliense.com.br/politica/2020/11/4887822-apos-suspensao-de-vacina-chinesa-bolsonaro-diz-que-ganhou-de-doria.html ('After suspension of Chinese vaccine, Bolsonaro says he 'beat' Doria' *Correio Braziliense*, 10 November 2020).

avoid the daily traffic jams by using private helicopters. The economic gains of the early 2000s, which saw many Brazilians lifted out of poverty and the state investing in numerous expensive health, educational, and research facilities, have been reversed.

In 2003, for example, Brazil inaugurated its first million-dollar NB3 (Level 3 Biosecurity) lab at the University of São Paulo's Institute for Biomedical Sciences, part of an 8-million dollar state investment in a network of virology labs intended to study emergent viruses. Once the Brazilian 'patient zero' with COVID-19 had been confirmed at the Einstein Hospital, he was sent to the NB3 lab at USP-IBS so that the virus could be isolated and sent for investigation to other labs around the country (Angelo 2020, p. 46). More recently, however, federal interest in and funding for science and public education have been drastically reduced. An Interministerial Executive Group (GEI-ESPII) was founded in 2005 to deal with public health emergencies of national and international importance. GEI-ESPII brings together the Minister for Health and other pertinent ministers of state, alongside the National Health Surveillance Agency (*Agência Nacional de Vigilância Sanitária*) and it coordinated the national response to the Zika outbreak in 2015. However, the group was later disbanded and had to be reactivated by a presidential decree in January 2020[2] when the COVID-19 epidemic threatened.

A recent report into medical research in Brazil (Negri and Koeller 2019, p. 11; my translation) observes of the sharp decline in federal funding:

> Its collapse means that a Brazilian researcher investigating new treatments for cancer or dengue, for example, is virtually without a source of funds to finance his/her research.

This sentiment is echoed in a report in the magazine *piauí,* in which an epidemiologist at USP, Naomar Monteiro de Almeida Filho, comments, on the federal government's disinvestment in research, 'It's almost a miracle of voluntarism that Brazilian science still exists'. (Angelo 2020, p. 51, my translation)

The COVID-19 pandemic, then, arrived in Brazil at a point at which a brief period of prosperity had been succeeded by an economic downturn, which in turn had led to a defunding of universities and their scientific institutions, and the sudden rise of a populist government. The authority of the president was weakened the fact that he led a minority party, which he later left, in a government of shifting alliances, and by the relative autonomy of state and municipal levels of government. In this context, the president's public pronouncements, characterizing the threat and the means of responding to it, became a crucial instrument in addressing the pandemic.

3 'A Mild Dose of the Flu'

The onset of COVID-19 in Brazil found the country in only a partial state of preparedness. There was a legacy of scientific expertise and facilities, and a fund of knowledge and skills accumulated from recent outbreaks of other viruses. On the other hand,

[2] http://www.planalto.gov.br/ccivil_03/_ato2019-2022/2020/decreto/D10211.htm.

there was recent sharp defunding of scientific research, the disbanding of an inter-ministerial coordinating group, and bitter partisanship amongst a large and volatile set of political groups at different levels of government. Before 2020, there was some awareness of the possibility of a large-scale epidemic caused by a coronavirus; unfortunately, plans were laid to deal with the wrong one. In 2019 the Ministry of Health published a contingency plan for a public health emergencies relating to the seasonal occurrences and possible epidemics of influenza (Brazilian Ministry of Health 2018). As Henriques et al. (2020, p. 30, my translation) observe:

> Given the apparent similarity between the clinical manifestations and mechanisms of transmission of the infection and those of influenza, much of the preparation that had already been made for these epidemics could be used as the basis for the response.

At the outset, then, the official response to COVID-19 was framed in terms of influenza, although the viruses that cause each disease are different. Both viruses cause varying degrees of respiratory disease amongst diverse populations and both are apparently transmitted by the diffusion of droplets through contact. However, the speed of infection, the way in which the respiratory system is attacked, the reproductive number and the mortality rate differ between COVID-19 and influenza (WHO 2020a).

On March 24th, 2020, a full month after the arrival of COVID-19 in Brazil, President Bolsonaro appeared on radio and television, downplaying the impact of the new coronavirus by referring to the virus in terms of influenza. The context of his announcement was the repatriation of Brazilian citizens from China, a site perceived as the source of the infection, although the Brazilian 'patient zero' had, in fact, caught the virus in Milan, Italy. Bolsonaro praised the role of the armed forces in returning the Brazilian citizens, before going on to urge his fellow citizens not to panic in the face of what he described as "media hysteria." In the midst of the 7-minute broadcast, he made the following claims (UOL News 2020; my translation):

> In my own case, thanks to my history as an athlete, if I was infected by the virus, I wouldn't have to worry, I wouldn't feel anything or I would be, at most, suffering from a mild dose of the flu [*gripezinha*] or a little cold [*resfriadinho*], as that well-known doctor from that popular TV program said. While I am speaking, the world is searching for a treatment for the disease. The American FDA and Albert Einstein Hospital, in São Paulo, are seeking proof of the effectiveness of chloroquine [*cloroquina*] in the treatment of COVID-19. Our government has received positive news about this medicine manufactured in Brazil and widely used to fight malaria, lupus and arthritis.

President Bolsonaro's dismissal of the degree of the threat came a month after the arrival of what was, even as he spoke, a major health crisis in the country. An indication of the spread and seriousness of the threat is evident in the report of the early impact of the virus on the healthcare system in the north-eastern state of Ceará (Lemos et al. 2020):

> The first 45 days of the COVID-19 epidemic in Ceará showed an explosion in the number of cases and deaths, reaching more than 1,000 confirmed deaths. In the first days after the detection of the first cases, infections spread most rapidly in the city of Fortaleza and municipalities with higher HDI [Human Development Index], mainly among users of the

> supplementary health network. In the following month, infections began to spread to the interior of the state, reaching the periphery of large cities and the most vulnerable social and economic populations. These populations have a higher prevalence of comorbidities, and often have living situations that make effective social isolation unfeasible. This likely contributed to the early exponential increase in the number of cases and deaths.

The contrast between these two characterizations of the epidemic is stark and illustrates why COVID-19 began to play an increasingly prominent role in the turbulent culture wars in Brazil. President Bolsonaro's announcement, typically, stresses the virtues of individual prowess (athleticism) as opposed to a collective response. He goes on to display his ideological affiliations when he touts chloroquine, a treatment promoted by US President, Donald Trump (cf. Lowe & Barber, this volume) and manufactured in Brazil, as a likely cure that he predicts would be endorsed by the US Food and Drug Administration as well as the most prestigious private hospital in the country.

In the same broadcast, seeking to minimize the evidence of the threat of the epidemic, President Bolsonaro describes Italy, which at that point in time was the epicenter of the COVID-19 crisis, as a country 'with a large number of old people and a climate unlike ours' (UOL News 2020, my translation). By contrast, the report by physicians working in Ceará shows the extent to which the President's announcement misrepresented the healthcare crisis. The report tells of an 'explosion' of cases far from São Paulo, the location of 'patient zero,' and rapid transmission from the high-income groups in the urban centers to the socially and economically vulnerable communities on the urban peripheries and in the interior of the state. If COVID-19 began as an illness of the Brazilian 'elites'—particularly those who could afford air travel for business or leisure—then it rapidly spread to the other classes, proving to be much deadlier than flu.

As evidence of the human cost of the COVID-19 quickly mounted in the wake of President Bolsonaro's broadcast on 24th March, the battle for narrative control of the political response to the epidemic intensified. On 16th April, President Bolsonaro sacked his Health Minster, Luiz Henrique Mandetta, for refusing to back chloroquine and for promoting measures such as physical distancing. At the same time, the desire to announce an accessible quick-fix to the crisis continued when the Minister for Science and Technology, ex-astronaut Marcos Pontes, hinted that one of several drugs that Brazilian scientists were experimenting with had shown some potential as a treatment for COVID-19. This drug was quickly revealed to be nitazoxanide (*nitazoxanida*), a treatment against intestinal worms. The Brazilian public promptly rechristened the drug 'Annita' (in likely homage to 'Anita,' a popular Brazilian singer in the style of Beyoncé) and such was the demand for it in pharmacies that the government sought to ban its sale without prescription. President Bolsonaro added to the demand for wormicides when he announced, on 11th June, that another such drug, ivermectin, would probably be even more effective than chloroquine 'because it kills all the worms' (Angelo 2020, p. 48, my translation). By this time, after just a month in office, Mandetta's replacement as Health Minister, Nelson Teich, had also resigned, citing to his own disagreements with the President. Teich's replacement, nominally on an interim basis, was to be Eduardo Pazuello, a general with no medical experience (Shalders 2020).

The President's championing of chloroquine followed that of US President Trump, and this endorsement, in turn, originated in the announcement by a French doctor, Didier Roault, that a derivative, hydroxychloroquine, had been used successfully on those infected with the COVID-19 virus, eliminating the disease within five days in all of his patients. When this claim was tested in Brazil, and elsewhere, however, the findings were not reliably replicated, and, indeed, after a heated debate amongst the scientific community regarding its possibly harmful impact on certain patients (Funck-Bretano et al. 2020) the WHO discontinued research on its alleged benefits for hospitalized patients at the start of July (WHO 2020b). Undeterred, President Bolsonaro affirmed the efficacy of chloroquine when he acknowledged, on 7th July, that he had been infected with COVID-19 and that the medicine had provided a cure or, at least, had a curative effect.

The public endorsement of chloroquine as a COVID-19 preventative and treatment by Presidents Bolsonaro and Trump was challenged by the Brazilian doctor, Marcus Vinicius Lacerda, who found himself caught in the tangle of opposing scientific and political discourses. Ektorp (2020) and Angelo (2020, pp. 48–49) report on Lacerda's attempt in the Amazonian capital, Manaus, to verify Roualt's results. When the study failed to corroborate Roualt's findings, there was an international backlash; Ektorp (2020, p. 661) explains:

> Micheal Coudrey, an American political activist with 256 700 Twitter followers referred to [Lacerda's] study as "a left-wing funded study that intentionally administered extremely high doses and used a less-safe version of the drug hydroxychloroquine, then used this as a pretense to indicate that chloroquine was ineffective and dangerous". Soon after, Brazilian president's son Eduardo Bolsonaro (who has 2 million Twitter followers) called it "a fake study aimed at demonizing the drug."

The twitterstorm resulted in Lacerda receiving death threats, and his family being placed under police protection for two weeks. With the publication of the findings of the clinical trial in a prestigious North American medical journal (Borba et al. 2020) the death threats ceased. Even so, an inquiry was opened into the scientific procedure followed in the clinical trial by three public prosecutors openly supportive of Presidents Bolsonaro and Trump. Lacerda concludes of the chloroquine episode (Angelo 2020, p. 49, my translation):

> I fell for the biggest *fake news* in history,' said the doctor, regretting his interest in the supposedly healing properties of chloroquine. 'We put all our research energy into it and put things with more promise aside.

A critical discourse analysis of the Brazilian experience of the miracle cures of chloroquine, ivermectin and 'Annita' demonstrates the mutual push and pull of political and scientific discourses and practices that in many ways rely on each other but which in other ways are incompatible. Populist leaders such as Presidents Bolsonaro and Trump continue to appeal to the apparent objectivity of science to support their authority, even when their tone is hyperbolic and their conclusions are flawed. However, the claims for the efficacy of chloroquine and 'Annita' did not originate with Bolsonaro or his political soul-mate, Donald Trump, but in claims, strong and weak, that originate from within the scientific community. One problem is that the testing, verification and refinements of knowledge claims that characterize scientific discourse do not suit a form of political discourse in which retraction is seen as weakness, and apparent mixed messaging is assumed to erode public trust. On the other hand, the political and public championing of one or another potential treatment, such as chloroquine or 'Annita,' amplifies its significance for the scientific community whose members are inclined to attend to the political agenda—after all, politicians hold the key to public funding.

The problems that arise from symbiotic but incommensurate practices and discourses are acknowledged in the conclusion of Priscilla Wald's study of 'cultures, carriers and the outbreak narrative' (Wald 2008. p. 262):

> The danger [...] lies not in scientific research or epidemiological investigation per se, but in stories, in the conventions of representation that infuse the images, phrases, and narratives through which we make sense of the world. They inflect – and yes, infect – every aspect of the scientific and epidemiological processes from the collection and interpretation of data to the social and medical diagnoses of the problem.

Wald goes on to discuss the potentially negative consequences of 'medicalizing' a pandemic by focusing solely on narratives of outbreaks, carriers, networks and treatments, and neglecting to consider what Malcolm Gladwell (2000, p. 261) called 'the beliefs and social structures and poverty and prejudices and personalities of a community.' Wald follows Gladwell in suggesting that epidemics might also be addressed by engaging more directly with just those beliefs and social structures, alongside issues such as poverty, prejudices and personalities. One of the roles that the humanities and social sciences can continue to play in Brazil, then, is to counterpoint political and scientific discourses (and how they are reported in the media) in order to uncover the ways in which competing ideologies bid for public attention and approbation. The critical analysis of political, media and scientific discourses can support a broader understanding of how different players interact and compete to characterize the health crisis in the public imaginary. What the case of Brazil dramatically demonstrates, however, is that academics in the humanities and social sciences are dependent for funding on institutions directed by politicians who are increasingly resistant to the social critique that such scholars are charged with providing.

4 Going Viral: COVID-19 on Twitter

The critical analysis of public discourse around the pandemic is perhaps the most obvious response of the humanities and social sciences to the health crisis, but it far from the only one. Many scholars working in the humanities in recent decades have adopted digital technology associated with data collation, visualization and mining. While these techniques can be used in marketing and other applied disciplines, those in the humanities have adopted them for other purposes, such as displaying in new ways those covert ideological positions and conflicts that are embedded in different forms of discourse. The digital humanities offer ways of mining 'big data' around global events such as the COVID-19 epidemic, not only to expose conflicting ideological positions, but also to complement healthcare responses.

The impact of social media on shaping and circulating the COVID-19 'outbreak narrative' has been pervasive. We have seen in the above discussion examples of politicians taking to twitter and medical experts invoking 'fake news' as a malign influence on scientific practices. Meanwhile the 'actual' news picks up on the international buzz of scientific announcements, reports, retractions and refinements, as journalists and pundits disseminate official and unofficial advice, comments, witness statements, investigative reporting, editorializing and opinion pieces. Fragments from a multiplicity of sources are recycled, framed, packaged, illustrated, and delivered online to smartphones and tablets, with regular updates. An analysis of the part played by social media in constituting and disseminating these stories reveals what Wald might describe as the 'ideological ecosystem' of a pandemic. A twenty-first century problem for the analyst is dealing with the sheer volume of textual storytelling.

Xavier et al. (2020) suggest a method for analyzing Portuguese-language posts on Twitter, primarily as a means of 'health surveillance': that is, as a way of assessing public reception of both official guidelines and 'fake news' to support healthcare responses. Using the COVID-10 epidemic as a case study, they combined linguistic analysis with data science to design a machine-learning algorithm that extracts information from samples of big data circulating on social media. Their immediate purpose in doing so was to address the following questions (Xavier et al. 2020, p. 264, my translation):

> What is public opinion with regard to the virus and suggested ways of controlling infection?
>
> How many people are reporting a symptom?
>
> What fake news is being disseminated on the internet?
>
> What are the locations in which people are reporting a symptom?

To address these questions, a multi-disciplinary team collected 7,720,408 Portuguese-language tweets posted between 16th April and 16th May 2020, a period in which Brazil saw confirmed cases of COVID-19 rise from 234 to 233,142. A program was developed to download the tweets automatically for analysis. The data was then filtered by a search for keywords related to COVID-19 symptoms and treatments that were identified by healthcare researchers (Table 1). Some of these keywords were hashtags (identified by #) that expressed the topic of the tweet.
After the analysis of the data, the results were presented in the form of graphs and tables, for discussion by specialists across disciplines. Tables 2 and 3 illustrate some of the salient data that can be made available to different agents. Table 2, for example, shows the degree of interest in chloroquine (*cloroquina*) in relation to other potential treatments.

Further analysis of the tweets shows that over the two months in question, mid-March to mid-May 2020, posts that mentioned chloroquine rose from fewer than 10 to 10,000 per day by 6th April, a level that was sustained and indeed exceeded by the

Table 1 Keywords used [+ *English translation*] (cf. Xavier et al. 2020, p. 268)

Group	Terms used
Sickness	COVID19, corona, COVID-19, #COVID19brasil, #CoronavirusPlantao [*#CoronavirusOnCall*], coronavirus, COVID
Symptoms	febre [*fever*], tosse [*cough*], falta de ar [*breathlessness*], coriza [*runny nose*], dor [*pain*]
Treatments	cloroquina, hidroxicloroquina, atazanavir, remdesivier, ivermectina, azitromicina
Actions	isolamento [*isolation*], lockdown, quarantena [*quarantine*]

Table 2 Tweets about symptoms related to COVID-19 (Xavier et al. 2020, p. 271)

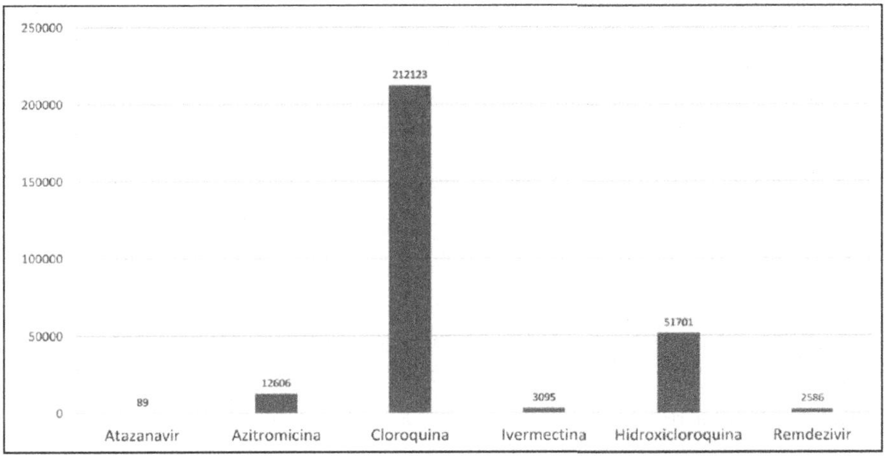

Table 3 Word-cloud of tags with the 50 most-used words in the tweets (Xavier et al. 2020, p. 272)

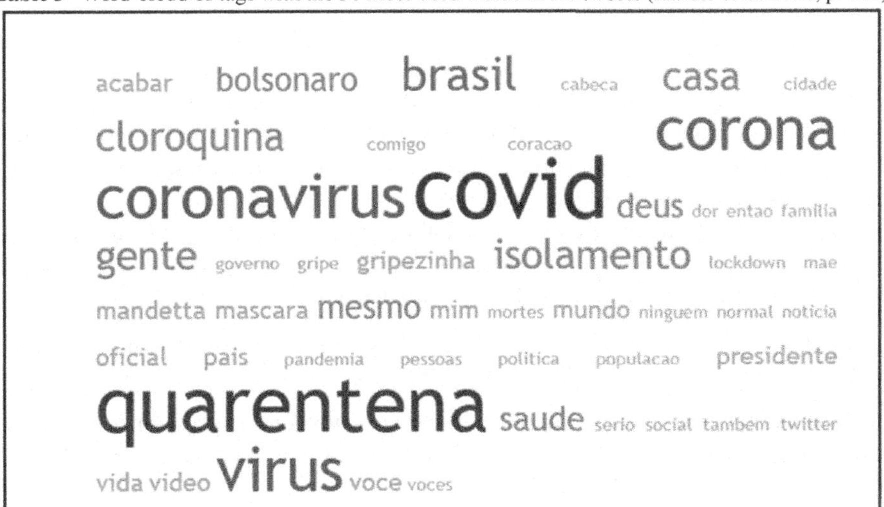

end of the study. The word-cloud shown in Table 3 is a convenient visualization of salient topics in the tweets; the cloud shows the 50 most-cited words in the data set: the larger the word in the cloud, the more frequent its use. Synonyms for COVID-19 naturally figure prominently, but so do expressions such as *cloroquina* (chloroquine), *quarantena* (quarantine), *bolsonaro*, and *gripezhina* ('a mild dose of the flu').

What a simple frequency analysis of expressions cannot indicate, of course, is the stance of the sender and receivers to the tweets. N-gram analyses of word clusters suggest more detail about the elaboration of the concepts expressed by the terms; for example, among the most common 3-word clusters involving *cloroquina* and its associated treatments were *efeitos colaterais clorquina* ('collateral effects of chloroquine;' 455 occurrences) and *morrido usando hidroxicloroquina* ('died using hydroxychloroquine;' 341 occurrences). These clusters, as Xavier et al. (2020, p. 273) affirm, suggest a lively public debate about the possible side effects of using chloroquine and its derivatives.

Even so, the degree to which Twitter users are affirming or challenging what they hear and see elsewhere on the news and social media is difficult to ascertain. Xavier and his colleagues term this aspect of their data analysis 'noise' and relate that they sought to filter out joking and sarcastic references, for example, to *quinine* and *cloro* ('chlorine,' the chemical used in cleaning products with brand names such as *Clorox*) on the grounds that these occurrences muddied the data. They note (2020, p. 274, my translation):

> This factor of the repercussion of a certain type of news on the internet is the biggest noise generated in this analysis. When an item of fake news appears and is widespread, it begins to be quoted ironically (as with the association of quinine [*quinina*] with chlorine [*cloro*] that was filtered during the experiment), which represents a challenge to the awareness of the real extent of the reach of the original news.

While the propensity of social media to disseminate false information with self-serving, malicious or joking intent is repeatedly raised as a problem by commentators, the presence of ironic counter-narratives on social media, and their reception are clearly worth further investigation. Similarly, Xavier and his colleagues deleted images such as emojis that offered clues to the attitudinal perspective of the users, and how given tweets might be read. For other analysts, they acknowledge, this kind of information would be insightful, although it is admittedly difficult to code and analyse in conjunction with the verbal text.

As well as the frequent use of non-verbal means of communication such as GIFs and emojis, Xavier et al. identify particular challenges to those who wish to use big data from Twitter to engage in health surveillance in real time (ibid, 277–278):

> Each tweet is constrained by being limited to 280 characters and so its short length demands a high level of inference on the part of the readers.

The immediacy and brevity of tweets privileges informal expressions, slang and abbreviations. The analyst needs to decide whether or not to include or exclude such items from the keywords being analyzed.

Some posts are automatically boosted by 'bots.' While platforms such as Twitter attempt to minimize the automatic generation of tweets, the analyst must be aware of the possibility that certain tweets might have a non-human origin.

The analysis of social media data for epidemiological purposes must attend to the truthfulness or accuracy of the data; for example, in the COVID-19 data, epidemiologists must ask whether or not the 33,369 instances of the expression 'died' relate to actual deaths. If so, the tweets may indicate the extent of under-reporting of COVID-19 deaths in official statistics.

Xavier et al. (ibid, p. 278) observe that 365,331 (4.73%) of the more than 7 million tweets analyzed mentioned President Bolsonaro, and so it is reasonable to assume that they express an ideological position, whether in favor of or against his handling of the crisis. Those purely interested in epidemiological data might consider the data 'contaminated' by ideological bias; other analysts might be interested in how the public (or at least that part of it with access to social media) is responding to government actions and announcements.

While Xavier et al. present their analysis of social media posts primarily as a means of supplementing epidemiological data available to healthcare professionals in the midst of a pandemic, it clearly has implications for the humanities and social sciences beyond its immediate potential for such use. Indeed, some of the 'noise' filtered out of the analysis might be used by others to determine more clearly the kinds of narratives that Wald envisages as being important to 'non-medicalized' aspects of epidemic management. For example, alternative choices of keyword might probe more deeply why 'family,' 'mother,' 'home,' and 'God' are so frequently mentioned in COVID-19 tweets (Table 3), and interrogate the sentiments that cluster around the frequent mention of 'isolation' (*isolamento*). Oddly, little of the data sampled and presented addresses the economic impact of the COVID-19 crisis, particularly on Brazil's economically marginalized communities, a fact that also raises the question of how those without access to Twitter or other social media might raise their concerns in public forums. Clearly, in a country such as Brazil, there are profound issues around not just access to the means of engaging with social media, but there are large sections of the population still struggling with basic literacy. The question remains how their voices can be heard.

Xavier et al.'s study is suggestive of a multi-disciplinary approach to epidemic management and the possibility of extending beyond positivist approaches to medical crises. Their analysis draws on expertise not only from healthcare specialists but also data scientists and linguists who are interested in methodologies that mine big data and analyze aspects of narrative. More broadly, there are clearly ongoing issues around privacy, consent and the ethics of 'health surveillance' that are of interest to lawyers and philosophers, as well as to the users of social media. Transdisciplinary approaches to the management of an epidemic go beyond medicine and public healthcare, and the humanities and social sciences can also draw upon information technology and data mining to develop innovative approaches to understanding how narratives are constructed and interpreted.

5 Rethinking Internationalization During and After COVID-19

So far we have considered how the humanities and social sciences might respond to the circumstances of a global health crisis in a nation struggling with an economic downturn, and led by a populist political leader whose authority is constrained by a fragmented political system that functions at different levels of government. President Bolsonaro's television broadcast on March 24th, in which he described the symptoms of COVID-19 as a mere *gripezinha,* also praised the successful repatriation of groups of stranded Brazilians from what were suddenly perceived as being dangerous overseas sites of infection. One of the most immediate impacts of the COVID-19 epidemic for higher education – not just in the humanities and social sciences but more generally – has been the threat to the 'internationalization' of top-ranking world universities. 'Internationalization,' while it has multiple definitions, has, at its core, the flow of intellectual, human and economic capital facilitated by the increased global mobility of academic staff and students. The proportion of 'international' staff and students that an HE institution could boast was one of the key indicators that boosted or depressed the institution's position in the world rankings. The global pandemic curtailed the international travel that sustained the flow of faculty and staff across national boundaries.

In relative terms, Latin American universities had a poor record in internationalization, even before it was threatened by COVID-19. For example, according to the 2021 Times Higher Education World Rankings, the highest ranked university in South America, the University of São Paulo, which lies in the 251-300 band, has only 4 percent international students, and, while it is rising, its 'international outlook' lags well behind its ratings for teaching, research, citations or industry income (THE 2020). For comparison the current No. 1, the University of Oxford, has 41 percent international students, and its 'international outlook' exceeds its income from industry.

Before the pandemic, Brazilian universities had attempted to address the pressure to internationalize in several ways. In her survey of successful Brazilian graduate programs, Ramos (2018) identified numerous strategies then being undertaken. The most popular of these schemes was outward student mobility under the government-funded 'Science without Borders' (*Ciências sem Fronteiras*) initiative, which was discontinued in 2017. Since outward mobility programs, even when they were being subsidized, only reached a minority of Brazilian students, some institutions began to advocate 'internationalization at home,' a central pillar of which is the delivery of courses using English-medium instruction (Martinez 2016; Carvalho Fonseca, Corbett & Costas, forthcoming). The broader range of elements of internationalization include (Ramos 2018, p. 9):

> *Mechanisms or strategies* (international mobility, international scientific cooperation, international networks and collaboration, curriculum internationalization, international engagement in science policy/governance), *academic output* (international publications, international co-authorships, attendance to international scientific meetings and conferences),

enabling factors (institutional, organizational and administrative support) and *access to resources* (sharing of cutting-edge research facilities and technology, international funding) to *desirable outcomes* (global competence development and scientific capital accumulation).

The full impact of the COVID-19 epidemic on these kinds of activity is yet to be understood. However, given that Brazil higher education was hitherto largely a provider of exchange students to other countries, and that, alongside other actors in the education sector, at all levels worldwide, Brazilian university education has swiftly moved to an online mode of activity; there should be, at least in principle, greater opportunities in Brazil for 'virtual internationalization' as universities elsewhere address the accelerated move towards online delivery of programs, networking, collaboration in publishing, conference participation and sharing of research resources. Public universities in Brazil, as throughout Latin America, will be less adversely affected by any reduction in overseas university fees than their counterparts in Europe and elsewhere, at least until the effects of the pandemic have receded.

Similarly, international conferences and seminars are now largely being conducted virtually, and online participation in such events, while possible for some time before the epidemic, may well now become routine. In sum, since the obstacles to academic travel are now similar for students and staff everywhere, there may well emerge an increased appetite and opportunities for online internationalization. The shock that COVID-19 represents to Brazilian universities' economic viability and cultural practices, not to mention their sclerotic bureaucracies, coming as they do during a period of federal belligerence, might paradoxically force institutions to adopt some positive structural changes that could only occur in the face of a severe social crisis.

These possibilities have been recognized by some senior staff in major Brazilian universities. In one of a series of webinars on the 'New Normal' in higher education in the post-coronavirus era, the USP Dean of Research, Professor Carlos Graeff, identified key points learned so far from the Brazilian experience of the epidemic (USP 2020). He outlined the need for more flexible teaching, both online and blended, as universities go forward. He praised higher education for its swift response, and, while reaffirming the importance of face-to-face encounters for building trust, he confirmed the utility and value of virtual meetings and online/blended conferences for future research activities. Not least, he restated the way in which global scientific collaboration around the response to COVID-19 had demonstrated the need for 'Open Science', which can be defined as the free dissemination of knowledge, subject to aspects of ethics and intellectual property, by means of Open Access to publications, Open Data (access to raw data from the initial stages of research, models and documentation), and Open Computational Process (software and algorithms). FAPESP, a public agency for the promotion of research in the state of São Paulo (FAPESP 2020) outlines its contribution to Open Science in relation to COVID-19 thus:

> In June 2020, it [FAPESP] launched COVID-19 Data Sharing/BR, an open repository containing health data on patients who had undergone COVID-related testing in Brazil since the pandemic outbreak in the country.

> This repository was created as a result of the collaboration of FAPESP with the University of Sao Paulo, and three prestigious Brazilian healthcare institutions - Instituto Fleury, Hospital Sírio-Libanês and Hospital Israelita Albert Einstein.
>
> In its first stage, the repository made available curated data on 177,000 patients, together with information on primary endpoints and patient transfers, corresponding to almost 5 million records that were pre-processed to meet Brazil's data protection laws. It will subsequently contain medical images of COVID-19 patients, and associated reports. Periodically updated throughout the pandemic, this represents an exemplary open science effort launched within a public-private partnership.

While Open Science is clearly in the public good and it facilitates research collaboration between scientists in Brazil and elsewhere, the prospects for the humanities and social sciences, already bleak before COVID-19, seem bleaker. Squeezed by an unsympathetic federal government, typically more individually oriented in their research agendas than their collaborative colleagues, less positivist in their theoretical frameworks and methods, and often valuing modes of dissemination that are not subsidized by project funding (e.g. traditional formats such as printed books), those who work in the humanities and social sciences will need to be creative in order to thrive in the difficult months and years ahead.

6 Conclusions

One of the ways in which those in the humanities and social sciences might reaffirm their value in a society that is dealing with a pandemic is, as suggested above, to contribute to the debates around the 'over-medicalization' of responses to COVID-19 and other epidemics by offering alternative narratives. As Wald (2008, pp. 269–270) insists:

> Disease emergence ineluctably evinces human interconnections on a global scale, but the stories of disease emergence fashion the terms in which those connections make sense. It is possible to revise the outbreak narrative, to tell the story of disease emergence and human connection in the language of social justice rather than of susceptibility.

In the case of Brazil, as we have seen in the foregoing sections, the language of susceptibility has, for generations, tended to drown out that of social justice. Consequently, it is perhaps not altogether shocking that, when asked about his country's high infection and mortality rate at the beginning of May, 2020, President Bolsonaro reportedly responded, 'So what? What do you expect me to do about it?' (*The Lancet* 2020). A cynical population, 13 million of whom live in slum conditions, can have few expectations that their elected representatives, tainted by years of deal-making, infighting, scandal and corruption, will take effective action on their behalf. As noted above, rather than taking to political activism, many seek solace in evangelical Christianity, a doctrine that suggests that plagues are a sign of divine anger and that there is dignity in suffering.

Those in the humanities and social sciences might be tempted to engage in a strategy of resistance to the language of susceptibility, drawing on theoretical frameworks such as critical discourse analysis to decry, for example, President Bolsonaro and his government's regular attempts to shore up their authority by recourse to militaristic metaphors (Pfrimer & Barbosa Jr. 2020). However, as well as demystifying public discourse, the humanities and social sciences can draw upon their intellectual reserves to offer complementary alternatives to medical positivism. The development of a medical cure for COVID-19, whether in the form of 'Annita', chloroquine or an as yet unapproved vaccine (whose viability might be popularly judged by whether the word 'Oxford,' 'Chinese,' or 'Russian' precedes it) will not address the deeper issues that have allowed the virus to spread. In an article on COVID-19 and urban management in the megacity of São Paulo, Buckeridge and Philippi Jr (2020, p. 150, my translation) observe:

> It seems evident that the urban structure, consisting of elements such as transport, crime, sanitation, the environment, habitation, and population, has some role in the spread of COVID-19 in the city of São Paulo.

The authors' recommendation, given the multi-factorial nature of the issues that contribute to the spread of the virus is to think of the city as an ecosystem (what they call an *urbsystem*), and address the issues in parallel, systemically, acknowledging that the scale and range of the challenges mean that substantial improvement in the living conditions of the majority will take generations to achieve. Those of us in the humanities might call the *urbsystem* a 'culture' and see such as system as a metaphor for Brazilian society in general.

There is no single or swift treatment for the poor leadership, abject poverty, experiences of trauma, and profound social injustice that characterize lives, livelihoods, education and scientific research in Brazil. There are, certainly, individuals and groups who are calling for politicians to adopt a systemic approach that will actively address the social ills that allow disease to spread—the outcome of one such initiative is the 'Pact for Life and Brazil,' a manifesto presented to the three branches of government in April 2020, signed by over 100 Brazilian organizations. As reported on a human rights news site (Connectas 2020), the intention of the manifesto is to:

> Call on governments, the branches of the Republic as well as Brazilian citizens to come up with solutions, in this time of crisis, to enable a better quality of life for those most in need, both during and after the pandemic.

It is the responsibility of the humanities, in particular, to foster the sense of 'human connection' between all the members of the ecosystem that makes up Brazilian society. We need to attend to the countless narratives of loss and resilience, despair and hope, isolation and community that emerge from this epidemic, to understand how these stories frame the experiences of Brazilian citizens, and to show how such stories play their modest but necessary part in the long-term process of resistance and healing.

References

Angelo, C. (2020) Contra a besta-fera. *piauí*, July, Issue 166, 46–51.

Bonin, R. (2020) *O projeto de João Doria para 2020* [Online] Available at: https://veja.abril.com.br/blog/radar/o-projeto-de-joao-doria-para-2022/ (Accessed 25 August 2020).

Borba, M. G. S. et al. (2020) Effect of high vs low doses of chloroquine diphosphate as adjunctive therapy for patients hospitalized with severe acute respiratory syndrome coronavirus 2 (SARS-CoV-2) infection: a randomized clinical trial. *JAMA Network Open*, 3(4), pp. e208857–e208857.

Borges, H. (2019) *Bolsonaro defende cortes em cursos de Humanas e diz que dinheiro do contribuinte deve ir para 'leitura, escrita e fazer conta'* [Online] Available at: https://oglobo.globo.com/sociedade/bolsonaro-defende-cortes-em-cursos-de-humanas-diz-que-dinheiro-do-contribuinte-deve-ir-para-leitura-escrita-fazer-conta-23623980 (Accessed 13 November 2020).

Brazilian Ministry of Health. (2018) *Plano de Contingência para Resposta às Emergências de Saúde Pública: Influenza - Preparação para Sazonalidade e Epidemias.* Brasília: Secretaria de Vigilância em Saúde, Departamento de Vigilância das Doenças Transmissíveis.

Buckeridge, M. S. & Philippi Jr, A. (2020) Ciência e políticas públicas nas cidades: revelações da pandemia da COVID-19. *Estudos Avançados*, 34(99), 141–156.

Carvalho Fonseca, L., Corbett, J. & Costa, J., forthcoming. Enhancing academic literacies through EMI training: Three perspectives on teaching towards the Certificate of EMI Skills at the University of São Paulo. *Letras.*

Connectas. (2020) *Nearly 100 organizations sign Pact for Life and for Brazil* [Online] Available at: https://www.conectas.org/en/news/nearly-100-organizations-sign-pact-for-life-and-for-brazil (Accessed 24 August 2020).

Correio Braziliense. (2020) *Após suspensão de vacina chinesa, Bolsonaro diz que 'ganhou' de Doria* [Online] Available at: https://www.correiobraziliense.com.br/politica/2020/11/4887822-apos-suspensao-de-vacina-chinesa-bolsonaro-diz-que-ganhou-de-doria.html (Accessed 13 November 2020).

Ektorp, E. (2020) Death threats after a trial on chloroquine for COVID-19. *The Lancet. Infectious Diseases*, June, 20(6), 661.

FAPESP. (2020) *Open Science @ FAPESP* [Online] Available at: http://www.fapesp.br/openscience/en (Accessed 24 August 2020).

Financial Times Editorial Board (2020) *The Self-Destruction of the 'Tropical Trump"* [Online] Available at: https://www.ft.com/content/72bed346-888b-11ea-9dcb-fe6871f4145a (Accessed 13 November 2020).

Funck-Brentano, C. & al. (2020) Retraction and republication: cardiac toxicity of hydroxychloroquine in COVID-19. *The Lancet*, 396(10245), e2–e3.

Gladwell, M. (2000) *The Tipping Point: How Little Things Can Make a Big Difference.* New York: Little Brown.

Henriques, C., Pessanha, M. & Vasconcelos, W. (2020) Crises dentro da crise: respostas, incertezas e desencontros no combate à pandemia da COVID-19 no Brasil. *Estudos Avançados*, 34(99), 25–44.

Hunter, W. & Power, T. (2019) Bolsonaro and Brazil's illiberal backlash. *Journal of Democracy*, 30(1), 68–82.

Lemos, D. R. Q. et al. (2020) Health system collapse 45 days after the detection of COVID-19 in Ceará, Northeast Brazil: a preliminary analysis. *Revista da Sociedade Brasileira de Medicina Tropical*, Volume 53.

Martinez, R. (2016) English as a Medium of Instruction (EMI) in Brazilian higher education: Challenges and opportunities. In: K. Finardi, ed. *English in Brazil: Views, policies and programs.* Londrina: EDUEL, 191–228.

Negri, F. d. & Koeller, P. (2019) *O Declínio do Investimento Publico em Ciência e Tecnologia: Uma Análise do Orçamento do Ministério da Ciência, Technologia, Inovações e Comunicaçoes até o Primeiro Semestre de 2019*, Brasília: s.n.

Pfrimer, M. H. & Barbosa Jr, R. (2020) Brazil's war on COVID-19: Crisis, not conflict—Doctors, not generals. *Dialogues in Human Geography*, 1–4.

Ramos, M. Y. (2018) Internationalization of graduate education in Brazil: Rationale and mechanisms. *Educação e Pesquisa: Revista da Faculdade de Educação da USP*, Volume 44, 1–20.

Shalders, A. (2020) *Quem é Eduardo Pazuello, o general que assume interinamente o Ministério da Saúde* [Online] Available at: https://www.bbc.com/portuguese/brasil-52686114 (Accessed 24 August 2020).

Skidmore, T. E. (1999) *Brazil: Five Centuries of Change*. Oxford: Oxford University Press.

The Lancet. (2020) Editorial: COVID-19 in Brazil: 'So what?' *The Lancet*, Volume 395, 1461.

THE. (2020) *University of São Paulo* [Online] Available at: https://www.timeshighereducation.com/world-university-rankings/university-sao-paulo (Accessed 24 August 2020).

Traumann, T. (2020) *A nova guerra da vacina* [Online] Available at: https://veja.abril.com.br/blog/thomas-traumann/a-nova-guerra-da-vacina/ (Accessed 13 November 2020).

UOL News. (2020) *'Gripezinha': leia a íntegra do pronunciamento de Bolsonaro sobre COVID-19* [Online] Available at: https://noticias.uol.com.br/politica/ultimas-noticias/2020/03/24/leia-o-pronunciamento-do-presidente-jair-bolsonaro-na-integra.htm?cmpid=copiaecola (Accessed 21 August 2020).

USP. (2020) *Heading to the New Normal—How coronavirus is changing higher education perspectives for university research and teaching* [Online] Available at: https://youtu.be/OydiX9UXMmw (Accessed 18 August 2020).

Wald, P. (2008) *Contagious: Cultures, Carriers, and the Outbreak Narrative*. Durham and London: Duke University Press.

WHO. (2020a) *Q&A: Influenza and COVID-19—Similarities and differences* [Online] Available at: https://www.who.int/westernpacific/news/q-a-detail/q-a-similarities-and-differences-COVID-19-and-influenza (Accessed 21 August 2020).

WHO. (2020b) *WHO discontinues hydroxychloroquine and lopinavir/ritonavir treatment arms for COVID-19*. [Online] Available at: https://www.who.int/news-room/detail/04-07-2020-who-discontinues-hydroxychloroquine-and-lopinavir-ritonavir-treatment-arms-for-COVID-19 (Accessed 22 August 2020).

Worldometer. (2020) [Online] Available at: https://www.worldometers.info/ (Accessed 25 August 2020).

Xavier, F. et al. (2020) Análise de redes sociais como estratégia de apoio à vigiliância em saúde durante a COVID-19. *Estudos Avançados*, 34(99), 261–282.

New Order and Impacts in Business, Culture and Society

Translating Against COVID-19 in the Chinese Context: A Multi-agent, Multimedia and Multilingual Endeavor

Mengying Jiang

Abstract In the COVID-19 crisis, multilingual and multimodal translation services, provided by both professional translators and volunteer communities, have greatly facilitated the communication between different parties. This chapter gives an overview of how diverse agents have engaged in this large-scale translation endeavor and draws attention to the importance of translation planning in crisis contexts. It not only discusses the operations of volunteer translators, highlighting their contribution in providing language assistance in crisis situations, but also analyzes the significant role played by government-sponsored institutions in mobilizing language professionals and organizing translation projects, such as Language Service Group Against COVID-19 and China International Publishing Group. Moreover, this chapter focuses on the relevance of translation to *waixuan* (often translated as international publicity) in this crisis situation and investigates how translation is strategically adopted by the government as a medium of communicating the Chinese experience of fighting COVID-19. After analyzing all these disparate efforts, it argues for the significance of translation in overcoming language barriers in crisis contexts and concludes with suggestions on how to enhance translation planning for health emergencies.

Keywords COVID-19 · Translation planning in crisis contexts · Volunteer translators · Government-sponsored translation · *Waixuan* (international publicity)

1 Introduction

The communication of public health information has been a major aspect of the ongoing COVID-19 pandemic. Never before have so many people globally engaged with the same topic. During the pandemic, the availability of effective and timely high-quality information has been vital not only for the general public, but also for health professionals and decision makers at all levels (Xiang et al. 2020). Therefore, effective communication during a crisis is of strategical and operational

M. Jiang (✉)
BNU-HKBU United International College, Zhuhai, China
e-mail: mollymyjiang@uic.edu.cn

S.X.B. Zhao et al. (eds.), *COVID-19 Pandemic, Crisis Responses and the Changing World*, https://doi.org/10.1007/978-981-16-2430-8_14

importance (Seeger 2006; Fischer 2008). As language barriers to accessing and sharing public health information pose a pressing concern to different linguistic and cultural communities, the need to translate COVID-related information into as many languages as possible figures prominently in crisis communication. Gretchen McCulloch (2020) has even claimed that "COVID-19 is history's biggest translation challenge" and cautioned against the threat of a communication emergency, or what the WHO calls an "infodemic". Access to information in a crisis setting is a human right for all members of affected populations (Federici et al. 2019a). To facilitate the communication of COVID-related information, a large number of translation projects have been springing up all around the world.

Though the multilingual composition of foreign residents in China is not as diverse as that in European countries, there was still an urgent demand to translate public health information from Mandarin into multiple other languages during the early phase of the COVID-19 outbreak in February and March 2020. The demand was even more urgent in large metropolitan cities such as Beijing, Shanghai and Guangzhou which are popular destinations for foreign visitors. For example, Shanghai is said to have 172,000 foreign residents among its total population of 24 million (Shanghai Statistics Bureau 2020). Even in Hubei Province, 19,000 foreign nationals were officially registered as business-purpose residents in 2018 and 81% of them lived in Wuhan, the first epicenter of the pandemic (The Hubei Government 2018). Local foreign affairs offices as well as students majoring in foreign languages at local universities in these places became active agents in coordinating and managing translation-related resources and activities. They were communicating important information about disease control and prevention measures to foreign residents and visitors. In addition to translation activities that accommodated domestic needs, some transnational volunteer translation alliances also emerged. One example is 中伊防疫互助小组 (China-Iran Alliance Against COVID-19), founded by Chen Binbin to share Chinese experiences to help Iran fight the pandemic. Chen is a PhD student in Peking University who lived and taught Chinese in Iran for over one year. This translation team not only collected and translated pandemic information, but also made videos and posters which were to be distributed among the Iranian public. Moreover, the significance of translation reached beyond the function of information communication and was strategically adopted by the Chinese government as a means of *waixuan* (外宣, often translated as international publicity). As the COVID-19 pandemic originated in China, it has brought anti-Chinese and anti-Asian racism to the fore (Zhang 2020). The pandemic has become not only a health crisis but also produced a global political crisis. In response to this situation, government-sponsored institutions, headed by 中国国际出版集团 (China International Publishing Group), launched different translation projects to disseminate Chinese stories, notably the bilingual book series "China's Battle Against the Coronavirus". The aim was to address prejudices and promote mutual understanding between China and other countries.

As can be seen from the above discussion, the significance of translation in the context of pandemic communication should not be overlooked. The potential of translation to contribute to positive outcomes in crisis situations has been acknowledged by researchers in crisis translation studies (Federici 2016; O'Brien and Cadwell 2017; Federici and Cadwell 2018; Federici et al. 2019b). Recognizing that language is a vital part of the COVID response, linguistic scholars have been calling for studies on linguistic diversity and language planning in this time of crisis (Shen and Kan 2020; Piller et al. 2020). Nevertheless, such linguistic studies have only mentioned in passing the role of translation in addressing the language challenges of the COVID-19 pandemic. Against this backdrop, this chapter focuses on the two major functions of translation in China's response to COVID-19: communicating public health information and sharing Chinese stories to the international community. This descriptive study aims to provide an overview of how multiple agents have engaged in this large-scale translation endeavor. Below I mainly analyze three levels of crisis communication through translation: starting from grassroots-level volunteer translation, to institution-level translation and finally to the top state-level translation. Ultimately, I attempt to integrate these disparate efforts and conclude with suggestions on how to enhance translation planning for health emergencies.

2 Grassroots-Level Translation: Volunteer Translation for Broader Information Communication

Although there are abundant official materials circulating on official channels globally, these materials may not be made available broadly and they may also not suit the specific needs of different users. For example, the official multilingual public services could not provide timely assistance to hospitals and communities when they had to communicate important information about disease control and prevention measures to foreign residents and visitors. The insufficiency of professional translation services, especially translation into languages other than English, has resulted in an outpouring of grassroots volunteer translation worldwide from large numbers of highly diverse community groups. A large amount of multilingual information such as posters recommending handwashing, instructional videos for face covering, and interpretation services hotlines was translated and produced by volunteer translators. Volunteer translation was carried out both online and offline and in various forms such as sign language interpreting and community translation. According to McCulloch (2020), "grassroots efforts have, in a few months, created resources in almost twice as many languages as Wikipedia has in 19 years, in almost five times as many languages as Google Translate has in 14". Therefore, the scope and intensity of volunteer translation should by no means be underestimated.

In the Chinese context, barely any attention had been paid to volunteer translation in crisis communication until the outbreak of COVID-19. Internationally, a well-known non-profit organization called Translators without Borders (TWB) has been providing language assistance in disaster settings. It was originally founded in 1993 in Paris to deliver translations free of charge to humanitarian organizations. In response to COVID-19, TWB, in collaboration with academic and industry partners and the

World Health Organization, made key content related to COVID-19 available in many languages. The stated aim has been to provide machine-readable translation data related to the COVID-19 pandemic. TWB has been "working towards filling some of the linguistic gaps in the services provided by more traditional humanitarian organizations active in danger zones. Through its work, the organization has made significant efforts to raise awareness of the importance of languages in crisis contexts" (Tesseur 2019, p. 285). The stated objectives of TWB can serve as a timely reminder to policymakers in China: states need not work alone to produce language policy. Top-down language planning should be complemented by timely and flexible volunteer work from the bottom up. This critical point was noted by Qi Shen, a well-known academic from Tongji University, who acknowledged the efforts made by volunteer translators, especially 帮帮湖北义务翻译群 ("Help Hubei" Volunteer Translation Group) when devising his framework of language governance planning for a PHEIC (Public Health Emergency of International Concern).

The inaccessibility of emergency language services in the initial two months of the COVID-19 outbreak in Hubei Province posed a severe challenge for language professionals. Among the multiple efforts to handle the language emergency and develop multilingual public communication services, the "Help Hubei" Volunteer Translation Group (hereafter "Help Hubei") merits particular attention. This translation group even featured in a report by China Network Television (CNTV), a national web-based TV broadcaster, and received considerable media attention. I contacted a volunteer in this group and obtained some inside knowledge of their operation.[1] The interviewed volunteer was an MTI (Master of Translation and Interpreting) student from Central South University in China and he was recommended by his teacher to join this translation group. According to him, this group was comprised of two sub-groups: the European and American language group and the Asian language group. There were 280 members (Chinese, overseas Chinese and foreigners) in total, including translators, purchasers, suppliers and distributors (most of them were students majoring in foreign languages). The volunteer translators worked via WeChat and served as mediators for the provision of medical supplies, mainly translating documents such as customs declaration and certification. Team leaders organized the translators and distributed translation tasks which were usually texts in the format of Word and PowerPoint. The first and foremost difficulty was the urgency of the task. The group upheld accuracy and promptness as overriding principles and would use machine translation coupled with post-editing. Translators would discuss key words and technical terms which require professional knowledge to ensure accuracy. There were no reviewers for the translation and the team leaders collected the translations and acted as supervisors. In this situation, translation quality may be undermined owing to the need for promptness. How to balance the urgency of the task and the quality of volunteer translation is an important issue to address in crisis translation.

[1] On May 1, 2020, I talked with the volunteer translator Cai Zhiqiang via Wechat about the operation of the translation group "Help Hubei". All the following references about the translation process are from our personal communication.

As the composition of members of the "Help Hubei" group shows, foreign language students were a major force in multilingual crisis translation and could be mobilized and assembled in prompt response to the needs of multilingual communication in the time of crisis. A prime example is the students and teachers at Tianjin Foreign Studies University who completed a video collection of health tips in 28 languages. Yongyan Zheng (2020) studied the multilingual translation efforts of a group of 67 volunteer translators from Fudan university during the COVID-19 outbreak in Shanghai. These volunteers translated and compiled a *Community Visiting Questionnaire* to communicate quarantine measures to local community workers. They also translated and compiled *Frequently Asked Questions in the Inquiry of COVID-19 Suspected Cases* for the local hospitals' Fever Clinic and *The Notification for Foreign Visitors*. These works were undertaken in 10 languages and proved to be very useful. Similar to the information provided by the student translator from "Help Hubei", Zheng identified "time constraints, limited language proficiency, and limited technical knowledge" as the major challenges confronting the university volunteers (ibid., p. 587). In contrast to other forms of translation, translation in crisis contexts requires a high level of national emergency language competence—the competence of a state to use language to cope with domestic and international public emergencies (Li et al. 2020). To form a more effective mechanism to mobilize foreign language students as multilingual resources for emergency language service, the universities need to pay more attention to medical translation training and translation technology development. They can also consider establishing a national emergency language service training center.

Another active volunteer translation team is the "全球看武汉 Global View of Wuhan" founded by an editor of 澎湃 *The Paper*, a Chinese digital newspaper run by the Shanghai United Media Group. This team translated and edited a widely circulated multilingual document entitled 致外国友人的生活防疫指南 (Pandemic Prevention Tips for Foreign Friends) into eight languages. Its members included students, professors, overseas Chinese and foreign residents in China. Starting on January 23, 2020 when COVID-19 broke out in Wuhan, this team was translating and editing useful information from foreign languages into Chinese, such as "A World at Risk: Annual Report on Global Preparedness for Health Emergencies". Their translation was edited and published on *The Paper* to ensure wider circulation. Besides translating public health information, the team also showed particular concern for the mental health of their readers and translated several articles addressing this concern. After around one month's translation from other languages into Chinese, the team shifted their focus to translating Chinese into other languages as COVID-19 cases started rising in other countries. Such a shift of focus demonstrated that volunteer translation in China can reach beyond national boundaries and be of assistance to a wider international audience.

In addition to the self-organized volunteer translation teams, local government also recruited volunteer translators to complement its professional translation team. Peng Wang, a crisis manager at the Office of Foreign Affairs in the Municipal Government of Wuhan, provided first-hand experience in coordinating the efforts of professional and volunteer translators in the Crisis Translation Team established at the Office of Foreigner Affairs on 8 January, Wuhan. As the crisis translation went beyond the capacity of professional translators at the office, Wang recruited two groups of volunteer translators "within 2–3 days through the alumni network of local universities and recommendations from local language service providers" (Wang 2020, p. 91). Not all volunteer translators were untrained or inexperienced: some of them were in the final year of their MTI study from local universities, while others were professional translators who already had experience working in the language industry (they were also called volunteer translators in Wang's study). Unlike the translation volunteers discussed above, volunteers working for the government were "provided with health insurance and paid with the same remuneration as civil servants working for the local government" (ibid., p. 92). They also had 120 minutes of online training offered by the crisis manager. Their priority was to translate containment measures and make basic protective and control measures accessible to affected foreign nationals in the response phase from 8 January to 7 April, 2020. The operation of the government-sponsored volunteer translation and the self-organized volunteer translation were similar in the sense that they both relied on translation technology and post-editing and their translated products were disseminated free of charge via multiple platforms such as TV, social media and official websites.

3 Institution-Level Translation: The Case of 战疫语言服务团 (Language Service Group Against COVID-19)

In addition to the multiple grassroots efforts, more professional translation was organized at the institutional level. This section focuses on the multilingual and multimedia translation of the state-sponsored institution Language Service Group Against COVID-19. After the outbreak of COVID-19 in early 2020, multiple agents, including but not limited to government-sponsored institutions, universities, translation companies and volunteer translators, have been dedicated to providing emergency language services to multilingual communities. When COVID-19 broke out in Hubei Province, China mobilized a range of national resources to assist this initial epicenter. However, although Mandarin has been promoted as the national language of China, dialects in different provinces remain communication barriers that impeded the progress of the transprovincial rescue missions. To overcome these barriers, China's Ministry of Education and the State Language Commission assembled more than 40 experts from universities and enterprises to form the Language Service Group Against COVID-19. This Group developed a series of language service materials, such as *The Handbook of Hubei Dialects for Medical Assistance Teams*, *Plain Chinese for Epidemic Prevention and Control*, and *A Guide to the Prevention and Control of the COVID-19 Epidemic in Foreign Languages*. According to Yuming Li et al. (2020, p. 618), "these linguists made a positive contribution to facilitating doctor-patient clinical communication in Hubei dialects as well as international medical services in multiple languages". The establishment of the Group is an eloquent example which epitomizes the state's endeavor to accumulate resources for emergency language competence. This Group is the first large-scale organization of its kind and has contributed significantly to the development of emergency language services.

The language service materials developed by this Group were made as broadly available as possible by national ministries and commissions and were widely acclaimed (Li 2020). It is worth mentioning that these materials are all presented in multimodal forms. *The Handbook of Hubei Dialects for Medical Assistance Teams* is presented in videos and can be accessed via WeChat, website and translation software. *A Guide to the Prevention and Control of the COVID-19 Epidemic in Foreign Languages* (hereafter "*A Guide*") is translated into 41 languages and is presented in the form of pamphlets, website and videos. The making of these products required translators to think beyond verbal forms of linguistic transference and consider the meaning-making mechanism of multimodality, especially in terms of colors and images. Weinian Zhang et al. (2020) analyzed different forms of *A Guide* based on visual grammar and suggested enriching the content of the multilingual videos by adding some animation so as to increase the efficiency of communication. Zhang's suggestion again highlights the necessity for translators to develop skills required in media communication.

Reflections upon the operation of this Language Service Group were mainly made from the perspective of linguistics, for example, multilingualism, rather than translation studies. Translation constitutes only a small component of the framework of language planning in China (Shen and Kang 2020). Nevertheless, as discussed above, translation is the key to ensuring high-quality multilingual crisis communication: many aspects of emergency language services are related to translation. Both professional and volunteer translators are valuable resources to be mobilized short-term in emergency situations. Translation scholars can draw insights from linguists' studies of language policies and planning for PHEIC. They can study how multi-agent, multilingual and multimedia translation during the pandemic can inform translation studies in the areas such as translation planning, translator training, translation software, translated terminology and translation memories, among others.

4 State-Level Translation: An Emphatic Chinese Perspective

The grassroots-level and institution-level translation serves primarily for the communication of information. Another special function that translation has performed during the pandemic is the provision of *waixuan* (often translated as international publicity). Since its founding in 1949, the young People's Republic of China has fully recognized the importance of translation and considered it to be a significant resource for international publicity. In October, 1949, 国际新闻局 (International News Bureau), the predecessor of 中国外文局 (China Foreign Languages

Publishing Administration), also called 中国国际出版集团 (China International Publishing Group, CIPG), was established to publicize New China globally. CIPG has become the largest foreign-language publishing organization in China and has been dedicated to translation and international publicity up until the present day.

As mentioned earlier, this pandemic has brought about not only a health crisis but also a political crisis. Accusations abound in the international arena that China mishandled aspects of the initial outbreak. The President of the USA, Donald Trump, even sought to make political capital out of the crisis by labelling COVID-19 "the Chinese virus". *The Coronavirus Prevention Handbook*, written by Dr. Wang Zhou and his colleagues at the Wuhan Center for Disease Control and translated into English by university teachers, was criticized by many readers as Chinese Communist Party propaganda (Amazon customer reviews 2020). Advertised as a must-have guide for preparing for an outbreak of the coronavirus, the publication prompted polarized reviews on the Amazon website, with some readers acknowledging the usefulness of its contents while others voiced skepticism about its provenance and legitimacy. Against this backdrop, CIPG has undertaken different translation projects in an attempt to make Chinese voices heard globally. Shen and Kang (2020) claimed that translation planning under COVID-19 should not only emphasize "inward translation", translating and introducing useful information and advanced technology from abroad, but also should make efforts to promote "outward translation" to share "Chinese stories", "Chinese plans" and "Chinese wisdom". The multilingual magazines affiliated to CIPG such as *Beijing Review, China Pictorial, China Report and China Today* all featured stories about the Chinese people's fight against COVID-19, using slogans such as "An All-Out War", "Contagious Courage", "China Faces up to COVID-19" and "Uniting Against a Common Enemy". CIPG has not only published bilingual books and magazines related to China's fight against COVID-19, but also released videos about China under COVID-19. For example, China Matters and Angshi Culture Communication (Guangzhou) released the first documentary film on the fight against COVID-19 in the Chinese megacity Guangzhou, which was said to have 8.5 million views abroad.

In the following section, I will provide examples of translating pandemic-related terms into English and emphasize the semantic subtlety required in translating for international publicity. More importantly, I will analyze the introduction of the bilingual electronic document entitled *Key Words to Understand China: The Fight Against COVID-19* and the bilingual book series "China's Battle Against the Coronavirus", both launched by CIPG. I will also analyze the introduction of *Fighting COVID-19: China in Action* released by the State Council Information Office of the People's Republic of China. Through both textual and paratextual analysis, I hope to highlight the importance of adopting a Chinese perspective in translating for international publicity.

4.1 Political Implications in Translating COVID-Related Terms

外宣翻译 (international publicity translation) has been a frequently discussed topic in translation studies in China. It is distinguished from other types of translation in that international publicity translation requires a high level of political sensitivity, or more specifically, a Chinese standpoint. The following three examples demonstrate that the translation of COVID-related terms is not just about linguistic transference and information communication as it places a heavy emphasis on political implications.

Example 1 我们举全国之力予以支援, 组织29 个省区市和新疆生产建设兵团、军队等调派330多支医疗队, 41600多名医护人员驰援。
Version 1 We organized the dispatch of more than 330 medical teams comprising over 41,600 members from all geographical areas.
Version 2 We organized the dispatch of more than 330 medical teams comprising over 41,600 members from 29 provinces, autonomous regions, centrally-administered municipalities, Xinjiang Production and Construction Corp and the military. (Huang 2020).

According to Youyi Huang (2020), former vice president of CIPG, the foreign expert suggested generalizing the translation of "29 个省区市和新疆生产建设兵团、军队" (literally, 29 provinces, autonomous regions, centrally-administered municipalities, Xinjiang Production and Construction Corp and the military) into "all geographical areas". However, Tibet is not one of these areas and if the original text is generalized into "all geographical areas", it implies that Tibet is not a part of China. Consequently, this phrase should be translated literally even at the expense of fluency.

Example 2 方舱医院.
Version 1 Cabin hospitals.
Version 2 Temporary hospitals.
Version 3 Fangcang shelter hospitals (Huang 2020).

This commonly seen term in the pandemic is translated into "modular hospitals", "cabin hospitals", "mobile hospitals", "compartment hospitals", "makeshift hospitals" or "capsule hospitals". According to Huang (2020), such a literal translation may imply that China's 方舱医院 is not well equipped. To avoid such a negative implication, it can be translated into "temporary hospitals or temporary treatment centers". Even so, the translation does not convey the Chinese characteristics. This is why some Chinese scholars translated it into "Fangcang shelter hospital" in which the Chinese characteristics were maintained through the transliteration Fangcang.

Example 3 要严格落实对所有入境人员都实施 14 天集中隔离的要求.
Version 1 Inbound passengers will be placed under centralized observation at centralized/concentration places.
Version 2 Inbound passengers will be placed under medical observation in designated facilities (Chen 2020).

Mingming Chen (2020), a diplomat and renowned expert in translation, argued that in Version 1, the word "centralized" or "concentration" could be associated with "concentration camp" and therefore was not a good choice. "Placed under medical observation in designated facilities" in Version 2, though not a literal translation of the original, is more appropriate in this context. Through these three examples, we can see that literal translation and semantic equivalence sometimes cannot serve the political needs of international publicity translation.

4.2 Publishing Translations to Communicate Chinese Experience

CIPG has been playing a critical role in responding to negative international comments on China and has been dedicated to making Chinese voices heard globally through translation. Besides trans-editing multilingual news through convergence media, CIPG also launched a series of bilingual books on China's battle against the coronavirus, including *Stories of Courage and Determination: Wuhan in Coronavirus Lockdown* (武汉封城: 坚守与逆行) and *China's Battle Against the Coronavirus: A Daily Log* (2020: 中国战"疫"日志). Another important translation project undertaken by CIPG is the release of the multilingual electronic document entitled *Key Words to Understand China: The Fight Against COVID-19*, co-presented with Academy of Contemporary China and World Studies and the China Academy of Translation. *Keywords to Understand China* is a selection of the "China Keywords" entries included in a national-level multilingual platform. This book series is labelled as required reading for all novice and avid China-watchers who are interested in its progress since liberation in 1949. Another significant translation project is *Fighting COVID-19: China in Action* (《抗击新冠肺炎疫情的中国行动》白皮书) released by the State Council Information Office of the People's Republic of China. These translations, on the one hand, are very representative of the Chinese experience in fighting COVID-19 and on the other hand, signify China's strong desire to make itself heard globally.

A look at the introduction reveals that these translations are framed explicitly for international publicity. The introduction of both *Key Words to Understand China* and *Fighting COVID-19* emphasizes the notion of "a global community of shared future", claiming that China has acted as a responsible member in the community and contributed significantly to global public health security (The State Council Information Office 2020). It also highlights that "China has great empathy with victims all over the world, and has done all it can to provide humanitarian aid in support of the international community's endeavors to stem the pandemic" (ibid.). While stating an emphatic Chinese standpoint, these books are people-focused, which document the Chinese people's united efforts in combating the virus. There is no hard evidence about whether or not these free e-books can influence target readers' perception of China, but at least they represent the Chinese government's firm intention to make Chinese voices heard in the global community.

5 Conclusion

COVID-19 posed unexpected and formidable challenges to emergency language services. According to Wang, "a cursory look of *Guidelines for Responding to Natural Disasters, Environmental Hazards and Health Emergencies of China* reveals that translation or related concepts (language barriers and language mediation) are not mentioned at all in national-level approaches to crisis response" (2020, p. 89). Many linguists have now realized the necessity of promoting language diversity and multilingualism in order to respond to the language needs of culturally and linguistically diverse communities in crisis contexts. Nevertheless, crisis translation, understood as "a broad concept that includes written translation, oral interpretation and sign language interpreting in all phases of a crisis" (ibid., p. 88), remains an underdeveloped tool and under-researched topic in crisis management, particularly in China. Although the spontaneous grassroots volunteer translation and the state funded institution-level translation responded to the crisis in an effective and forceful manner, more work needs to be done to better understand, plan and carry out crisis translation.

Without delving into more details, this chapter intends only to draw a large picture of different translation activities being undertaken in China to fight the COVID-19 pandemic. The three bottom-up levels of communication can be better coordinated to build trust among foreigners in the time of a crisis. Broadly speaking, translation planning in emergency language services needs to consider who can be mobilized as a major actor in crisis translation and provide relevant training for them accordingly to avoid inconsistency and chaos. The planning should also include management and communication strategies to coordinate the efforts of different actors and translation-related resources. More importantly, it should not focus solely on the response phase, but also on the preparedness and recovery phases of a crisis. More specific suggestions include: volunteer translation teams can learn from TWB and make their service more sustainable; universities, language institutions and language service companies need to enhance medical translator training, translation technology development and translation terminology management. Institutions can also establish language service and translation centers to train qualified translators for health emergency translation, both full-time and part-time. Besides, translator training should not be largely limited to English, the so called "big language" (大语种) and more attention should be paid to other foreign languages. Although Beijing International Studies University has established the China Academy for Public Policy Translation, crisis translation, considered to be a special branch of public service translation, is still not well-recognized in China. To conclude, translation planning for health emergency needs both a macro framework and some concrete and sustainable policies that support the development of health emergency translation.

References

Amazon customer reviews. (2020) Available at: https://www.amazon.com/Coronavirus-Prevention-Handbook-Science-Based-Could-ebook/dp/B085DKMXGY (Accessed 10 July 2020).

Chen, M. (2020) 如何进行抗疫情涉外翻译 [How to Translate for Foreign Affairs During COVID-19: The Case of Beijing]. June 7, SPIRIT, Online lecture.

Federici, F. M. (2016) *Mediating Emergencies and Conflicts: Frontline Translation and Interpreting*. Basingstoke: Palgrave Macmillan.

Federici, F. M. and Cadwell P. (2018) "Training citizen translators: design and delivery of bespoke training on the fundamentals of translation for New Zealand Red Cross." *Translation Spaces*, 7: 20–43.

Federici, F. M. et al. (2019a) *The International Humanitarian Sector and Language Translation in Crisis Situations: Assessment of Current Practices and Future Needs*. London; Dublin; Phoenix, AZ: INTERACT The International Network on Crisis Translation.

Federici, F. M. et al. (2019b) "Crisis translation training challenges arising from new contexts of translation." *Cultus*, 12: 246–279.

Fischer, H.W. (2008) *Response to Disaster: Fact Versus Fiction and Its Perpetuation*. 3rd edn. Lanham: University Press of America.

Huang, Y. (2020) 通过实例看公共政策翻译的意义和难度 [Learning the Significance and Challenges of Public Service Translation Through Examples]. June 6, Beijing International Studies University, Online lecture.

Li, S. (2020) "战疫语言服务团"用语言利器助力抗疫 [Language Service Group Against COVID-19 Uses Language to Fight COVID-19]. 世界汉语教学 [Chinese Teaching in the World] 2: 231.

Li, Y. et al. (2020) "Conceptualizing national emergency language competence." *Multilingua*, 39 (5): 617–623.

McCulloch, G. (2020) COVID-19 Is History's Biggest Translation Challenge [Online]. Available at: https://www.wired.com/story/covid-language-translation-problem/ (Accessed 27 July 2020).

O'Brien, S and Patrick C. (2017) "Translation facilitates comprehension of health-related crisis information: Kenya as an example." *Journal of Specialised Translation*, 28: 23–51.

Piller I., Zhang J. and Li J. (2020) "Linguistic diversity in a time of crisis: language challenges of the COVID-19 pandemic." *Multilingua*, 39 (5): 503–515.

Seeger, M. W. (2006) "Best practices in crisis communication: an expert panel process." *Journal of Applied Communication Research*, 34: 232–244.

Shanghai Statistics Bureau. (2020) Shanghai Statistics Year Book [Online]. Available at: http://tjj.sh.gov.cn/tjnj/nj19.htm?d1=2019tjnje/E0211.htm. (Accessed 21 August 2020).

Shen, Q and Kang M. (2020) 面向重大突发公共卫生事件的语言治理能力规划 [Towards a Framework of Language Governance Planning Against Public Health Emergency of International Concern]. 新疆师范大学学报(哲学社会科学版) [*Journal of Xinjiang Normal University (Edition of Philosophy and Social Sciences)*] 5: 64–74.

Tesseur W. (2019) "Communication is aid—but only if delivered in the right language: an interview with Translators without Borders on its work in danger zones." *Journal of War and Culture Studies*, 12: 285–294.

The Hubei Government. (2018) 1.9万外国人在湖北常住 81%在武汉 汽车行业从业者最多 [19,000 Foreign Residents Live in Hubei Province (81% in Wuhan) and Most of Them Work in the Automobile Industry] [Online]. Available at: https://www.hubei.gov.cn/zwgk/bmdt/201801/t20180108_1241099.shtml (Accessed 20 August 2020).

The State Council Information Office of the People's Republic of China. (2020) Fighting COVID-19: China in Action [Online]. Available at: http://www.scio.gov.cn/zfbps/32832/Document/1681809/1681809.htm. (Accessed 21 August 2020).

The Editorial Board. (2020a) *Stories of Courage and Determination: Wuhan in Coronavirus Lockdown*. Beijing: Foreign Languages Press.

The Editorial Board. (2020b) *China's Battle Against the Coronavirus: A Daily Log*. Beijing: Foreign Languages Press.

Wang, P. (2020) "Translation in the COVID-19 health emergency in Wuhan: a crisis manager's perspective." *The Journal of Internationalization and Localization*, 6(2): 86–107.

Wine, T. (2019) "Communication is aid—but only if delivered in the right language: an interview with translators without borders on its work in danger zones." *Journal of War & Culture Studies*, 12(3): 285–294.

Xiang, Y. et al. (2020) Timely research papers about COVID-19 in China. *The Lancet*, 395(10225): 684–685.

Zhang, J. (2020) Racism Hinders the Fight Against COVID-19 [Online]. Available at: https://www.languageonthemove.com/racism-hinders-the-fight-against-covid-19/ (Accessed 15 August 2020).

Zhang W. et al. (2020) 多模态视角: "疫情防控外语通"分析 [A Multimodal Analysis of *A Guide to the Prevention and Control of the COVID-19 Epidemic in Foreign Languages*]. June 5, 语言资源高精尖创新中心 (Beijing Advanced Innovation Center for Language Resources), Online discussion.

Zheng, Y. (2020) "Mobilizing foreign language students for multilingual crisis translation in Shanghai." *Multilingua*, 39(5): 587–595.

Imagining Online Exhibition in the Pandemic: A Translational Perspective

Ge Song

Abstract The lockdowns brought about by the COVID-19 pandemic have rendered many people unable or reluctant to go to museums, so online exhibitions with texts in more than one language and with visitor-friendly arrangement are in high demand. Translation functions in online exhibitions to convey one heritage to an audience that belongs to culturally and linguistically different communities. In order to create a satisfactory online visiting experience, the design of webpages, the aesthetics conveyed, the ways artefacts are presented, and the audiovisual devices installed, are obviously more important than ever before. Using the concept of multimodal translation as the theoretical underpinning, this study examines four offline museums in Singapore, London, Hong Kong and Vienna, with the aim of providing insights into how the COVID-19 pandemic can potentially inspire effective visiting experiences online. It reveals how elements of translation are embedded yet largely hidden in offline museum spaces, which are closely related to online ones. Connections are made between physical and online exhibitions, and the relevance and inspiration of the former to the latter is what this chapter attempts to demonstrate, thus this research is more deductive and analytical than empirical. From the perspective of multimodal translation, there is an integration of textual, visual, audio and digital information, as applied to online exhibitions. This perspective affords cross-cultural understanding of how to create a satisfactory online visiting experience.

Keywords COVID-19 · Online museum · Museum translation · Multimodal translation · Cross-cultural communication

1 Introduction

The lockdowns of cities, regions and countries on a worldwide scale during the COVID-19 pandemic starting in early 2020 have caused a geographical separation, the scale of which is unprecedented in the past several decades. Many scholars and

G. Song (✉)
BNU-HKBU United International College, Zhuhai, China
e-mail: gesong@uic.edu.cn

S.X.B. Zhao et al. (eds.), *COVID-19 Pandemic, Crisis Responses and the Changing World*, https://doi.org/10.1007/978-981-16-2430-8_15

critics view this incident as spelling the death of the decades-long process of globalization and heralding a new era marked by largely self-sustainable economies and societies. However, the advancement of digital technologies and the empowerment of the internet over the past decades have made this world tightly connected. People of different ethnicities and cultural origins have become accustomed to developing a mentality that fits in well with this globalized and globalizing world.

Undeniably, the internet has become a necessity in most parts of the world for business, learning, communication, information obtaining and sharing, etc. The centrality of the internet to contemporary life has not been challenged by the pandemic—rather it has been boosted and empowered by it. Despite varying degrees of lockdowns, we currently have no reason to doubt the momentum of (cultural) globalization, which is expected to continue to advance at least in aspects of people's cultural attitudes and ways of thinking via virtual reality and the internet. In many parts of the world during the pandemic, people have been brought even closer together than ever before, as many learning experiences and academic conferences have been realized through online platforms. However, in the past, only a selected group of people had the opportunity to join these activities, due to factors such as long-distance travel, visa application, financial situation, and schedule clash. Admittedly, online participation is different from and in some way incomparable with the offline, physical one, but we cannot deny the fact that easy access to and massive participation in virtual interactions and engagements have become the new norm.

The year 2020 showed that our world, at least for the broad realm created by the internet, is still a globalized one despite the severe impact of COVID-19, and translation is invariably required for global online communication. For example, as many museums are forced to close, their exhibits and artefacts may need to be presented through alternative outlets. One immediate possibility is exhibition via an online platform. However, online exhibitions are generally far from satisfactory at this moment. For example, many official museum websites are only intended to give a general introduction to some, not all, of their artefacts. In addition, insufficient interaction between the artefacts and online visitors makes this alternative less attractive, as people find it difficult to immerse themselves in a given cultural environment. Normally, people can only see one picture of one artefact from one fixed angle, and, despite its technical availability, virtual reality is still not widely used by individuals. Worse still, many online exhibitions are not foreigner-friendly. For instance, many fewer artefacts can be found if the user switches the language from the default (normally the language that is local to where the museum is located) to his or her most familiar or preferred ones. Furthermore, some functions are likely to be found lacking when the user chooses a non-default language. In response to these problems, curatorial teams can either upgrade the existing websites or create new and better ones. However, one can see from various sources during the pandemic that many museums have made all or part of their collections available online, and people of various cultural backgrounds can easily "go" and visit.

Given that no physical border-crossing is required on the internet, online visitors tend to be collectively more culturally hybridized and linguistically diversified than those in physical museums. Translation is not only called for to explain the exhibits, but is applied to the design of webpages (i.e. localization), because people of different backgrounds with different mentalities and cultural traditions are prone to interpret artefacts quite differently. While we acknowledge that any "fusion of horizons" (Gadamer 1997, p. 302) that emerges through intercultural engagement can bring newness to the world, we cannot ignore the possibility that it may cause failed cross-cultural communications. A failure to localize the webpages of online exhibitions risks undermining visitors' ability to understand and appreciate the exhibits. Thus, nonverbal or visual means of representation are expected to work with textual explanations (in multiple languages and/or in translation) to create a satisfactory experience for online visitors.

This chapter addresses different layers of translation in online exhibitions that have been presented against the backdrop of COVID-19. It examines four physical museums, namely the National Gallery Singapore, the British Museum, the Hong Kong Heritage Museum and Time Travel Vienna, with a view to seeking inspirations for better online exhibitions in a (post-)COVID-19 world. The four museums taken as case studies are still predominantly physical spaces and they have not as yet responded to the pandemic by offering their exhibitions online. However, they do all have the potential to promote online globalization in response to physical de-globalization, and, in doing so, even make a virtue of necessity by addressing some of the critiques of their current practices. The discussion below suggests how multimodal translation and digital technology might be used to enhance and de-center a range of exhibition types, from traditional to avant-garde. The chapter ends with a reflection on the potential impact and legacy of COVID-19 on online exhibitions, and the centrality of translation to the design of engaging and non-ethnocentric exhibition practices.

2 Multimodal Translation: A Practice Enhanced by COVID-19

This section aims to justify multimodal translation as the theoretical departure of this study. It is discussed in relation to COVID-19 in the broad context of "home office" and "home travel", which have been gaining prominence during the pandemic, as people are largely restricted from traveling physically.

Since the late 1990s, cultural studies began to expand and the cultural turn has lent translation studies many opportunities to transcend the dichotomy of source text and target text to address the conveyance of local significance, which is not text-restricted. Currently, linguistic transfer or equivalence is only one of the many aspects of translation studies. Multimodality, which may be defined as the "simultaneous engagement of multifarious modes, such as written language and image, within a given context" (Gibbons 2012, p. 8), potentially addresses how written words interact with nonverbal modes of cross-cultural communication. In a similar vein, multimodal translation explains "how translation plays a role in the interplay of different semiotic planes of representation" (Chiaro 2008, p. 141). As translation involves plenty of sociocultural, geopolitical and nonverbal circumstances, the concept of multimodal translation becomes capable of describing and explaining multilingual and multicultural issues in a "third space" (Bhabha 1994) where things are culturally hybridized. As online exhibitions potentially target visitors of different cultures, textual and visual means of translation (i.e. to translate the introductory panels and captions beside exhibits into several languages, and to translate one set of semiotic codes into another) are intertwining to evoke cultural associations and create meanings.

In a nutshell, the focus of multimodal translation on the interactive mechanism of textual, visual and digital presentations, and on "sociological, functional, and medial aspects of the multimodal approach" (Kaindl 2020, p. 52), makes it a pertinent concept guiding the discussion of this chapter.

3 Staging Exhibits Online: Inspirations from Four Offline Museums

This section takes four exhibitions as case studies to show how meaning is created by the combination of verbal and nonverbal means of presentation. Each case emphasizes one particular aspect that leads to specific ideas about online exhibitions in relation to COVID-19. The four cases are ordered from the most traditional to the most avant-garde.

3.1 The British Museum

The British Museum is dedicated to the history, art and culture of the world. Its permanent collection was largely assembled during the era of the British Empire, and it documents the story of human culture from its beginnings to the present. Partly due to the fact that it is the first public national museum in the world, the mode of presentation is the most traditional among the four exhibitions under scrutiny, as it features paintings (hanging on walls) with introductory captions, using the fewest state-of-the-art technologies to "activate" and "contextualize" the exhibits. That is to say, multimodality does not feature prominently in this museum. Nonetheless, translation is manifested by the following two aspects that can inspire us as to how the translational aspects of the British Museum can be viewed critically as contributing to a model of how to deliver future online exhibitions.

Firstly, throughout the panels and captions in the physical space of the British Museum, English prevails. English is the one and the only language visible, telling stories of the world—thus it translates all the cultural realities and embodiments of non-Anglophone societies into English, presenting a form of "cultural translation" that is largely internalized and inconspicuous, not strictly based on the "ST-TT" formula (see Song 2020b, p. 778). The word "translation" is used metaphorically here to mean the state of interculturality—to "carry or bear across cultures" (Trivedi 2007, pp. 4–5). Despite the existence in the physical museum of a self-service audio guide that enables the choosing of languages, textual information in English is still dominant due to its visibility and prominence. This exercise of exhibiting multicultural arts largely monolingually "shows (alarmingly) how easily several different languages and cultures could be translated into English", partially because English, as a century-long colonial language, is currently the international *lingua franca* (cf. Song 2017, p. 82). As Rushdie said, "having been borne across the world, we are translated men" (1991, p. 18). This is particularly true for the exhibits in the British Museum which come from across the world and are thus "translated". The state of being "translated" is realized in a culturally hybridized museum space. To a large extent, visitors are experiencing different layers of "translation" when they engage with the exhibits of the British Museum in person.

Secondly, since the museum is located in the core of London, the capital city of a country where most of the exhibits do not originate. Understandably, to bring together objects representing worldwide cultural heritages in a specific place is fraught with issues of translation, as it presents a situation whereby local culture is resituated in a global context. In view of Rushdie's argument, all the non-local artefacts are translated, and are thus perceived anew by a new audience and in a new place where the original cultural contexts of the artefacts are erased. As an emphatically global city, London meets the condition of what Homi Bahbha called the "third space", where the chemistries, brought about by various ways of cultural hybridization and how visitors interpret the artefacts, emerge and function.

The implications of the translational factors embedded in the British Museum for the pandemic are twofold, and, while they are drawn upon in my discussion above, they are stimulated by the lack of multimodal elements in the physical museum. On the one hand, the analysis reveals how translation functions in a context woven by the interaction of texts and exhibits, and indicates a well-established method so as to apply the embedded yet hidden translation practices to online exhibitions. For example, buttons linking to multiple-language audio guide can be created on certain webpages to give online visitors an opportunity to experience "translated" artefacts so that the visit takes less effort. On the other hand, online visitors' cross-cultural interpretation of the exhibits can boost the process of cultural hybridization and thus potentially create more meanings than that in a physical setting. Online exhibitions might potentially "decolonize" the Anglo-centrist visiting experience by bringing more voices and perspective into a dialogue. To sum up, the British Museum inspires us to respond to the pandemic by putting exhibits online: An online exhibition can open up more space for cross-cultural interaction, as it can potentially bring together a large number of visitors from all over the world.

3.2 The National Gallery Singapore

The National Gallery Singapore goes one step further, compared with the British Museum. It gives us a much more recent case of a national collection, which is, however, still fraught with struggles as to how to stage artefacts, or how traditional and innovative ways of staging artefacts can be balanced. The exhibition in question is one called "Between Declarations and Dreams", which was housed in the National Gallery Singapore in 2016, presenting twelve galleries of artworks collected from most Southeast Asian nations. Inside the galleries, there were paintings hung on the walls and large panels of written texts in English. The curatorial narrative critically examined the shared artistic impulse of Southeast Asia in one given period. The engagement of art in social change, especially anti-colonialism and nation-building, was highlighted as the underlying curatorial agenda (Song 2017).

Southeast Asia, as a geographical region and conceptual category, however, is "a contested entity shaped by diverse cultures and communities" (ibid., p. 72). Interpretations of these paintings are "language dependent" (ibid., p. 79), and thus the process of cultural representation is certainly "contingent, historical, and contestable" (Clifford and Marcus 1986, p. 13). In some cases, culture can intentionally "resist interpretation because of secrecy or forms of restricted knowledge" (Nakamura et al. 2013, p. 4), and "artists of non-Western origins in particular are often expected to represent or at least reference the cultures of their birthplace to be recognized in the global art world" (ibid., p. 7). However, the dominant language throughout the exhibition was English. The exhibits were thus only partially presented by the explanatory texts in English without their being sufficiently linked to their original cultural contexts. Similar to the British Museum, in the National Gallery Singapore, the English language was simultaneously translating and unifying a variety of cultures. However, the differences are twofold. First, though largely invisible, Southeast Asian languages are by no means nonexistent in this exhibition. A corner of each gallery was set aside for brochures in a variety of Southeast Asian languages. Visitors who are familiar with any of the languages can resort to specific brochures for further and more detailed information regarding the artefacts shown in this very gallery. The second difference is that these Southeast Asian arts are located in Singapore, arguably the most influential financial and cultural hub of Southeast Asia, and for this reason, this exhibition is essentially a localized one.

The analysis can also shed some light on, and is conducive to, the design of online exhibitions, especially as to how translation is implicitly manipulated, and how multiple narratives can be offered by a language that is most articulate in telling the stories of some particular exhibits. The cultural hybridity of the exhibits (i.e. various nations in Southeast Asia), as well as their being partially represented, calls for an in-depth exploration of the translational nature inherent in the relationship between the artworks and their English explanatory texts (Song 2017, p. 81). By extension, for online exhibitions, the curators do not necessarily need to translate every webpage into several languages. Instead, they can keep the dominant language as they see fit, provided that other languages, especially those directly associated with the exhibits on display, can be found somewhere on the webpages. It is envisaged that once clicking a button, visitors can be greeted with a webpage that may not be a faithful replica of the one in the default language, but is an independent one leading to a more focused, localized, and nuanced story about certain artefacts that are explained in their "mother tongue". In addition, visitors may be enabled to choose a virtual location of the exhibition: One location is linked to one specific webpage and one localized way of presenting artefacts. Curators need to localize one and the same webpage several times so that visitors from all over the world can virtually bring the same exhibit to different places and interpret it from cross-cultural perspectives. Furthermore, the lessons we draw from the case of the British Museum can potentially be inherited and passed on to this one, especially how multimodal means of representation, such as audiovisual devices, are used.

3.3 The Hong Kong Heritage Museum

Another case in point is the digital transplantation of Dunhuang art in the Hong Kong Heritage Museum in 2018. This exhibition, themed "Digital Dunhuang – Tales of Heaven and Earth", presents in a virtual format some Dunhuang caves that were built one thousand years ago. These caves were digitalized to offer Hong Kong visitors an overview of Dunhuang art. Located in western China, Dunhuang had guarded the "throat" of the Silk Road for centuries, and people belonging to different ethnic groups speaking different languages gathered there. It was therefore a place where diversified cultures converged and integrated. Although it has been reduced to an ordinary town nowadays, it still boasts many cultural relics. For Hong Kong visitors of today, Dunhuang art appears exotic, as its artistic forms and cultural attachments are tangential to the realities of present-day Hong Kong.

This exhibition is different from the previous two in that it is a "digital" one, which means that Dunhuang artefacts were not physically brought to Hong Kong, but were "reproduced" by digital installations. It covered eight halls in total, which were linked by a suggested visiting route. All texts in captions and panels were bilingual, namely Chinese and English—Hong Kong's two official languages. Inspired by Rushdie's metaphor mentioned earlier, this exhibition can well be treated as a part of the "translated" Dunhuang art set in a Hong Kong context. However, Hong Kong visitors, who share a multicultural ethos (see Abbas 1997) with Dunhuang art, may find the digitized Dunhuang artefacts to be less exotic than they might have expected. The Dunhuang exhibition exemplifies a situation where "imported" exhibits may well remind visitors' of their own living realities and mirror the "self" through the lens of the "other".

This exhibition informs online ones primarily in terms of how a foreign atmosphere is created, and how a chord may be struck between visitors and exhibits. In my observation, an authentic-looking foreign atmosphere is made possible by paying attention to three aspects. First, the visual decorations on walls and ceilings are symbolic of Dunhuang art. Second, the bilingual texts feature a large number of exotic terms that are not commonly seen in daily life. Third, the digital devices and animation installations present enlarged digital replicas of selected Dunhuang caves and murals. As Kress (2020, p. 42) put it, if we regard translation as "the process of making knowledge and understanding available and accessible to someone else by means of semiotic resources which that person does not yet possess (fully)", which is exactly the situation of this case, then "the process of demonstration here might well count as an instance of translation".

All these three aspects, each with its specific emphasis, work together to help visitors immerse themselves in an authentic-looking Dunhuang cultural atmosphere. Online exhibitors can draw on these three aspects by designing their webpage and sub-webpages. They can narrate the digital objects with more culture-specific items, and animate some (not all of the) objects to the effect that they can greatly impress the visitors who can examine the object in question from 360 degrees simply with the click of a mouse. It would be better if visitors can zoom in and enlarge the object and see its details as they navigate on the screen. Another value of the Dunhuang exhibition in Hong Kong Heritage Museum that is particularly relevant to online exhibitions is the extent to which the foreignness of the exhibits is domesticated so as to target a particular group of visitors. A good balance has been maintained between a "foreignized" atmosphere created via visual decorations and digital installations, and "familiar" multicultural realities demonstrated by the exhibits. For example, since Hong Kong visitors largely share a multicultural ethos with Dunhuang art, they are likely to develop a strangely familiar feeling towards Dunhuang art, hence the balance. Both the foreign and the familiar are designed to cater to the visitors' perspective. For online exhibitions, curators are advised not to localize the visiting experience too much. Otherwise the visitors would be deprived of the sense of the foreign. In the meantime, curators need to explore the psychological fabric of the particular groups of visitors they target, who may find some familiarity in the strangeness that the foreign artefacts suggest.

3.4 Time Travel Vienna

Time Travel Vienna is an exhibition in Vienna's underground, which is designed as a walking tour with a "multi-dimensional" cinema, animatronic shows, laser effects and virtual reality. The route begins in a 5-dimensional cinema that takes visitors back to the age of Roman Vienna. It moves on to the Black Death in Vienna, with plagues of rats, and the second Turkish siege of Vienna in 1683. Other themes include the two world wars and the signing of the State Treaty on 15 May 1955. It ends with an interactive horse-drawn carriage ride through Vienna. The carriage "flies" and rides over the Imperial Palace, Stadtpark, State Opera to Schönbrunn and the Prater. The total of eight stops are equipped with a state-of-the-art show enhanced by effects technology. The tour lasts around fifty minutes through the virtual world of history. It is branded as "an exciting way to discover Vienna".[1]

This exhibition is one hundred percent virtual, which means all the artefacts one can see and all the sounds one can hear are not found on "real" historical artefacts. However, the experience leaves visitors with a deep impression, as evidenced by their comments posted on the website of TripAdvisor.[2] The exhibition tour embodies an innovative means of presenting the essential parts of Vienna's history. Very little textual information is provided in the exhibition space, and visitors have to be highly dependent on their personal audio guides on which they can choose from several languages provided. With the audio guide, visitors are led to roam about the exhibition space and experience the animated settings. What they see is simultaneously linked with the audio explanations delivered in a language of their choice. Translation works on the following two levels.

First, the default language of the tour is German, but the special audio devices visitors wear provide a simultaneous interpretation of both the audio introduction and the shows and films that one can see every now and then throughout the exhibition (there are 10 languages to choose from).[3] Thus, verbal translation applies if the language chosen is not German. Second, translation is used metaphorically as a way to bridge gaps of various kinds, such as the temporal gap and the psychological distance between the historical scenes and the modern-day visitors. For those whose backgrounds are non-European, an intense cultural difference would be possibly felt. After all, all the historical events being vividly described in the exhibition were taking place in the past, and textual plus visual narratives can only offer visitors a static, detached, and archaeological record of what happened in the past. The variety of digital devices revived the history of Vienna, as if it is unfolding just in front of the visitors' eyes. In this sense, the exhibition translates the past into the present as if visitors travel back in time to bridge the temporal gap. Besides that, visitors are put in an "authentic" historical Vienna where they can virtually roam around, immersing themselves in a "foreign" atmosphere, as if they are from places where a different set of value systems, customs and mentalities prevails.

Time Travel Vienna informs the design of online exhibition in the following three ways.

First, its interactive virtual reality installations inspire online exhibitions to offer functions such as rotation of exhibits and zooming in and out, together with audio guides equipped with artificial intelligence that offers interpreting services and enables interaction with visitors.

The second lesson we can learn from this case is the authentic-looking atmosphere being created, where visitors, regardless of their ethnicities and cultural backgrounds, can enjoy "living" in and "feeling" the historical Vienna. Instead of an extensive foreign flavor that curators strive to achieve in the Hong Kong Heritage

[1] https://www.timetravel-vienna.at/en/, accessed 26 August 2020.

[2] https://www.tripadvisor.com/Attraction_Review-g190454-d3316866-Reviews-Time_Travel_Vienna-Vienna.html, accessed 26 August 2020.

[3] https://www.wien.info/en/sightseeing/sights/time-travel-vienna, accessed 26 August 2020.

Museum, Time Travel Vienna offers a visitor-friendly and visitor-oriented atmosphere where one is granted the chance to be briefly exposed to the "real" Vienna while being led by a personalized guide. By extension, this model is more suitable to those online exhibitions that are dedicated to the narration of history. Curators of this type of online exhibitions can innovate some localized webpages where visitors can appreciate the exhibits by making full use of their prior knowledge. For example, a historical event in Vienna may be presented to a Chinese visitor as something that is comparable to an event that is familiar to the general Chinese. Although this mode of presentation may lead to some distortions in cross-cultural communication, it at least attracts visitors in a "sincere" manner and gives the online exhibits more possible cross-cultural interpretations.

Thirdly, there is a real staff member who guides the tour in German throughout the routes in Time Travel Vienna, and simultaneous interpreting services are ostensibly offered via visitors' earphones. However, the fact is that the staff member is professionally trained to speak verbatim according to the pre-set script, and speaks in the fixed speed and stops at fixed intervals, exactly corresponding to the previously recorded soundtracks in different languages delivered through the earphones. For online exhibitions, we might as well create some buttons linking to an audio guide, and similarly, we might model the effect of simultaneous interpreting, as it gives visitors a kind of authentic interpreting experience, which enhances their sensory input to make them "believe" that they are positioned in a "real" historical setting, authentic and non-mediated. It is unnecessary to take pains to translate all the webpages into different languages. Instead, they can be kept in their original forms, including the language by default, the design and the possible cultural associations they evoke. When visitors click relevant buttons, interpreting services are activated. This is demand-oriented, individually-tailored, as if visitors are really "exploring" something by themselves, rather than being passively led to "learn" something that is principally based on written narratives and visual depictions.

It should be noted that although virtual reality applications have not been widely used by individuals at home at this moment, the analysis of Time Travel Vienna inspires us to place our attention to high quality audiovisual elements, and provides a possible direction for the future development of online exhibitions.

4 Reflection on the Impact of COVID-19 on Online Exhibitions

The COVID-19 pandemic urges us to establish alternative ways to present and appreciate exhibits, especially when curbing our activities has become a part of our normal life. The alternatives are expected to be able to recreate and restore, as much as possible, the visiting experiences before COVID-19 hit the world. At best, they can bring online visitors some extraordinary feelings which normally can only be obtained by visiting museums physically.

The restricted entry to museums and exhibitions because of COVID-19 is undoubtedly a severe blow to museum-enthusiasts, scholars and general visitors alike. With a worldwide closure of borders, the demand for visiting museums in a traditional way can by no means be met. In response, online exhibitions are greatly desired and much welcomed. Predictably, surfing the internet for exhibitions has become a new habit and a new way of life for many. However, during the pandemic, at least since the year 2020, it is common to hear grievances that online exhibitions can never be compared with physical ones. Indeed, there is a great amount of truth in this complaint, because people want or need to see the real artefacts on the spot and with their own eyes. However, I generally cannot agree with this view. Instead, I argue that, given useful design, online exhibitions can even be more engaging than physical ones.

In fact, one can find "reality" in "virtual reality", as multimodal translation can facilitate cross-cultural communication and understanding by giving full play to its potentials to integrate multiple means of presentation. First of all, online exhibitions can present more exhibits to visitors than physical exhibitions. Many museums, such as the British Museum and the Palace Museum of China, boast countless treasures and exhibits, which cannot all be displayed in a physical space. Most of the time, visitors can only see a tiny part of the museum collections, and the selection that they are presented with depends on chance. However, this problem is not inherent to online exhibitions, as long as curators and their team members take the effort to digitalize all the treasures and put them online. Secondly, online exhibitions are not time and space restricted. People across the globe can browse and study online exhibits wherever they are and whenever they want. It is very convenient for global visitors to access exhibits from various cultural origins, thus the threshold for cross-cultural accessibility is significantly lowered. Thirdly, virtual reality finds many applications and is likely to become a trend in today's society for people to "really" experience something that presently lies beyond the reach of their daily life. As COVID-19 will continue to haunt human beings for maybe two decades, as the World Health Organization warns, the first idea that pops up in people's mind when they want to go to a distant museum may be a recourse to online alternatives. People's mentality regarding museums has thus been changed. With a variety of modes to present foreignness (i.e. staging exhibits to visitors with different backgrounds) which are integrated into the practice of translation, online exhibitions are empowered by the wide reach of the notion of translation, and able to give rise to a plethora of cross-cultural interpretations regarding exhibits that were once known to or significant for only a small number of people.

During the time when COVID-19 is rampant, physical, digital and online exhibitions are expected to be equally important, with the latter two gradually gaining momentum and becoming the dominant forms of staging exhibits in the context of global migration of cultural heritage. In this evolving process, what we usually call "cross-cultural" communication will become an "intercultural" one (see Sun 2017, pp. 56–57; Song 2020a, pp. 895–896). The word "cross" carries the meaning of going or jumping from one place to another. When someone is positioned, physically or otherwise, in a new cultural atmosphere, his or her mind may linger on the familiar. This person thus turns out to be unable to adjust to the new environment and be culturally static. That is to say, this person is simply there, without being "translated". For example, when some Chinese tourists are in Rome, they may only notice the cultural difference but do not try to put themselves in local people's shoes. Similarly, visitors in the Dunhuang exhibition, which was positioned in a Hong Kong museum to present the authenticity of Dunhuang, may only be present in a museum space without being culturally, mentally and psychologically influenced. Their systems of culture and belief, acquired in their native cultural environment(s), remain unaffected and intact. In this situation, we can only say that they simply "crossed" the cultural borderline, without being hybridized. By contrast, if they become constantly and multiply hybridized through the experience of visiting museums that stage cultural heritages unfamiliar to them, and they invariably empathize with the foreign others every time they confront alterity, they are adulterated, hybridized, and thus "translated". Online exhibitions, as suggested by the above commentary on the four existing offline ones, potentially offer visitors a "translational" and "intercultural" experience, as they may be equipped with textual, audiovisual, and multi-dimensional means of communication that enable visitors an immersive experience. Moreover, with an interactive means of presentation, visitors are granted the opportunities to choose exhibits and listen to (simultaneously interpreted) explanations. They are offered an opportune atmosphere to develop critical thinking and plunge into otherness.

5 Conclusion

While the COVID-19 pandemic poses a threat to free movement of people, it nonetheless calls for a world that is intensely connected by, and heavily relied on, the internet. Online exhibitions constitute and exemplify the relentlessly advancing trend of globalization, albeit in a virtual way. Admittedly, it is not easy to launch satisfactory online exhibitions in the short period of time after the outbreak of COVID-19, but lessons drawn from some prestigious offline museums and exhibitions will prove beneficial to establishing better online ones. The four case studies give us a clue as to how to draw inspirations from offline museums that feature varying degrees of multimodalities and constitute multilayered representations. More importantly, multiple modalities need to be integrated into one coherent and systematic mechanism that can create adequate opportunities for various interpretations.

As people of diverse cultural backgrounds can easily access one and the same online exhibition, a particular local culture is granted the opportunity to be constantly resituated in a global online context. Multimodal translation breaks free of the perpetual conceptualization of translation as a variety of dichotomies, such as source text and target text, adequacy and acceptability, domestication and foreignization, etc., and takes into account things located between cultures that are composed by interactive multiple modalities. The practice of a cross-cultural museum visit requires various kinds of translation that mediate cultures, languages, perspectives and experiences. Clearly, translation does not only work on textual and verbal level, but also functions on audiovisual and multi-dimensional levels. On the one hand, a sense of authenticity, mainly created by a careful design of webpages, can transport distant visitors to the cultural environment where the exhibits belong. On the other hand, a sense of familiarity, motivated by a wish to cater to a specific group of visitors, can relieve visitors from possible feelings of alienation. Back in 1991, Lavine and Karp observed that "every museum exhibition, whatever its overt subject, inevitably draws on the cultural assumptions and resources of the people who make it" (1991, p. 1). Now we have more technologies of digitalization and virtual reality that can help us tell better stories about exhibits in an immersive and interactive way, and visitors from various cultures are empowered to align exhibits with particular narratives.

References

Abbas, A. (1997) *Hong Kong Culture and the Politics of Disappearance*. Hong Kong: Hong Kong University Press.

Bhabha, H. (1994) *The Location of Culture*. London and New York: Routledge.

Chiaro, D. (2008) *Between Text and Image: Updating Research in Screen Translation*. Amsterdam and Philadelphia: Benjamins.

Clifford, J. and Marcus, G. E. (1986) *Writing Culture: The Poetics and Politics of Ethnography*. Berkeley, Los Angeles and London: University of California Press.

Gadamer, H.G. (1997) *Truth and Method* (English translation revised by Joel Weinsheimer and Donald G. Marshall). New York: Crossroad.

Gibbons, A. (2012) *Multimodality, Cognition, and Experimental Literature*. London and New York: Routledge.

Kaindl, K. (2020) 'A theoretical framework for a multimodal conception of translation' in Boria, M., Carreres, Á., Noriega-Sánchez, M. and Tomalin, M. (ed.) *Translation and Multimodality: Beyond Words*. London and New York: Routledge, pp. 49–70.

Karp, I (1991). 'Culture and presentation' in Karp, Ivan and Steven D. Lavine (ed.) *Exhibiting Cultures: The Poetics and Politics of Museum Display*. Washington and London: Smithsonian Institution Press, pp. 1–11.

Kress, G. (2020) 'Transposing meaning: Translation in a multimodal semiotic landscape' in Boria, M., Carreres, Á., Noriega-Sánchez, M. and Tomalin, M. (ed.) *Translation and Multimodality: Beyond Words*. London and New York: Routledge, pp. 24–48.

Nakamura, F, Perkins, M. and Krischer, O. (2013). *Asia Through Art and Anthropology*. New York: Bloomsbury Academic.

Rushdie, S. (1991) *Imaginary Homelands: Essays and Criticism 1981–91*. London: Granta Books.

Song, G. (2017) 'Voices of art: Cultural translation in the exhibition of "Between Declarations and Dreams: Art of Southeast Asia since the 19th-Century" in National Gallery Singapore', *Translation Quarterly*, 2017(85), 71–96.

Song, G. (2020a) 'Conflicts and complexities: A study of Hong Kong's street signs from the functional perspective on translation', *Journal of Multilingual and Multicultural Development*, 41(10): 886–898.

Song, G. (2020b) 'Re-conceptualizing foreignness: Strategies and implications of translating Chinese calligraphic culture into English since the twentieth century', *Perspectives: Studies in Translation Theories and Practice*, 28(5), 777–791.

Sun, Y. (2017) 'Cosmopolitan translation and cross-cultural paradigms: A Chinese perspective', *Telos*, 180(fall 2017), 47–66.

Trivedi, H. (2007) 'Translating culture vs. cultural translation' in St-Pierre, P. and Kar, P.C. (ed.) *Translation—Reflections, Regractions, Transformations.* Amsterdam: John Benjamins Publishing Company, pp. 277–287.

The Role of American Journalism During a Pandemic: Uncertainty and Lessons not Learned

Jesse Owen Hearns-Branaman

1 Introduction

Flaws in the structure of a system are often not evident until there is a crisis. Emergencies, such as disasters or pandemics, lay bare the weaknesses of various structures that people rely on to live a normal life, be it the medical system, politics, or journalism. While holding on to the ideal version of a system, structure, or profession is tempting and seductive, the breakdown in those standards and practices caused by a breakdown in normality can also better show us their intrinsic flaws and give us an opportunity to better reflect on how to improve on the system. Indeed, it is often only through the exposure of the inherent weaknesses of systems that we can make major progress instead of simply proffering surface-level, temporary adjustments.

How journalists reported on the outbreak of COVID-19 should be viewed as one of those inflection points, allowing us to look at journalists' professional practices and failures in a new light. This is not to point out specific failings of specific news outlets or specific journalists, but weaknesses in the professional norms and epistemological standards of journalism. This essay will attempt to address these weaknesses by examining (1) how US journalist covered COVID-19, specifically the Coronavirus Taskforce press conferences, (2) epistemological issues around balancing experts and politicians as well as fact-checking, (3) the reporting of statistics, and (4) issues with the lack of sufficient medical reporters.

I will not examine right-wing or conspiracy theory media outlets, such as *Fox News*, *One America News Network*, Brietbart.com, or *Infowars*. Their coverage is problematic in much more obvious ways as they casually spread debunked conspiracy theories, have 'medical expert' guests who are not qualified doctors or epidemiologists, and, with Trump, co-construct a feedback loop of bad information. Instead,

J. O. Hearns-Branaman (✉)
Beijing Normal University-Hong Kong Baptist University United International College, Zhuhai, China
e-mail: johearnsbranaman@uic.edu.cn

S.X.B. Zhao et al. (eds.), *COVID-19 Pandemic, Crisis Responses and the Changing World*, https://doi.org/10.1007/978-981-16-2430-8_16

the focus here will be on the coverage by the more mainstream or left-leaning media outlets such as CNN, MSNBC, and *New York Times*. It is expected, to a much greater extent, for these outlets to not be influenced as much by politics in their coverage of natural disasters and medical crises, and to report in a fully professional manner. It is a critique of those professional standards in and of themselves that is needed, not a critique of when these norms breakdown.

Journalism critics need to use their foresight, not hindsight, when exposing the weaknesses of reporting on certain events. For example, we now know there were no so-called ‘weapons of mass destruction’ in Iraq, yet we cannot criticize journalists for promoting the idea that the Iraq War was caused by the threat of those weapons being used on the USA and UK. A proper critique would be to examine why journalists so easily accepted such a pretense for war without critically fact-checking information given by the government and intelligence agencies. The problem is that journalists were to beholden to those in power and relied too much on elite framing of events, which is viewed in the journalism field the correct, professional way to be a journalist. Instead, a criticism should come from the perspective of problematizing those relationships which are the backbone of journalism (Hearns-Branaman 2018).

We also need to be mindful not to criticize journalists and journalism for things that they cannot control. COVID-19, as with all novel viruses, was a complete mystery at the beginning of the outbreak. Our knowledge about the disease, such as how it is transmitted, what the symptoms are, how long the incubation period is, and other aspects of epidemiology, is constantly changing and growing. Epistemologically speaking, our knowledge is very contingent (Hearns-Branaman 2016) in that old information will be replaced by new, more correct information as we learn more, and at any given moment we must remember that our knowledge is only temporarily correct. The continuing investigations by scientists and medical experts around the world, and the lack of scientific consensus that often occurs, are out of the hands of journalists; they should not be criticized, for example, for not promoting the usage of masks when there was no consensus about the efficacy of that practice. Journalists also cannot entirely control how honest or knowledgeable their sources are, and at the beginning of a new years-long news event like this it would take journalists several weeks or even months to establish a network of trustworthy, well-informed experts to provide the specialist knowledge needed to better inform their news reports.

2 Coronavirus Taskforce Press Conference Coverage

The White House Coronavirus Taskforce was setup on January 29, 2020, first under the direction of the Department of Health and Human Services before adding additional members, including the Vice President, in the following weeks and months. Press briefings started to be given out of the White House beginning Mar 16, with the White House press corps in attendance.

One of the more infamous cases of dangerous misinformation to emerge from these press conferences occurred on April 24, 2020, when President Trump mused for several minutes about the possibility of using ultraviolet light and disinfectants to treat COVID-19. The reaction of journalists was mixed, but occasionally just as dangerous as Trump's own statements. For example, on April 24, *NBC News* (2020) ran the headline 'Trump suggests "injection" of disinfectant to beat coronavirus and "clean" the lungs,' uncritically repeating what Trump had said. If readers had not gone beyond the headline they might have thought that Trump's suggestions were proper advice from officials. The *New York Times* originally tweeted a tweet which framed Trump's comments in a 'he said-she said' style, noting that "some experts" viewed his comments as "dangerou[s]" (quoted in Ellefson 2020). Only "some experts," apparently, yet support from experts who promote the injection of disinfectants or UV light into the human body to treat viruses was sorely lacking, bringing into question such framing. They eventually deleted that tweet and issued an apology of sorts, adding "To be clear, there is no debate on the danger" (*The New York Times* 2020). It is concerning that there was an apparently automatic reaction to frame patently dangerous medical advice as a legitimate debate via the routine of false balance, which will be discussed more later.

CNN took Trump's comments in its stride, publishing an analysis by Stephen Collinson (2020) who likened his comments to an "old West traveling medicine show" and equating them with Trump's previous marketing of "stakes and real estate, board games and vodka," and casting his potentially deadly ramblings on treating COVID-19 as Trump simply being an "incorrigible salesman." This is an entirely irresponsible take as it diminishes the power that Trump's words have to endanger the lives of those who listen uncritically to them.

As *First Draft News* (2020) argues, headlines should "lead with the truth" instead of repeating someone's lies, myths, or bad advice. News outlets such as *BBC News* (2020) and *Al Jazeera English* (2020) performed better, the former's headline being "Outcry after Trump suggests injecting disinfectant as treatment," and the latter being "Experts react with horror to Trump coronavirus disinfectant idea." In this case, the story is about the reaction to Trump's musings and not Trump's words themselves. They "don't repeat myths" (ibid.) and begin with a debunking instead of hiding the debunking later in the story.

In the end, the White House briefings imploded after this specific case and did not resume until late July and only sporadically thereafter. Journalists are in a tough position in this case; it would be irresponsible to *not* attend the briefings and to *not* report on what Trump says, yet attending and reporting are also irresponsible, but in a different way which I will discuss shortly. Treating anything Trump or another political leader says as automatically newsworthy gives them too much power to set the agenda, especially when they are dispensing dangerous and deadly 'advice' about a pandemic. Yet the furthest that journalists and commentators would go was advocating not covering the press conferences live, MSNBC's Rachel Maddow (2020) doing so on Mar 21, and the *St Louis Post-Dispatch* Editorial Board (2020) doing so on Apr 2. Jay Rosen (2020) advocated for not covering it live much earlier, starting on Mar 19, advising that news outlets should, instead, attend and listen to what is said, then verify the information before publication.

I would argue covering Trump's taskforce press conferences was irresponsible because it fell into Trump's trap. He knows when he has a press conference the press will come and he also knows that journalists have lost a lot of the power to set the news agenda in the age of social media. As Weimann and Brosius (2015: 37–38) argue, news audiences "select the story itself" instead of simply relying on a specific "news source," and that "a vast range of produsers and active bloggers" can more actively push items onto the agenda, which the journalists will follow if it has enough clicks and shares on social media. The more journalists give prominence to the crazy or bizarre statements he makes in the press conferences, the less prominence they will give to how disastrous the federal government's response to the pandemic is. He knows the White House correspondents will never *not* cover his press conferences, he knows that they will never band together to boycott his speeches, and he knows that controversial statements he makes will become fodder for social media, thus elevating his presence even more.

We must also consider that one reason reporters kept coming to the daily briefings is that it makes their jobs a lot easier and gives them a lot of content to write about. Press conferences in general are already subsidies for news organizations. Trump's briefings present extra opportunities when Trump makes dangerous or misleading statements, one of the task force members disagrees with something Trump said, or if Trump directly challenges a journalist by insulting them or calling them 'fake news' or something similar. Being the target of Trump's attack automatically raises a journalist's profile, invitations to talk about their confrontation with Trump pour in from CNN and other new organizations, and they are able to write several more articles about their experience to help fulfill their daily quota or stories.

After a certain point political leaders need to be able to lose all credibility and thus not automatically warrant coverage for all their statements, even if they are Presidents and Prime Minsters. Mechanisms which have tended to enforce deplatforming leaders in such a way are often internal, such as pressure from within their party and from their supporters, yet the vast majority of Republicans and Trump's voter base continued to legitimate and even defend him. Nixon was able to be removed because he became unbearable to both his party and his supporters, and this counter-pressure against Trump was simply too weak.

Journalists have to consider that framing statements from leaders in a way that promotes safety, public health, and science is far more important than routinely amplifying whatever a powerful person says, be it dangerous or helpful, only because they are powerful. Journalists have to ask themselves, do we cover Trump because he's powerful and thus inherently newsworthy? Or is Trump powerful because we cover him no matter what he is saying, thus amplifying him and reinforcing his newsworthiness?

3 False Balance Between Politicians and Experts

Balancing sources to present a 'wide' picture or give 'both' sides to a story is a fundamental practice of journalism (Hearns-Branaman 2016). Yet as many have argued, we don't necessarily need to balance all sides, for example climate change deniers should not be balanced with climate scientists, the NAACP should not be balanced with neo-Nazis. Yet in coverage of COVID-19 many journalists fell into this trap again, often balancing statements made by Trump and other politicians with those of scientists, epidemiologists.

A prime example of this comes from the March 30 *New York Times* headline "Trump suggests lack of testing is no longer a problem. Governors disagree" (Martin et al. 2020). Presented in this way, neither party seems to be telling the truth. Testing is either not a problem or it is a problem, and the final determination is left to the audience, who are, especially in this case, woefully unable to determine if testing is or is not a problem. Those who support Trump maybe would side with him and those who oppose wouldn't. Yet is it impossible to find evidence to support either side in this case and make the headline stronger?

An annotated version of the *NYT* headline was circulating online, changing it to "Lack of testing is still a problem, governors, experts agree. Trump refuses to accept it." This adjustment still gives 'both' sides, yet adds important information to better contextualize Trump's position. At that time, most governors and medical experts, including those on Trump's taskforce, were arguing for increased testing, both in scale and in efficiency, while Trump was against it because increased confirmed cases made his handling of the situation look worse. However, at the same time such a headline would appear to be unprofessional as it contains too much of the journalist's own opinion and judgement.

USA Today (2020), on May 6, tweeted a link to their story about Sen. Rand Paul, who was one of the first major US politicians to contract COVID-19. The tweet read 'Sen. Rand Paul said since he already had coronavirus, he could not contract it again or spread it to others—claims that experts say are still unproven.' Again, the journalists are balancing the claims of a politician with those of medical experts. At that time, details about immunity and COVID-19, if and to what extent those recovering from it receive enough antibodies to be immune to getting it again, were unknown. No studies had shown either that people do or do not get immunity, and epidemiological principles state that if that information is unknown then you still must treat everyone as possible carriers who could be re-infected. Sen. Paul was still unwilling to wear a mask or take other precautions, and his position goes against medical advice. Yet the headline is still presented as if both sides' arguments are equally valid. A more adequate headline would be 'Sen. Rand Paul ignored medical advice and wrongly assumes he has immunity, potentially engendering those around him.' But this headline would seem to be too judgemental and opinionated and would be deemed 'unprofessional' for journalism.

This is a structural weakness of journalism, more accurate headlines that debunk lies and are socially responsible can also be viewed as being unprofessional and not objective. Journalists, editors, producers, and their social media experts need to be more bold and courageous and take a firm stand on these kinds of stories. They have to differentiate between cases which are simple political scuffles or about differences of opinion with those which are a matter of life and death. The concern should be about amplifying reliable medical advice and not every political disagreement about a pandemic.

4 Fact Checking Disingenuous Sources

"[Y]ou're in the middle of a pandemic and you're trying hard to address all the appropriate issues, it is truly a waste of time to have to debunk nonsense. But you know, unfortunately, we've had to do that," said Dr. Anthony Fauci during a webinar on Sept 11 (quoted in Watts 2020). That sentiment holds true not only for public health communicators like Fauci but journalists covering the pandemic as well. Despite Trump having been a major player the US political sphere for over 5 years, if not more, and despite the steady stream of lies, misinformation, misinterpretation, exaggeration, and obfuscation from the Trump camp, his position as a lead agenda setter and main source for journalism across the board has remained steady.

In the same way journalists are trapped in the 'false balance' paradigm, they are also trapped in a fact-checking loop with the Trump Administration. That is to say, Trump or one of his accomplices will tell a lie, the lie will be fact-checked, and when asked about the lie they will obfuscate and prevaricate until the journalist gives up and moves on. Then the cycle begins again and again. This would be one thing in the normal course of politics as Trump is not the first, nor last, intellectually and ethically dishonest politicians, it is another during the worst pandemic in centuries. Yet the journalistic routine is the same: fact-check a lie, get a disingenuous response from Trumpland, rinse and repeat.

Fact checking in and of itself is not new and can form a counter-point to the 'he said-she said' style discussed above. It is less often used than 'balancing statement' because the journalist could "be accused of [their] fact checking being their 'opinion' and such an activity being unprofessional" (Hearns-Branaman 2016: 30), no matter how concrete the evidence the fact check is based upon. The Trump Administration is famous for rejecting fact checks in increasingly ludicrous ways, for example Kellyanne Conway's oft maligned 'alternative facts' statement. Yet journalists continue to fact check, probably out of a sense of public duty, and despite their fact checks being ineffective in convincing Trump supporters about his inherent dishonesty.

In regard to coverage of COVID-19, fact-checking becomes simultaneously more important and more useless. In many ways this is due to the way in which the fact checking is framed, in that generally the false statement is given first, in the headline or tweet, with the actual fact-checking occurring inside the article. This framing causes the false statement to be given additional unwarranted credence, as a statement of such inherent value that we need to spend our precious time to decipher its validity.

For example, a CNN headline read "Trump says he did wear a mask in Arizona—you just didn't see him" (Carvajal 2020), with the rest of the article basically summarizing Trump's exchange with reporters questioning him on his mask usage. As it is unverifiable if Trump did or did not wear a mask, it is questionable why the reporters spent so much time questioning Trump about this, and questionable why his answer should be taken on face value. He could be lying to save face, he could be obfuscating to confuse the reporters, or he could have actually worn the mask, but in the end the audience knows no more than they did at the beginning and may even be more confused.

As discussed above, Trump's April 24, 2020 musings about using dangerous and potentially lethal methods to 'cure' COVID-19 (injecting bleach, UV light, etc.) is an example of a kind of statement that does not deserve to be dignified with a fact check. Reports about his statement should not begin by re-stating what he said and then fact checking it. The story should be that the president is giving deranged and deadly advice about 'cures' and 'treatments' for COVID-19 and is 'discussing' these ideas during a press conference with his medical advisors. No time should be spent 'debunking' these kind of senseless ramblings, journalism should not be used to amplify them simply because they are newsworthy as they should only be noted as part of a story about lies and disinformation about public health.

A source, no matter their place in the political hierarch, needs to eventually lose their credibility and de facto legitimacy if they persistently act as suppliers of dangerous disinformation. The public needs to trust journalists, and journalists also need to trust their sources. How can the former happen when the latter does not?

5 Hose Race Reporting of Statistics

Reporting of statistics during COVID-19 also left a lot to be desired. Reporting should, but rarely does, say 'confirmed cases,' instead simply saying 'cases.' This is problematic on many levels. Statistics of infections and deaths are unreliable everywhere, yet they are presented as facts. Comparing data gathered with different standards (i.e. Deaths at home? Care facilities? With or because of the virus?) would lead to inaccurate reports and ultimately would mislead the public and politicians who follow such reports.

Confirming if someone is positive for the virus is only one indication of how far the virus has spread and is not the ultimate gauge. Yet CNN routinely has breaking news reports simply stating that, for example, "Virus has now infected more than 1.34 million people." Stating "more than" does not cover the unknowable numbers of people who have been infected, which is many more times higher than those who have been tested.

For example, the CDC's recommendations were that only "deaths that have COVID-19 listed on the death certificate" as a contributor to death should be counted (quoted in Elis, Hicken, and Frantz, CNN, Apr 7, 2020). Yet are those who died but did not have a COVID-19 test included? Tests for those who have already passed away are not common. There is also no standard to say if someone really has COVID-19 or not as the symptoms and where the disease actually occurs vary widely from patient to patient. Different coroners with different experiences in different areas working for different hospitals would arguably have different standards for listing COVID-19 on the death certificate.

Another aspect is the way in which these statistics are reported. CNN has nearly consistently had a side bar on all of their broadcasts listing "TOTAL CASES" and "DEATHS" both "GLOBALLY" and "IN THE UNITED STATES." This is continually updated and is based on Johns Hopkins University Statistics. While it is important to keep up to date with these statistics, it can also create a sense of desperation or depression in the audience to be continually reminded of the negativity of the situation. The reliability of these statistics is also questionable, as the 'actual' rate may be lower or higher than the Johns Hopkins' data.

Other measures of the scale of the pandemic are available but not used as often. For example, it has become increasingly useful to compare the overall death rate of 2020 with that of previous years. Data specific about deaths directly or indirectly caused by COVID-19 can be inconsistent, yet the total death rate taken in aggregate can be more illustrative. As data journalist John Burn-Murdoch (2020) tweeted, "a lot of data on reported COVID deaths is highly suspect, so we've been looking into excess mortality." The report (Burn-Murdoch et al. 2020) from the *Financial Times* on Apr 26 collated data from over 14 countries "show[ed] 122,000 deaths in excess of normal levels across these locations, considerably higher than the 77,000 official COVID-19 deaths," which indicated that the so-called 'cases' reported by other news outlets is likely very inaccurate.

Greater care needs to be given in reporting such grave statistics, and contextualizing the reliability and validity of the data needs to be increased. Simply reporting 'cases' here are greater than 'cases' there really means very little and gives a false impression to the audience of the extent of the pandemic and a comparison of how different countries are dealing with it. It is a classic case of comparing apples and oranges, and without consistently mentioning this divergence will only complicate and mystify audience understanding of the pandemic.

6 Lack of Experienced Medical Reporters

What kind of journalists are needed to cover a story as massive as a global pandemic? In an ideal media ecosystem, there would be plenty of well-trained medical or science journalists. Medical journalism is important because reports "can increase or diminish the willingness of individuals to seek medical care [...], may raise expectations (some-times falsely), may dash hopes, or may provoke alarm (sometimes unnecessarily)" (Larsson et al. 2003: 324). All of these aspects of medical journalism are especially pertinent during a pandemic where public health communication is instrumental in both lowering risk of infection for people and containing the outbreak as early possible. Yet the lack of sufficient medical journalists unfortunately leads to coverage being done by general assignment journalists or, even worse, political journalists. There are issues and limitations to both.

General assignment journalists are skilled at learning quickly, and learning just enough about a subject or event to create a basic report about it. This can often be no problem as many news stories happen again and again; car crashes, airplane disasters, protests, robberies, the basic fodder for news. Yet when more rare events happen, the general reporter's training can often be insufficient, such as with the COVID-19 pandemic. While reporters, much like the general public, have basic knowledge about how diseases spread, the specific terminology used by heath care officials, doctors, and epidemiologists can take a while to understand fully. This lack of sufficient or partial understanding then spreads to the anchors, editors, and producers who rely on the specialists for such background information.

For example, the World Health Organization (2020) on Jan 14 tweeted "Preliminary investigations conducted by the Chinese authorities have found no clear evidence of human-to-human transmission of the novel #coronavirus (2019-nCoV) identified in #Wuhan, #China." This was widely and inaccurately interpreted as WHO stating clearly that the virus *cannot be* or *is not* transmitted human-to-human, and was used later as 'evidence' of WHO and the Chinese government misleading the public. The *Washington Examiner*, for example, wrote that: "Two months after that tweet, the world was met with a pandemic that had hit most countries on Earth and put the global economy in a free fall, with human-to-human transmission playing a major role in the spread of the virus. Many questioned the WHO and its parent organization, the United Nations, for sharing a study that turned out to be inaccurate." (Dibble 2020). Yet the study was not 'inaccurate' as the critics claim, it was being scientifically rigorous and was misinterpreted by many. As Aaron Blake from the *Washington Post* points out, "the WHO didn't say on Jan. 14 that there was no human-to-human transmission—just that there was 'no evidence' of it at that point" (Blake 2020). Once there was better evidence the WHO updated its recommendations. Scientists can only operate on the best evidence they have at hand, and calling into question their integrity for not knowing then what we know now is highly inappropriate.

Another issue is the usage or preprints, or early drafts of medical research that have yet to go through an editorial and/or peer review process that are released publicly. As Haelle (2020) notes, "coverage of them in medical/health/scientific journalism has been growing and has become particularly pronounced during the COVID-19 pandemic." Many non-specialist journalists rely on these as sources of information and story ideas, yet they often do not have the training or expertise to fully interpret these preprints. As the results are not peer reviewed, their validity is questionable, yet at the same time certain preliminary results are very newsworthy. Many early studies of therapeutics to treat COVID-19 "are so small—39% are enrolling or plan to enroll fewer than 100 patients—that they are unlikely to yield clear results" (Herper and Riglin 2020). Yet when a preprint of an early study with a small sample size that appears to show *some* effectiveness of a treatment, such as the now debunked hydroxychloroquine, is picked up by a journalist and amplified inappropriately, the impression can be given that the treatment is effective. While later studies showed the drug was highly ineffective, and even dangerous, the danger had already been done and the perception of hydroxychloroquine as a potential miracle cure persists.

The reasons of these limitations can probably be boiled down to economics; it's cheaper to hire several general reporters who can cover a variety of stories in a basic but sufficient depth, while having a full-time health journalist is only economically feasible for the largest of news outlets. It is very positive that CNN or the *New York Times* do have high-quality, experienced medical journalists, like Sanjay Gupta, and further efforts should be made to train former doctors in journalism or, more likely, experienced journalists in specific courses about science and medical reporting. It may not be the best economic decision, but it serves the public interest, saves lives, and will enhance the reputation and standing of any news organization that makes the effort.

7 Conclusion

The basic structure and operating methods of US journalism served and, in many cases, continue to serve the country very poorly during the COVID-19 pandemic. This is not to blame journalists personally for their individual failings, nor is it to criticize them for not having hindsight on details about the epidemiology of COVID. This is to highlight how the system of American journalism is broken in fundamental ways that have failed to serve the people in the way that is needs during such a crisis.

Simply because a powerful person gives a press conference claiming to be informative about a pandemic does not mean it needs to be covered live, nor even reported on unless scientifically valid information needed to mitigate a public health crisis has in fact been collected from the pseudo-event. Such events can even be ignored or delegated to a single sentence. Yet journalists are attracted to press conferences because it is an easy source of words and video they can use to fill their daily quotas, and the powerful know this and use it to serve their own ends. Editors and producers in different organizations need to work together to ensure press conferences are covered to gain useful, life-saving information to help the public during a pandemic, no more and no less. No politics, no mixing of political infighting with health information, no grandstanding by indignant reporters, no capitalizing on attacks on journalism to play the victim.

Secondly, the paradigm of false balance needs to be broken. It should be more widely accepted for journalists to say a source is lying, especially if they are an influential political figure. Journalists do not need to 'balance' falsehoods given for one's own political benefit with the informed, well-researched, and trusted information given by experts in a specific field. Balance has to be of equally trustworthy sources, for example two experts who disagree about the effectiveness of masks to prevent spread of the virus when the data was still unclear about their utility. After the scientific consensus has been reached then there is no need for more 'balance.'

On the other side of the coin, sources known for being untrustworthy and disingenuous should not have their lies amplified by well-meaning fact-checks. *That* they are lying *is* the story, *what* they are lying about *is not*. Amplifying a false statement in order to debunk it has the opposite effect of validating the lie as something that could potentially be true. Those who do not trust the 'fake' mainstream news media will thus, through a process of reverse psychology, have more credence in the false statement.

How many people have been infected or died during a pandemic is not a competition and journalists should be careful about how such data is presented. It is not a matter of politics, a matter of polling, it is human life, not votes. Political framing of such data, while probably inevitable, is very inappropriate. Journalists also need to be careful about the precision of their language. A 'case' is not the same as a 'confirmed case,' data that is not compatible due to differences in the way that sampling is done, and the reliability and validity of the data collection methods should not be compared directly.

Lastly, there needs to be a greater emphasis on training reporters specialized in medicine and health issues. Early on in the pandemic journalists were still educating themselves on basic epidemiology and trying to find proper sources who can talk authoritatively on the subject. After several months many major news organizations, like MSNBC and CNN, did end up having a good stock of doctors and immunologists to bring on TV and talk about COVID-19 in an appropriate and informative matter, yet this process still took several months. It is also not uniform, with smaller organizations financially unable to hire such specialist journalists. For the public interest, such reporting needs to be just as fundamental as sports or the weather, and the investments made in inculcating such talent should be expanded, not retracted, when the pandemic wanes.

It should also be noted that, despite all the structural limitations mentioned above, a lot of good reporting did take place, and journalists were often able to overcome these constraints to inform the public effectively. There is always room for improvement at the individual and institutional level. Journalistic routines themselves need to be reformed, especially in regard to sourcing of information, giving of credibility to sources, and how dangerous information is framed, and it is only though the work of individual journalists in their discussions with each other and their superiors can changes actually take place and become formalized as new routines.

References

Al Jazeera English. (2020) Experts react with horror to Trump coronavirus disinfectant idea. April 24. Available at: www.aljazeera.com/news/2020/4/24/experts-react-withhorror-to-trump-coronavirus-disinfectant-idea.

BBC News. (2020) Coronavirus: outcry after Trump suggests injecting disinfectant as treatment. April 24. Available at: www.bbc.com/news/world-us-canada-52407177.

Blake, A. (2020) Trump vs. the WHO: Breaking down the president's claims and the WHO's actions. *Washington Post*, April 10. Available at: www.washingtonpost.com/politics/2020/04/09/trump-vs-who/.

Burn-Murdoch, J. (2020) NEW: a lot of data on reported Covid deaths is highly suspect, so we've been looking into excess mortality—how many more people than usual have been dying around.... Available at: www.twitter.com/jburnmurdoch/status/1254461123753054209twitter.com/jburnmurdoch/status/1254461123753054209 (Accessed 26 April 2020).

Burn-Murdoch, J., Romei, R. and Giles, C. (2020) Global coronavirus death toll could be 60% higher than reported. *Financial Times*, April 26. Available at: www.ft.com/content/6bd88b7d-3386-4543-b2e9-0d5c6fac846c.

Carvajal, N. (2020) Trump says he did wear a mask in Arizona—you just didn't see him. *CNN*, May 6. Available at: www.edition.cnn.com/us/live-news/us-coronavirus-update-05-06-20/h_8219213e1624f59335616d599b475d04.

Collinson, S. (2020) Trump is peddling dangerous cures for coronavirus. *CNN*, April 24. Available at: www.edition.cnn.com/us/live-news/us-coronavirus-update-04-24-20/h_fbbc3e66507ff72948db14dd67307616.

Dibble, M. (2020) WHO trashed for sharing Chinese study claiming humans can't spread coronavirus during outbreak's onset. *Washington Examiner*, March 19. Available at: www.washingtonexaminer.com/news/who-trashed-for-sharing-chinese-study-claiming-humans-cant-spread-coronavirus-during-outbreaks-onset.

Ellefson, L. (2020) *New York Times* deletes tweet saying 'some experts' warn against ingesting disinfectant. *The Wrap*, April 24. Available at: www.thewrap.com/new-york-times-deletes-tweet-saying-some-experts-warn-against-ingesting-disinfectant/.

First Draft News. (2020) Reporting on misinformation without amplifying falsehoods is hard. Here are some thoughts and tips on headline writing from speaking to [...] world. April 29. Available at: www.twitter.com/firstdraftnews/status/1255518886293909508.

Haelle, T. (2020) Beware the preprint in covering coronavirus research. *Association of Health Care Journalists*, April 17. Available at www.healthjournalism.org/blog/2020/04/beware-the-preprint-in-covering-coronavirus-research.

Hearns-Branaman, J.O. (2016) *Journalism and the Philosophy of Truth: Beyond Objectivity and Balance*. Routledge.

Hearns-Branaman, J.O. (2018) 'What the Propaganda Model can learn from the sociology of journalism' in Broudy, D., Klaehn, J., and Pedro, J. (eds), *The Propaganda Model: Filtering Perception and Awareness*, University of Westminster Press.

Herper, M., and Riglin, R. (2020) Data show panic and disorganization dominate the study of COVID-19 drugs. *StatNews.com*, July 2. Available at: www.statnews.com/2020/07/06/data-show-panic-and-disorganization-dominate-the-study-of-covid-19-drugs/.

Larsson, A, Oxman, A.D., Carlingà, C., and Herrin, J. (2003) Medical messages in the media—barriers and solutions to improving medical journalism. *Health Expectations 6*: 323–331.

Maddow, R. (2020), 'The Rachel Maddow Show,' March 21, *MSNBC*.

Martin, J., Haberman, M., and Baker, M. (2020) Trump suggests lack of testing is no longer a problem. Governors disagree. *The New York Times*, March 30. Available at: www.nytimes.com/2020/03/30/us/politics/trump-governors-coronavirus-testing.html.

NBC News. (2020) Trump suggests 'injection' of disinfectant to beat coronavirus and 'clean' the lungs. April 26. Available at: www.nbcnews.com/politics/donald-trump/trump-suggests-injection-disinfectant-beat-coronavirus-clean-lungs-n1191216.

Rosen, J. (2020) Today we are switching our coverage of Donald Trump to an emergency setting. *PressThink.org*, March 19. Available at: www.pressthink.org/2020/03/today-we-switch-our-coverage-of-donald-trump-to-an-emergency-setting/.

St. Louis Post-Dispatch Editorial Board. (2020) Editorial: It's time for the networks to stop live broadcast of Trump's briefings. *St Louis Post-Dispatch*, April 2. Available at: www.stltoday.com/opinion/editorial/editorial-its-time-for-the-networks-to-stop-live-broadcast-of-trumps-briefings/article_5754dc67-bcfc-5638-a0c4-012a92598998.html.

The New York Times. (2020) We've deleted an earlier tweet and updated a sentence in our article that implied that only 'some experts' view the ingestion of household disinfectants as dangerous. To be clear... Available at: www.twitter.com/nytimes/status/1253719616603541504).

USA Today. (2020) Sen. Rand Paul said since he already had coronavirus, he could not contract it again or spread it to others [...]. May 6. Available at: www.twitter.com/USATODAY/status/1257829430355001351.

Watts, A. (2020) Fauci: "It is truly a waste of time to have to debunk nonsense". *CNN*, Sept 11. Available at: www.edition.cnn.com/world/live-news/coronavirus-pandemic-09-11-20-intl/h_ae091cf790c0a1ec65c4fe408cd818f7.

Weimann, G. and Brosius, H. B. (2015) 'A new agenda for agenda-setting research in the digital era' in Vowea, G. and Henn, P. (eds), *Political Communication in the Online World: Theoretical Approaches and Research Designs*, NY: Routledge.

WHO. (2020) Preliminary investigations conducted by the Chinese authorities have found no clear evidence of human-to-human transmission of the novel #coronavirus (2019-nCoV) identified in #Wuhan, #China. Jan 14. Available at: www.twitter.com/who/status/1217043229427761152.

Farther Apart, Closer Together: How the Use of New Technologies During COVID-19 May Forever Alter the Face of Journalism

Jesse Owen Hearns-Branaman and Johnny Bliss

Johnny Bliss, born in the Canadian city of Vancouver in the early 1980s, has spent the last fifteen years living in Austria's capital Vienna and working as a journalist for the radio station FM4, which is the bilingual youth, subculture and alternative station of the Austrian Broadcasting Corporation (ORF). He has spent the better part of the last decade travelling around the world for his radio column 'Johnny's Journeys' and collecting stories from interesting characters he met along the way. This came to an abrupt end in March when the pandemic started as his life as a professional globe-trotter was threatened by international travel bans and other pandemic prevention controls.

Johnny explained that, despite being largely confined to his bedroom studio since the beginning of the pandemic, he nevertheless continued to conduct interviews with many interesting characters and experts internationally, and even managed to do some of the best work of his career. The challenge of COVID, it turned out, was also a great opportunity for radio journalism as a medium to learn how to adapt in the face of a global catastrophe and tight controls on international travel. We discussed downsides as well, such as the ways in which the fidelity of the end product audio had been compromised and the many types of interviews that became difficult or impossible to conduct virtually. But in the end, there was a spirit of excitement in these times, in breaking with outdated constraints and habits, and exploring the new opportunities for international journalism afforded by virtual production techniques and practices.

J. O. Hearns-Branaman (✉)
Beijing Normal University-Hong Kong Baptist University United International College, Zhuhai, China
e-mail: johearnsbranaman@uic.edu.cn

J. Bliss
FM4, Austrian Broadcasting Corporation, Vienna, Austria

S.X.B. Zhao et al. (eds.), *COVID-19 Pandemic, Crisis Responses and the Changing World*, https://doi.org/10.1007/978-981-16-2430-8_17

1 Travelling Journalist Without the Travel

Jesse Owen Hearns-Branaman

Previously in your job you travelled a lot. Originally it was more travelling around Europe covering cultural events and music festivals, but eventually you were travelling around the world for 8 or 9 months at a time, including Europe, Africa, the Americas and Asia. The biggest change to your job during the pandemic must be that you have basically stopped travelling. On one hand, travel can make you exhausted and worn out, it's expensive, it's time-consuming, but at the same time that is what many journalists have to do in order to cover a wide range of stories in a variety of areas around the world.

How do you feel about this change? Can you still be a 'travel' journalist if you're not travelling? Can you still do your job in these conditions?

Johnny Bliss

I feel like one of the main things that I have learned, and that people are learning in general right now, is the extent to which some of these labels can be professionally detrimental in a constantly changing world. This applies both from the standpoint of the content producer, having the personal flexibility to change or alter your own medium, and from the standpoint of an external observer, even and especially if that observer is in the same field or company as you are.

To unpack that, the term 'travel journalist' and even the title of my column 'Johnny's Journeys' imposes artificial limits on my work, ones that really have very little to do with the work itself. In fact, these artificial limits were personally and professionally detrimental to my work long before COVID-19 forced everything to change.

In your question, you reference my exhaustion, my feeling of burn-out that I'd been suffering from for years. I've been desperately exploring what it could mean to do my job without having to physically board planes, trains, buses, or boats, without having to get visas, find accommodation, and so forth. Nothing would have made me happier than being able to stop doing all that stuff!

But the fact is, I kept hitting an invisible wall, firstly because many of my colleagues at the radio made no secret of being sceptical of the quality of recordings that get collected remotely and digitally. Secondly, because I was guilty of making some of the same assumptions. Thirdly, because the people I would contact for stories often did not take the idea of doing a remote interview seriously themselves either.

This is based on an old paradigm and many years ago that assumption would have been true. Smartphones really weren't reliable enough, people around the world were not technologically literate enough, the fidelity of whichever smartphone or laptop's internal microphone was not good enough. The fact is, we did try these things in the past and they didn't sound very good. But times have changed, and, if I've learned anything during this tumultuous, traumatic year, it is that we have to change our approach with the times.

That doesn't mean that there aren't situations where you'll need to travel personally of course. If, for example, you are monitoring elections in a place like Belarus or, less seriously, you're providing coverage of an offline festival or conference somewhere, then yes, there will still be the need for some journalists to personally travel sometimes. But I think in the future we will ask more questions about the necessity of putting bodies on planes for this or that story, if for no other reason than that it is much more expensive to do it offline.

Jesse

Working for the radio, your features often do have a very 'intimate' sound to them because people are showing you their artwork, you're in the same physical space with them walking around while interviewing them, you're talking to them during a conference or festival. Space and place seem to be vital in that context. Are you saying that this aspect of your work will not suffer from you recording it all from your bedroom?

Johnny

No, of course not. Obviously, there is no way to digitally take a physical tour of a remote village over Zoom or another digital medium—although that hasn't stopped the Faroe Islands tourism board from trying! Which I'll get into a little bit later. But no, some of what I'll call the more 'gimmicky' aspects of the travel part are of course sacrificed. But the heart and soul of my work has always been collecting the stories, the personal, intimate anecdotes of real people who open up to me, and I've unexpectedly found that video chat platforms have even managed to lend a newfound intimacy, and immediacy, to my recordings that may have been sometimes lacking in-person.

I think part of this stems from the fact that both people concerned, the interviewer and the interviewee, have to make a physical effort to find a quiet place and focus if the interview is going to actually take place. I've been astonished that sometimes the virtual interviews end up sounding better than the real-life ones, because whoever it is that I'm talking to seems to be taking the exercise more seriously than they would otherwise!

One example of this happened this summer when I visited Iceland. At the time, their COVID numbers were very low, nearly non-existent in fact, and the country was operating very much like normal. Astonishingly, this meant that annual summer festivals were still taking place in Reykjavik. I chose to cover one of the festivals taking place there, and had to chase one of the organizers around all afternoon to find a moment she was free to do the interview, which we ended up doing in a windy park surrounded by drunk people, a very noisy audio environment to do my work in. While it worked out eventually, it reminded me of how much trouble doing these interviews in 'real life' sometimes could be. And really, if we'd just organized an appointment over Zoom, it would have been logistically a lot easier for me.

Jesse

In the end you, like many other people, are back to working from home due to the pandemic, travel restrictions, and concerns for your health and the health of those close to you.

Johnny

Yep. I've often thought about it this year, that the situation of this pandemic really gave me a chance to take a break from some of the most exhausting aspects of my work. In the past, not only have I had to record in loud audio environments, I've also had to edit my audio in uncomfortable places, due to being on a very tight broadcast schedule; better working spaces were often simply unavailable at short notice. I remember editing an entire feature in a heavy metal band's rehearsal space in Mexico City—while they were playing! I had to turn the audio up on my headphones that day to some seriously uncomfortable level of decibels, let me tell you.

My career was full of moments like this; I remember walking around out on a remote Icelandic lava field in the middle of the night, trying to get a strong enough internet signal to send a feature for the next day's early morning show. Or hiking up a steep hill in the middle of a jungle on an island off the coast of Indonesian Borneo because otherwise I couldn't get a strong enough signal to send my radio program on time. And let me tell you, the rainforest was itself an obstacle to recording. Such places are seldom very quiet!

I could easily spend the entire interview talking about situations like this, but suffice it to say I regularly struggled to meet my deadlines and send my stories in time. I always did manage, but it was a huge stress factor. And while I may not presently have access to the same types of people or stories that I found when traveling by plane to a remote village in Papua New Guinea, there is an upside. The fact that I now can also very easily collect a story from somewhere I am not enables me to record and broadcast stories that are a lot more 'timely,' a lot more connected to what's going on in the day's news cycle, than the material I was collecting from wherever.

If I'm in Papua New Guinea, then I'm going to be entirely focused on what's in front of me, right? It won't be a factor that there are Black Lives Matter protests happening on the other side of the globe, or that Donald Trump is saying he wants to buy Greenland from Denmark, or whatever. 90% of the time, the stories I was collecting were timeless, broadcast-able anytime, because they were usually a world away from the news headlines. That's been the biggest shift: Almost everything I'm collecting from my little bedroom studio in Vienna now is related to what is 'trending,' what people everywhere seem to be concerned about.

2 Timeliness and the News Cycle

Jesse

You mentioned suddenly having to consider the timeliness and pay attention to the news cycle. You must feel more constrained by this because previously it was not a major pressure for you. And if you follow timeliness and the news cycle, it means that you now have to work on tighter deadlines instead of having more freedom and flexibility. You can no longer cover a story, record interviews, edit it together, and then release it weeks later.

One major criticism of journalism is that it is too fast, too concerned with the news cycle and deadlines, and this leads to journalists not fact-checking as well as they should due to lack of time. Doing long-form feature journalism, be it print, internet, or radio, does not fall into this trap and for that reason is highly praised for being able to have more time to, for example, fact-check their pieces. Has this been an increasing concern for you?

Johnny

Funny you bring up fact-checking. In fact, fact-checking has seldom been an issue for me in the past, but it's become a much bigger topic this year. Part of that is due to the nature of my radio work, as you noted.

Radio is by nature a much more limited medium, in the sense that you have to make broader strokes and it's more difficult to take a "deep dive" into the arcane details of a story. If you do a dry radio story full of numbers and data, your listeners will tune out or fall asleep. Therefore, radio is largely about personal stories, and if somebody is telling you about their father's life, or their own career, or a personal adventure they had, the idea of fact-checking it nearly feels perverse. Or, because of the timeless quality of most of these stand-alone features, it's been easy to just put a particular story off until the fact-checking was done.

But now, if I spend the afternoon talking to an Amnesty International expert about BLM protests in the city of Chicago, I also have to read what other journalists are saying *today*, see what headlines are coming out of Chicago, find out if anything's changed since we did the interview. That's not just a hypothetical, we actually did have a story that we had to cancel last minute after the Chicago police cracked down heavily on a particular protest. While the things I had been told by the Amnesty guy were still technically true, if we'd broadcast his comments at that moment, they would have come across as tone deaf.

Fact-checks aside, another new thing I've discovered that I have to be concerned about this year, is how quickly the public mood changes. For example, in late May I recorded an interview with a marine biologist who'd just returned from Antarctica. We talked about how the pandemic was altering life at the bottom of the earth, and it was really interesting. Ten days later, however, the story already felt dated because of BLM protests rocking America and spreading across the world. Talking about what marine biologists in Antarctica thought about the pandemic no longer felt 'timely' or even appropriate. This can be true about just about any topic: nearly anything I record nowadays has a much faster rate of turnover, because big shifts happen very quickly, and no one cares much what happened five minutes ago.

3 Maintaining Quality of Product

Jesse

Another change due to using internet-based reporting technology is that the quality is not as easy to maintain as before. Traditionally it's up to the journalists to maintain the quality or the audio and video footage, yet now you sometimes even have to rely on your interviewee to record their own audio. Has the quality really been affected in a negative way? Do you think the audience cares about it?

Johnny

It's more that I *used to* think I had to rely on my interviewee to record their own audio, early in the pandemic, that is. Lately, I haven't been asking that at all. When I interviewed you right at the beginning, I still asked you to do this whole song and dance of installing a recording app on your smart phone, and then we both recorded our own voices separately whilst wearing headphones; later, I put the two tracks next to each other in a multi-track editor, enabling it to sound like we were both in the same room. The thing is, that approach to doing remote interviews belonged very much to the old paradigm.

What I've discovered since is that the recording set-ups on the other end have often been either inferior to the Zoom/Skype recording quality, or even actively detrimental. For example, I recently did an interview with an Icelandic public figure. Her technician set up a recording device upon my request, but what I didn't realize was that, for some reason, it was beeping the entire time while we were recording. This meant that not only was the recording they made low-quality, it leaked into the Skype recording too. To hide the ever-present beeping, I eventually had to put a sound-bed of glitchy electronic music underneath our whole interview. But if I hadn't asked them to set up a recording device, that never would have happened!

Another eye-opening moment was an interview I did with a friend in Sydney, Australia. She had a high quality, working smart phone and installed the software I asked her to. For all intents and purposes, her local recording device acted nearly the same as my professional microphone would have. The problem? The room she was in was quite small and, it turned out, had an echo. This is something I would have realized in person, but was totally unaware of on the other side of a screen. Her professional-quality microphone picked up the echo and I ultimately didn't use her recording. Yet on the Skype recording we didn't hear that echo at all!

As far as the audience goes, I don't think radio listeners care unless something's wrong. So, if the interview sounds messed up because the internet on one end is bad, *then* listeners care. Or if there's a profound echo or random background beeping. But generally, so long as the voices are clear and not distractingly low quality, I don't think it matters at all most of the time.

However, let's say it's fundamentally important to sound like you're in the same room, if you're doing a professional podcast and you really want listeners to be able to imagine the host and guest sitting across from each other, looking each other in the eye while they talk. In that case, if you know each other quite well, and you trust the other person to be both technologically literate, and aware enough of their environment to take care of all of this stuff, it will still sound better if you record with individual microphones. But it's a lot of hassle, and hardly necessary for a short radio interview that gets played once and never again.

I am looking forward to seeing how technology continues to develop over the years. I think with remote work being on the rise, tech companies will increasingly be motivated to improve the capacities of the internal microphone. One day in the not-too-distant future, I expect digital platforms like Zoom and Skype to be able to rival radio studios in this respect. Of course, the downside of that is, if a room has an echo, these new improved internal microphones will also pick that up.

4 Breaking the Limitations

Johnny

One thing that does end up happening is you realize how arbitrary some of these invented limitations actually were, how habitual, how utterly imaginary. One thing I definitely am grateful for this year is the opportunity to look with new eyes at what is possible, using the technologies we have at our disposal. In that respect, this is an exciting time and it's definitely been a silver lining to the dark cloud that is this pandemic!

Jesse

Some limitations are not imaginary, however, like being able to grow your network of contacts and sources. You cannot meet people in social settings, establish a rapport, and earn their trust in that way anymore, nor use those connections to get other connections. How you actually get in touch with and cultivate your sources must have changed a lot, can you talk about that?

Johnny

I won't deny that I did have an advantage going in here; almost everyone I interviewed for the first three months were people I'd known before, who I'd previously made contact with and interviewed and become friendly with in real life, years ago. Most of the time people were very happy to get together on our laptops for a chat, because there was trust already established.

The truth is, it *is* harder to make first contact now. Sometimes you send out multiple press requests to numerous organizations, and they all get ignored, or you have to call the general number repeatedly before anyone answers. Some reports I've tried to make in this new environment have fallen apart simply because I didn't have a good contact anywhere in, say, Greenland, and I couldn't find anyone willing to talk. Also, sometimes I've discovered that people who I'd been able to get to sit down for an interview by chasing them around in real life, simply are not able or willing to organize themselves for a scheduled online interview.

I was very disappointed by a contact in Darwin, Australia, who had scheduled an interview with me and then just didn't turn up. When she finally surfaced, we made another appointment, and she didn't turn up for that one either. For her, I got the impression that because I was not physically there in front of her, the interview wasn't 'real' enough to bother with or communicate about. And if remote interviews had not become the norm, I probably never would have realized this about that person, that she wasn't very reliable, because I would have only reached out to her if I was physically in Darwin. There are plenty of new issues and that can't be helped, just worked around.

Jesse

It must be interesting to still have contact with people around the world and learn about their lives and their jobs and how they have been affected during the pandemic. Have your ideas about what it means to be 'present' and how that affects your storytelling changed? Have you seen any interesting ways that people are dealing with the restrictions caused by the pandemic?

Johnny

I certainly know that the tourism industry has been massively affected. Broadcasting anything related to normal travel adventures would have felt inappropriate, for example, but on the other hand there have been some very interesting virtual initiatives going on. Vienna, where I live, has had a special bus going around the city to host spontaneous concerts all summer long, instead of the usual big open air festival hosted over one long weekend.

One initiative that I found really interesting came courtesy of the Faroe Islands Tourism Board, who have been conducting live virtual tours of different villages, mountainous landscapes, and coastal areas over the summer. People who joined in the live tour were able to direct the guide to go here or there, and really get the visual sense of what it would be like to be physically in that place at that time from the comfort of your bedroom.

Meanwhile, I know several musicians who would usually be touring all the time, and since March they have been forced to try different things. One of them has been quite successful with actively selling tickets for virtual concerts, making a reduced income with 'live' shows.

It's been really interesting to look at how people are altering their lives and jobs to work around the pandemic, you see this outpouring of creativity, and it's really interesting to watch the many ways this manifests, even if it doesn't always work one hundred percent.

5 Closing Pandora's Box?

Jesse

It seems like many different ways of doing your job have opened up. This is probably the same with a lot of other white collar office jobs or some IT work. I know many companies will take this into account in the future, reducing their office space and requiring more employees to work from home. This is a change that might not revert when the pandemic is over.

I also feel that it's much more convenient teaching online, for example, no commute, more flexibility in my day-to-day schedule. But at the same time, the students are almost like strangers to me, which is very disconcerting. One of the great things about teaching is getting to know the students and interacting with them, so I know most teachers will be more than happy to get back to in-person teaching when it is safe.

Perhaps it is different for different fields and industries. What about for journalism? Do you feel the same way about your job? Will you go back to travelling the world after, or keep doing it from your bedroom?

Johnny

One thing I can say for sure is that I will not go back to the old way of traveling the world to do my stories. I adore working from home, and this year has proven that I could do great work—arguably, some of the best work of my career—without all of that other stuff.

In a broader sense, I do agree with you that the biggest development is that everyone's idea of what is or is not possible will not simply revert back to 2019 standards when this is all over, as if none of this ever happened. This isn't to say that people won't, for example, be obliged to go to in-person meetings or classes in the future, but rather that people will have more information to run a cost-benefit analysis before they decide to do something offline. We'll ask questions like: "Do we actually need the whole team to travel physically to another city, each with their own flight ticket and a hotel room? Do patients really need to visit the doctor's office to update their regular prescription, when that on its own can be done more efficiently online?".

In my case, in the future I will always ask myself the question, "Will my story be better if I am actually in this place and able to physically interact with the surroundings? Or does this story not actually need *me* to be in it?" Because, after all, often I am just supplying the platform, and it's sufficient if the only person who is "on-site" is the interviewee, the one with a deep personal connection to the place in question.

What I would say to anyone and everyone who has ever questioned the necessity of certain parts of their job: take the opportunity of Pandora's Box being open to explore new possibilities, because the opportunity won't always be there. As tragic and traumatizing as this pandemic has been, it is also a great chance to get those you work with to consider alternative ways of doing business. It takes extraordinary circumstances to break a habit, and these are indeed extraordinary circumstances.

6 How Much Has Radio Journalism Really Changed?

Jesse

At the same time, some journalism has not really changed during the pandemic, such as written journalism newspapers or websites or blogs. It has traditionally been a criticism of that kind of journalism that the reporters just stay in the office, don't go out to get fresh sources, and rely on second-hand information like press releases. At the same time, for radio or TV journalism, and especially photojournalism, you really need to go out and get the sound and images yourself. It seems as if the different genres and types of journalism have been affected differently.

Johnny

Absolutely, what I've been talking about has very much been directed to those working in radio or podcasts. If you are working with a visual medium or with a text-based medium this will have a very different impact on how you conduct your work. Radio is interesting because this situation sort of stripped the medium down to its essentials.

Before the pandemic, I had the experience that there was often a lot of pressure to always have gimmicky, unnecessary sounds popping up through a feature. You're interviewing a person in a hostel? Let's hear a guest come in and ask for their key. You're talking about crocodiles in a swamp? You should hear something slithering around, a splash in the water, even if nothing like that actually happened! You are looking around a museum? Let's add some sounds of footsteps and turning doorknobs and whatever. There was this idea that a story couldn't just be a story on its own. It had to provide a sense of space, or so went the conventional logic, even if that sense of space did not add anything to the story itself. Now, because of the impact of the pandemic, this has really pared radio back down to being a purer storytelling format, which is not at all to the detriment of the medium, from my perspective.

7 Digital Divide Limiting Sourcing

Jesse

There's this concept of the digital divide, that access to technology and skills to use that technology is not even for different groups of people for different reasons. For example, older people without technical literacy, people in areas without good internet, people of certain socio-economic backgrounds. Many have pointed out that this crisis has exacerbated the digital divide, for example younger and more technologically literate people who can do their job via computers and the internet have not been impacted as much as those who cannot.[1] There's a major concern that the billions of people who cannot take advantage of new digital technologies will be left behind, not able to have their voices heard.

It's easy for you to contact people on *our* side of the digital divide, but the pandemic has cut off those on the *other* side for you. That is to say, now you cannot physically travel somewhere to meet sources or hear stories from people without internet access or digital literacy. Have you considered this before?

Johnny

This is one of the tragedies of these pandemic times. A lot of the work I've done over the years that I'm most proud of was with people I couldn't have reached just by sending a polite email and scheduling a Skype interview. For example, I went to Cuba back when internet was prohibitively expensive, and interviewed brave and charming people who I never could have contacted today. The same goes with freedom fighters who I spoke to in Indonesian Papua, or protester monks in Myanmar. Because of how dangerous it was to talk to the press in some of these places, it would have been impossible to reach people online for an interview. And unfortunately, there aren't really many solutions to that issue right now. A lot of the world has simply been cut off from speaking to people like me.

On the other hand, we have witnessed widespread protests in places like Belarus, and there are still journalists who are already there or are in the position to go, sending reports: just fewer of them than usual. But thank goodness at least those people are there.

[1] Sostero, Matteo, Santo Milasi, John Hurley, Enrique Fernandez-Macías, and Martina Bisello (2020), *Teleworkability and the COVID-19 crisis: A new digital divide?* Seville: European Commission.

8 Paradigm Shift

Jesse

It has occurred to me that this crisis, this pandemic, could be the start of a paradigm shift, at least for journalism but also for society in general. We're moving more things to be virtual, to be de-spaced, to be this kind of detached audio-visual lifestyle. When I used to watch science-fiction shows or movies and people can only communicate via video chat, it made me feel a bit sad that they're so disconnected physically from one another, yet it has become the fundamental way in which they communicate and socialize. But now it totally makes sense to me and hopefully to others; you *can* become comfortable in communicating in that way, and it will be more acceptable from now on.

We've already talked about the effect of this on media production, breaking limitations, and keeping Pandora's Box open. Do you think this is a paradigm shift moment in the larger sense as well?

Johnny

If not now, then when? This situation is bringing everything to the surface, meaning that if a person was unhappy in a job or a relationship, this may be the moment that they decide to make a big change. I know a stand-up comedian who decided he didn't want to be a comedian anymore after a few months of COVID—not because of the pandemic, but because the pandemic gave him time to reflect on what's important in life. I want to make it clear that I realize there are also downsides, that I've certainly been one of the lucky ones. Domestic abuse has spiked in many places because of people being locked down together. Many businesses which were just struggling to stay afloat are shutting, even if they didn't necessarily have to, just because it 'felt like time.'

My friend Andri Magnason called this period the Apausolypse (in a great multimedia piece he produced about it for Emergence Magazine[2]), because we all had to collectively hit the pause button, which I think is a nascent point. At the same time, I also think of this moment as a great *accelerator,* because entrenched habits and routines are the enemy of change, of progress, and we've been awoken out of the habit-hypnosis, so to speak. We often do things just because this is the way we always have done them, and in a world where glaciers are melting in human timescales, we really don't have time to mess about. Full disclosure: I'm echoing Magnason here, who I recently interviewed about his fantastic new book *On Time and Water*,[3] which looks at the issue of climate change through the lens of a storyteller.

Climate change and global heating haven't gone away, and the way we were operating as a global society has been thoroughly unsustainable. I hope therefore

[2] Magnason, Andri Snær, and Anní Ólafsdóttir (2020), 'Apausalypse: Dispatch from Iceland,' *Emergence Magazine* (emergencemagazine.org/story/apausalypse-dispatch-from-iceland).

[3] Magnason, Andri Snær (2020), *On Time and Water*, tr. Lytton Smith, (Open Letter).

that we take the opportunity to restart in a much more sustainable fashion. These may seem like lofty hopes from this 'small' pandemic, but there we go.

Reference

Sostero, M., Santo, M., Hurley, J., Fernandez-Macías, E. and Bisello, M. (2020). *Teleworkability and the COVID-19 crisis: A new digital divide?* Seville: European Commission.

Post-pandemic Literature: Force and Moral Obligation to the Other in Boccaccio's *Decameron* and Camus' *The Plague*

Benjamin Barber

In a recent study titled, "Psychosocial Reactions to Plagues in the Cultural History of Medicine: A Medical Humanities Approach," medical researchers draw on works of literature—notably Boccaccio's *Decameron* (completed in 1353) and Albert Camus' *The Plague* (first published 1947)—to help psychiatrists understand the pychosocial effects of the current COVID-19 pandemic on individuals and populations. In their reflections on the texts, the researchers note that plagues typically evoke contradictory reactions among those affected by them (Wigand et al. 2020, p. 444). The texts they reference demonstrate that, during a plague, the competition between the individual's impulse to help others and his or her impulse to see to one's own needs is intense. With this tension in mind, this paper will take up the two previously mentioned literary texts and examine their differing treatments of the two types of human response to plagues. In my reading of *The Plague* I first consider how proximity to—and the imminent threat of—death may cause us to turn inward and grapple with the specter of our individual and collective mortality along with our capacity to persist and endure. Turning then to the frame plot of the *Decameron*, I highlight the way Boccaccio emphasizes humanity's capacity—in times of crisis—to turn toward others and create beauty for each other. I hope to show that these two works' representations of differing human responses to epidemics reveal our potential to elude the imperatives of, what Simone Weil terms, "force" through the experience of the transcendence that accompanies a recognition of our ethical obligation to the Other, an experience which Emmanuel Levinas contends demonstrates that we are not simply controlled by the totalizing determinism of force. Finally, by referring to the thinking of two contemporary writers, I conclude by considering two ways this recognition of the transcendence inherent to the Other may allow us to characterize the key of emerging post-pandemic literature.

B. Barber (✉)
Beijing Normal University Hong Kong Baptist University United International College, Zhuhai, China
e-mail: benjaminbarber@uic.edu.cn

S.X.B. Zhao et al. (eds.), *COVID-19 Pandemic, Crisis Responses and the Changing World*, https://doi.org/10.1007/978-981-16-2430-8_18

Literature reflects the infinite complexity of human individuals and societies back to us and, thereby, causes us to repeatedly rediscover ourselves in the midst of forces over which we have very little control. Our creative consciousnesses—having arisen from such powerful, often destructive, forces—frequently take these very same forces for the ground upon which to cast our literary self-depictions. War is one powerful instance of how these forces shape and affect humans. The circumstances created by an epidemic have often been described as analogous to a war—an irresistible force that draws in all those it comes into contact with. Indeed, *The Plague* is intended as an allegory for the Nazi occupation of France during WWII, along with the various reactions of the French people to that occupation (Judt 2001, p. viii). I will return to this fact later on. I will now define "force" with reference to its theorization by the French philosopher Simone Weil, a concept which she elaborates through her reading of a foundational piece of Western literature, *The Iliad*. The purpose of the following discussion of Weil's is to show how force, operating in the *Iliad*'s description of the Trojan war, mirrors the force exerted on human beings in large-scale epidemics.

In "The Iliad, or the Poem of Force," which "was written in the summer and fall of 1940, after the fall of France" (1965, 'Introduction to "The Illiad, or the Poem of Force,"' p. 5), Weil elaborates a metaphysics of force, opening her essay in the following way:

> The true hero, the true subject, the center of the *Iliad* is force. Force employed by man, force that enslaves man, force before which man's flesh shrinks away. In this work, at all times, the human spirit is shown as modified by its relations with force, as swept away, blinded by the very force it imagined it could handle, as deformed by the weight of the force it submits to. (Weil 1965, p. 6)

Force, for Weil, is the necessity that the human is moved and destroyed by, and the *Iliad* becomes an extended reflection on the human in the midst of that necessity. Given the time in which she wrote her commentary on The Poem of Force, as she re-titles the *Iliad*, "[i]t may be read as an indirect commentary on that tragic event, which signalized the triumph of the most extreme modern expression of force" (1965, 'Introduction to "The Illiad, or the Poem of Force,"' p. 5): the Nazi occupation and enforcement of its genocidal policies. Considering how force governs the conflict between the Greeks and the Trojans in the Trojan War, Weil focuses on the way that the advantage shifts from one individual or army to the other and back again—on one day making some soldiers the carriers of force and other soldiers subject to it and the next day inverting the arrangement. "Force is as pitiless to the man who possesses it, or thinks he does, as it is to its victims," Weil writes (1965, p. 11). "The truth is, nobody really possesses it. The human race is not divided up, in the *Iliad*, into conquered person, slaves, suppliants, on the one hand, and conquerors and chiefs on the other. In this poem there in not a single man who does not at one time or another have to bow his neck to force" (1965, p. 11). The reciprocity of violence in war becomes a great leveler, which ensures that, in time, all will cringe in fear or grieve with loss or personal suffering. The plague of war spares no one. All those connected to the combatants—even if innocent of violence themselves—are subject to it. Within the *Iliad*, soldiers are carriers and victims of the force of violence, just as every human being is a potential carrier or victim of a virus. The *Iliad* represents this ubiquitous human vulnerability to the forces that animate and threaten us.

In this way, Weil shows how we humans are embedded in—or immanent to—our force-inundated context, but is there no possibility for transcendence? Are there no avenues to escape from this thralldom to force? Weil holds that the *Iliad* does suggest such a possibility:

> [T]he despair of the soldier that drives him on to destruction, the obliteration of the slave or the conquered man, the wholesale slAugusthter—all these elements combine... to make a picture of uniform horror, of which force is the sole hero. A monotonous desolation would result were it not for those few luminous moments, scattered here and there throughout the poem, those brief, celestial moments in which man possesses his soul. (1965, p. 23)

She goes on to identify such moments in the instances of "inner deliberations," as when "Hector [prior to engaging in single combat with Achilles] ... tries to face destiny on his own terms, without the help of gods or men" (Weil 1965, p. 23). However, "[a]t other times, it is in a moment of love that men discover their souls—and there is hardly any form of pure love known to humanity of which the *Iliad* does not treat" (Weil 1965, p. 23). In her reading, the love displayed in hospitality, parent–child relationships, sibling relationships, conjugal relationships, friendships between comrades, and friendships between enemies are—what Weil terms—rare "moments of grace" that "make us feel with sharp regret what it is that violence has killed and will kill again" (1965, p. 25). These "moments of grace" are representations of the human capacity to transcend—through acts of altruistic courage and generous movement towards the other—our nature as immanent beings. Thus, in her reading of the *Iliad*, Weil shows how humanity—through the medium of literature—is able to reflect the infinite complexity of our paradoxical human nature back to us, so we may recognize that we are simultaneously profoundly imprisoned *yet* radically free beings. Our ability to commune with the Other through the through language unveils the infinite.

This apprehension of the infinite that is revealed through language is what allows us to transcend the imperatives of force. Considering our tendency to imagine force as a totalizing inevitability, the philosopher Emmanuel Levinas maintains that we are in fact transcendent beings in that we, as individuals, are infinitely distant from one another, yet primordially obligated by the face-to-face encounter to exist in communicative relation to the Other (Levinas 1991, pp. 180–81). This reality is what literature has the capacity to highlight. Taking up literature's power to disclose the moral obligations incumbent on the physician, Craig Irvine discusses the usefulness of literature through Levinas's idea of transcendence, which Levinas understands as the infinitude we encounter in the face of the Other. Quoting from Levinas, Irvine writes "The Other that I encounter remains infinitely Other, transcendent, in the encounter. The name Levinas gives to 'the way in which the other presents himself, exceeding the idea of the other in me' is 'face'" (2005, p. 10). Irvine goes on to discuss how he himself uses literature to help physicians recognize their moral obligation to the Other, as it appears in their fleeting transcendent encounters with patients who are suffering the final stages of terminal illness (p. 17). Summarizing Levinas, Irvine states that literature shows us our moral responsibility to the Other: "Literature, like science, *discloses* the face of the Other (which, *as Other*, is invisible) by clothing its nakedness in forms" (p. 14).

Levinas makes a hard distinction between totality and the infinity of the Other, yet acknowledges that, in order to perceive the infinite, totality is necessary: the "'beyond' [that exists outside] totality and objective experience is... not to be described in a purely negative fashion. It is reflected *within* totality and history, *within* experience" (Levinas 1991, p. 23). The infinitude we perceive in the face of the Other is only perceptible because of the condition of totality we inhabit—the world of force or necessity. Totality, as Levinas defines it in *Totality and Infinity*, is synonymous with war in the way that Weil defines it in "The Iliad, the Poem of Force." Levinas writes, "[d]oes not lucidity, the mind's openness upon the true, consist in catching sight of the permanent possibility of war? The state of war suspends morality; it divests the eternal institutions and obligations of their eternity and rescinds ad interim the unconditional imperatives" (p. 21). In the grip of threatening force—as manifest in war or, similarly, in a global pandemic—the obligation to act decently towards the Other is seemingly suspended, yet, because of this state of exception, the sense of obligation is all the more pressing. The moral imperative elicited by the transcendent encounter with infinitude found in the face of the Other is on full display in works of plague literature such as the *Decameron* and *The Plague*.

In turning to Boccaccio's *Decameron* and Camus' *The Plague* to query what post-pandemic literature will look like, I will examine each work's particular representation of human responses to epidemics—ensconced, as we are, in force yet, nevertheless, capable of transcendent acts of grace. The differing ways that these two authors represent these capacities will, hopefully,—when brought to bear on our current literary moment—offer some sense of what types of creative response the literary voices of our time will bring to the way we make sense of our humanity in the aftermath of the COVID-19 pandemic. I should note here that the two works I will be discussing are from very different time periods. This disparity is, to my mind, a great advantage in carrying out my purpose. We who study and write literature tend not to assume that the knowledge we have of human nature is steadily accumulating. We tend to assume that literary representations of the human predicament are iterative explorations and vary to the extent the investigators' or creators' particular experiences have enlivened their minds to emphasize certain aspects of what and who we are. In light of this, comparing a literary work from the Italian Renaissance with a post-war French existentialist novel will afford me the opportunity to exhibit the ways that changes of perspective between the Middle Ages and modern eras affect our approach to the position we occupy when beset by a plague.

Camus' novel, *The Plague*, depicts an epidemic of bubonic plague that breaks out in the French Algerian city of Oran in the 1940s. The narrator and central character is Dr. Bernard Rieux, who details the virus's progress through reference to a cast of characters who are all confined to the quarantined city, and who—like Rieux himself—are confronted with the moral dilemma of how to behave as they confront the high probability of their own deaths. Camus' deeply moral philosophy is central to the novel. As Tony Judt (2001) notes in his commentary on the novel's ethical import, "Camus was a moralist who unhesitatingly distinguished good from evil but abstained from condemning human frailty. He was a student of the 'absurd' who refused to give into necessity" (p. xv). In a review of Sartre's *Nausea*, Camus himself asserted this view of how best to confront an apparently irrational and chaotic universe filled with meaningless destruction, writing that it is a "mistake ... to believe that because life is wretched it is tragic.... To announce the absurdity of existence cannot be an objective, merely a starting point" (quoted in Judt 2001, p. xvii). Thus, if the plague in the novel is a manifestation of the seeming absurdity of force in the form of meaningless death it is also a moment for people to take action and answer the call to act morally that emanates from the face of the Other.

The plague as a manifestation of force is clearly depicted in the novel. In a conversation with a young journalist, Raymond Rambert, who is desperate to escape the city's lockdown and return to his young wife in Paris, Dr. Rieux—who has devoted himself to carrying on with his seemingly futile attempt to stop the virus in spite of being separated from his own wife—explains his own response to the chaos of the epidemic: "I have to tell you this: this whole thing [his fight against the plague] is not about heroism. It's about decency. It may seem a ridiculous idea, but the only way to fight the plague is with decency" (Camus 2001, p. 125). Dr. Rieux does not condemn Rambert's decision to escape the city—a decision Rambert ultimately renounces in favor of volunteering to help fight the virus. Thus, as Judt (2001) explains, "Camus was a *moraliste* but he was no moralizer. He claimed to have taken great care to try and avoid writing a tract, and to the extent that his novel offers little comfort to political polemicists of any school he can be said to have succeeded" (p. xv). Ultimately, Camus' work presents the individual with the moral dilemma of risking one's life to take action to quell suffering and death or shrinking in the face of one's own apparent finitude, which—as Levinas asserts—is illusory given that each individual's face is an expression of the infinite and a portal to transcendence. To turn towards the infinitude in the face of the Other is each individual's choice to make, and it is a choice that each major character in the novel is confronted with. Like Hector before the gates of Troy, each character in *The Plague* has his chance at experiencing a moment of transcendence.

Before turning to Camus' characters and their shared dilemma, I'd like to consider how we encounter the moral obligation to the Other amid the totalizing force of wars or epidemics. As I have noted, Camus' novel was written as an examination of the French people's response to the invasion of France by the Nazis and the establishment of the Vichy regime. The virus in the novel is analogous to the Nazis' presence and influence in France, and the choices of the novel's characters to either collaborate or resist the virus aligns with the French people's choice to resist or collaborate with the Nazi agenda to control all of Europe and exterminate the Jews. This most extreme form of modern, historical force underlies the novel's description of a merciless virus, which—similar to the Nazi grip on France—cripples people's capacity to act decently (to experience the infinitude of the Other) either through fear of infection (analogous to fear of penalties for defying the Nazis) or death from the disease itself (analogous to fear of execution by the Nazis for resistance). Thus, Camus' representation of the human is that of a moral being who perpetually stands at an ethical crossroads and, second by second, chooses to graciously respond to the Other or capitulate to force.

Camus represents this dilemma in his characterization of two of the central characters from the novel: Joseph Grand and Cottard. Like Dr. Rieux, Grand works to resist the virus. He is a low level clerk in Oran's Hôtel de Ville, where—in addition to his duties assigned prior to the plague—he tabulates the statistical analysis of the plague's effect on the city's population. In this capacity, he works closely with Dr. Rieux, who writes of Grand:

> he was exhausted ...but he continued none the less to do the calculations and statistics that the health teams needed. Patiently, every evening, he sorted out the card index translated it into diagrams and slowly endeavoured to present the situation in as precise a way as possible. [...] [I]f men really do have to offer themselves models and examples who they call heroes, and if there really has to be one in this story, the narrator would like to offer this insignificant and self-effacing hero who had nothing to recommend him but a little goodness in his heart .... (Camus 2001, p. 105)

In addition to his heavy load of clerical work, part of the reason for Grand's constant exhaustion is that he stays up at night attempting to perfect a sentence that he is composing as a tribute to his long lost love. In this character, Camus represents both enduring love for the common good of the city's inhabitants and an enduring personal love, which manifests the human capacity to seek transcendence in the call of the Other's face amid the immanent disaster of the plague's force.

Cottard is Grand's foil. His first appearance in the novel is after a failed suicide attempt. Eventually, the reader learns that Cottard is under investigation for unspecified crimes and, until the advent of the plague, is certain that he will be imprisoned, but the authorities become too distracted by the crisis to follow up on their investigation. For this reason, Cottard has no interest in seeing the plague come to an end. He further benefits from the epidemic by amassing wealth through smuggling goods into the locked down city. Nevertheless, Camus' narrator, Dr. Rieux, does not paint Cottard as a villain, and the other characters— Rieux, Tarrou, Rambert, and Grand, who work on the health teams—remain friendly towards him. At one point, Tarrou invites him to join with them in the health teams' efforts to fight the plague (Camus 2001, pp. 120–21). Cottard responds by asserting that "It's not my job" and stating that "this plague is doing me a favour, so I don't see why I should be involved in getting rid of it" (Camus 2001, p. 120). This is his potential moment to experience transcendence, wherein he might have acted to fulfill the moral obligation to the Other, but he does not seize it, as the other characters do. Despite his refusal to take action against the plague, Tarrou does not condemn Cottard, but only asks that he refrain from knowingly spreading the virus (Camus 2001, p. 122).

The novel's focus on simple decency in the face of mass suffering and death is its moral core. This is clear in Rieux's response to the sermon given by Father Paneloux—a respected Jesuit priest. As the virus takes hold of Oran, a wave of religiosity sweeps through the populace, who attend a mass, during which Paneloux, delivers a fiery sermon declaring that the plague is God's just punishment for the city's sins. Later, in a private conversation Tarrou asks Rieux what he thinks of the sermon. Rieux says that he does not think Paneloux or most Christians really believe the sermon's rhetoric. Tarrou presses further asking Rieux whether or not he believes in God (Camus 2001, p. 96). Rieux responds: "I am in darkness, trying to see the light. I stopped a long time ago thinking there was anything unusual in that" (Camus 2001, p. 91). Continuing to elaborate the nature of this darkness by reflecting on his horror at the fact of death even, and especially, given his profession as a physician, Rieux states: "since the order of the world is governed by death, perhaps it is better for God that we should not believe in Him and struggle with all our strength against death, without raising our eyes to heaven and to His silence" (Camus 2001, p. 98). The force of death—relentlessly manifest in the plague—is what Camus' proxy Rieux understands as the counter force against which the human must define itself by trying to see the light through acts of decency directed towards the face of the Other. This is Camus' view of the human situation in the mid-twentieth century: the individual virtually alone, in the dark, and—almost pointlessly—attempting to act morally vis-à-vis the Other.

The darkness Rieux acts in is briefly broken up by dim rays of creative light that come from Grand's private literary aspirations. As noted above, when he is not tirelessly compiling data at the Hôtel de Ville, Grand works on a manuscript that has run to many pages in length. At first he is reticent to talk to the other characters about the manuscript, but eventually he reveals that he is attempting to perfect the first sentence, which runs: "On a fine morning in the month of May, an elegant woman was riding a magnificent sorrel mare through the flowered avenues of the Bois de Boulogne" (Camus 2001, p. 80). He is so obsessive that he is constantly changing the syntax, diction, and structure of the line, yet he is never completely satisfied. Eventually—when Grand catches the plague and asks Rieux to burn his manuscript—Rieux discovers that the manuscript is meant as a gift to Grand's lost love, Jeanne, and it is completely composed of his repeated attempts to perfect the first sentence. Working in utter solitude, and without substantive promise of finding Jeanne, Grand persists in creativity against all odds of even the slightest recognition. Thus, the will to create as a response to the face of the Other is cast by Camus as an individual's inward struggle to create beauty amid the play of destructive force.

As an instance of plague literature, Camus' novel represents humans grappling with the force of a catastrophic, and seemingly meaningless, event. The novel shows the disparate ways humans react to such events and—through the voice of its central character, Rieux—advocates taking the high moral route of working to respond with generosity to the needs of the Other in spite of the temptation to become paralyzed by despair. Written at an earlier time, the *Decameron* comes to similar conclusions through different means. The Christian humanism of Boccaccio's novel represents a different response to the temptation to selfish indifference through its description of youths, who—quarantining themselves during a time of plague—band together to affirm their sense of the moral obligation to act liberally towards the Other.

The framing narrative of the *Decameron* is a story of creation and restoration, with all of the import those terms have in the Christian society Boccaccio writes from within. The novel is the story of ten young men and women who leave the plague ridden Florence of 1348 and take refuge in beautiful villas in the countryside, where they entertain each other with song, dance, and—especially—story telling.

The tales they tell make up the bulk of the novel, but it is the background against which they are told—the horror and moral chaos caused by the plague—that gives these stories and their telling their greatest significance. As Jonathan Usher explains, Boccaccio promotes the form of the vernacular novel by showing its creative and regenerative capacities. Boccaccio's.

> [p]romotion starts with the title: *Decameron* ('Ten Days', in Boccaccio's approximate Greek), imitates *Hexameron*, St Ambrose's commentary on the six days of creation in Genesis. Whilst numerically indicative of the ten days of story-telling, the title's suggestion of the [biblical] Creation (and attendant Fall) cannot be ignored—a theme of inescapable topicality after the calamity of the plague, and a pointer to fiction's own power of regeneration. (Usher 2008, p. xx)

Boccaccio's allusion to the Genesis narrative of the Creation of the human and its Fall, which inaugurates Death's reign, highlights the profound tension that Weil illuminates in her rendering of the human as caught between its capacity for transcendence (or grace) and destructive force that humans, all too often, become agents of. Nevertheless, for Boccaccio, having been ourselves made by God in God's own image, we are inherently creative and, thereby, capable of fulfilling our obligation to the Other—who is also made in God's image—in spite of the grisly horror of the plague.

The Renaissance is known as the period in which the intellectual and cultural movement of humanism began to burgeon and flourish. Boccaccio is a luminary of this period, and, as we know, this movement would drive an enormous wave of creativity in every field of human endeavor. Attention to classical literatures of the past powered the creativity and innovation of the Renaissance (Robinson 2015, p. 3), wherein Boccaccio sets out—like his contemporaries, Petrarch and Dante (Usher 2008, p. xx)—to elevate and dignify vernacular works of literature, such as his novel *The Decameron*, which was written in Florentine Tuscan. It is because of his Renaissance humanist excitement over the possibilities of contemporary human creativity and development that the characters in Boccaccio's great work band together—in the midst of fear, loss, and grief—to create a retreat and a chance for moral renewal with the stories they tell.

In order to show these creative capacities to their greatest advantage, Boccaccio vividly illustrates the dehumanizing and demoralizing nature of the 1348 plague. After apologizing to his readers for the images he is about to present them with, he describes the circumstances created by the ravages of the bubonic plague in Florence:

> As there was not sufficient consecrated ground in which to bury the vast number of corpses that arrived at every church day after day … [little] effort had been made to give each person his own burial plot in accordance with age-old custom, enormous pits were dug in the graveyards, once saturation point had been reached, and new arrivals were dropped into these by the hundred; here they were packed in layers … and each layer would get a thin covering of earth until the pit was filled up. (Boccaccio 2008, p. 13)

The citizen's reactions to the contagion varied from person to person. Some people locked themselves up in their houses, isolating themselves from the possibility of contracting the virus and showing indifference to the suffering of their fellow citizens.

Others gave themselves over to excess, drunkenness, and sexual promiscuity. Parents abandoned their sick children and fled the city rather than risk contracting the plague. The disparate responses and mass death lead to a breakdown in the social order both within the city and in the surrounding countryside. As Usher puts it, "[u]rban desolation gives way to rural mortality, where humans, once the higher authority, have abdicated, leaving domestic animals to maintain their former routines as if endowed with human reason" (Usher 2008, p. xxii). It is against this desolate and horrifying backdrop that the reader is introduced to the novel's principal characters, who will band together to create an orderly society out of chaos.

Meeting in a church where they have come to pray and practice the pious rituals that they continue to observe, seven young ladies—whose immediate families have already died or fled—come together to discuss the possibility of giving themselves a respite from the ghastly and dangerous precincts of Florence. They are accompanied by three young men, who are kinsmen of two of the ladies—a detail intended to protect the group from the taint of sexual impropriety. All of the choices Boccaccio makes for the group of story-telling young people are calculated to depict them as reasonable and responsible (Usher 2008, p. xxiii). Even though many of the stories they tell will deal with bawdy subject matter the storytellers themselves remain above reproach, a fact which is borne out in the equitable society and set of rules they make for themselves to follow after they have left the city with their servants and taken up residence in a beautiful abandoned villa. As Usher (2008) explains, "the party legislate their existence, establishing daily routines, schedules for servants, and, most importantly, a rota of leadership. Each narrator is to rule for one day [...] ...the company has other diversions—music, dancing, chess" (p. xxiv). However, story-telling in paramount among these pastimes, "because its pleasures are mutual" (Usher 2008, p. xxiv). In this way, "Boccaccio alerts his readers to the ideal community not only between narrator and listener, but also between different listeners" (Usher 2008, p. xxiv). The creator may take pleasure in the act of story-telling just as the appreciator takes pleasure in experiencing the story, and the groups' discussion of the stories enriches each auditor's particular appreciation of them. Attending to the call of the Others' faces by creating a mutually beneficial and entertaining society, the story-tellers and listeners encounter the transcendent infinitude unique to each member of the group.

The stories, or novellas, that the ten story-tellers tell each other cover universal themes of human experience. Each day, save the first and ninth, has a theme assigned to it by the King or Queen in charge of the day. The daily themes are juxtaposed with each other. I will return to the exception of the first and ninth days in a moment, but—in Usher's summary (2008, pp. xxiv–xxv)—the theme for the second day is humanity's subjection to fate and, therefore, an oblique reflection on the circumstance of the plague. Day three considers how fate may ultimately benefit human beings. Days four and five take up the theme of love. First, showing how it can be destructive and then showing how one may profit from it. The sixth day takes up language, beginning with a story on the very problem of telling a good story. The seventh day addresses the way wives may dupe their husbands, and the eighth day predictably reflects on the ways husbands lie to their wives. The tenth and final day foregrounds the virtue of open handedness or generosity—otherwise known as liberality: a central value of Renaissance humanist thought.

The virtue of liberality is manifest in the decision of the monarchs for the first and ninth days, as they allow the story tellers to choose their own themes on those days thereby exhibiting a generosity of spirit that refuses to impose the agreed upon strictures of the story-teller's society too exactingly. In these gestures of liberality, Boccaccio signals that human creativity derives from a mixture of structure and freedom from the constraints of structure. Ultimately, by addressing universal human experiences of fate, love, sex, language, deceit, and virtue, the story-tellers go towards each Other in this spirit of liberal generosity to create a transcendent experience that abstracts them from the immanent force of the plague. This transcendent movement towards the Other is contingent on the communicative encounter between faces, as described by Levinas.

Summarizing, Levinas' understanding of such encounters Pierre Hayat writes, "The face of the other is the locus of transcendence in that it calls into question the *I* in its existence as a being for itself. There is in this something like a trauma of transcendence that prevents the *I* from remaining within itself, and carries it to the limits of itself" (1999, p. xiv). Boccaccio's youths' mutual accord and attendant moral renewal is based on their face-to-face encounter through the stories they tell each other within the liberal, yet decent, structure of their quarantine. They establish this quarantine through equitable deliberation, in which they are always ready to defer to each other's tastes, comfort, and needs.

This readiness to call the *I* into question appears in the conclusion of the *Decameron*, wherein the frame narrative of the novel recognizes the fragile and fleeting nature of transcendent experiences. Like the moments of grace that are scattered through the *Illiad*, the experience of abstracting oneself (as a reader, listener, or as a narrator) cannot go on indefinitely. The ten young people's sojourn in the country—like the stories they tell each other—must eventually come to an end. In the conclusion of *The Decameron*, the tenth day's monarch, Pamphilo, suggests that it is time for the group to return to Florence, lest they corrupt the community they have created through their natural moral frailty. Pamphilo explains: "Now, in case our present life should go stale with repetition and give rise to something noxious, and to allay criticism over our extended absence … it would seem to me … that we would do well to return whence we came" (Boccaccio 2008, p. 679). The following day, the group returns to the church where they began their journey in Florence and take leave of each other. For each of them it is necessary, ultimately, to attend to those other Others—the residents of Florence still struggling with the difficulties, miseries, and horrors of the plague.

In the comparisons and distinctions I am attempting to draw between *The Decameron* and *The Plague*, this idea that humans recognize that they are subject to force—in Weil's definition—is shared. While Camus foregrounds meaningless suffering and death, Boccaccio presents chaos as meaningfully comprehensible—and in the grand order of things transcendable—within the Christian narrative of history. However, Camus' novel differs from Boccaccio's novel in its recognition that human creativity appears first as an internal, personal activity—rather than a collective, outward-moving activity. Thus, its affordance of meaningful transcendent experience is a great personal struggle. As previously noted, Camus' characters Grand and Rieux—though part of a small disparately connected group—are hesitant to open themselves up to one another while they bravely and tirelessly suffer personal loss and grief, with little hope of restoration. However, Boccaccio's characters are fully engaged with one another in a matrix of collectively agreed upon order and through the effervescent, joyful generosity of each individual's creative contribution to the other members of the group. This polarity in emphasis in the two authors' respective representations of the human condition is what I wish to focus on in my concluding consideration of what post-pandemic literature may look like. Between these two configurations of how humans transcendently move to the limits of them self in spite of force, where will most literary works stand in the near future? Phrased another way, where will authors largely place the emphasis on the ways our capacity for transcendence expresses itself in private internal struggle and public, outwardly-oriented acts?

Having elaborated two past works of literature that represent human beings' to experience transcendence in the midst of both war and pestilence, I will briefly consider how contemporary authors are thinking about the human capacity to transcend the force of the ongoing COVID-19 pandemic. Two contemporary literary voices are Anne Enright (whose novel *The Gathering* won the 2007 Booker Prize) and author Marilynne Robinson (whose novel *Gilead* won the 2005 Pulitzer Prize for Fiction). As I'll show, Enright's response reflects Camus' depiction of the sense of meaninglessness that accompanies the shock that the pandemic has visited upon us, a shock which reminds us of our need for, and obligation to, the Other. Robinson's response tends to reflect the behavior of Boccaccio's youths, who turn towards each other and, in good will and respect for each other's infinitude, confer regarding what type of society they would like to create in response to the force of the plague. Thus, both authors offer the hope of making the force of the pandemic an opportunity to experience transcendence by going to the limits of the *I* and answering the call towards the infinite inherent in the face of the Other.

In late March, in a dispatch piece for *The New York Review of Books*, Enright relates her first impressions of how news of the pandemic hitting the U.S. affected her as she was on a book tour on that country's Northeastern Seaboard. She comments initially on the political backdrop—specifically her own attempts to parse the president's contradictory responses to the emerging crisis. She then relates the radical simplification of her perceptions and understanding as the magnitude of the crisis swept over her. Overhearing people expressing heated opinions in a hotel bar, Enright (2020) writes:

> I deal in words for a living, but I have had difficulty forming them, since that moment, whether to describe or analyze. I don't really understand them anymore. I understand touch, breath, contact. I understand plane tickets—I booked one as the price rose under me, the morning after Trump's address. I took a car toward Cambridge and turned left for Logan airport. I understand the word "home."

The impression her dispatch gives is one of a person stunned to silence by an overwhelming, incomprehensible force that drives her towards her loved ones. Speaking candidly, Enright admits her sense of incapacity to affect a transcendent experience through language. Rather, she needs to see the faces of those she loves. Like that of Grand struggling to find just the right word in his first sentence or the young people at a loss before they leave plague ridden Florence, she acknowledges the essential human need to move towards the embodied other with "touch, breath, contact" (Enright 2020). This concern for the obligation to, and need for, the Other is echoed in her final statement: "The U.S. was not testing people, because America values private medicine over communal health. That is why the numbers were low, because Trump said, 'I like the numbers being where they are.' I don't even have the wherewithal to feel stupid about all this. I cannot find a tone" (Enright 2020). Implicit in this statement, I think, is the intention to write about the collective human capacity to meet the responsibility that the face of the Other imposes upon us. Thus, it functions as an indictment of the self-interested indifference to human suffering that Trump's words represent. Enright echoes Rieux's sense of appalled incomprehension, while—by implication—advocating a turn towards others in practical, material, and—eventually, when deep analysis is again possible—creative acts of generosity.

On June 11th, Marilynne Robinson's piece—"What Kind of Country Do We Want?"—appeared in *The New York Review of Books.* Robinson (2020) writes from quarantine, which she refers to as "my odd solitude." Her solitude—mitigated, as it is, with the means of communication and media of our time—amounts to a twenty-first century *Decameron* experience. She begins her essay by reflecting that present day America has fallen short of the possibilities its founding ideals, intellectual achievements, and wealth might have afforded it and then—turning to the pandemic—reflects:

> Before there was a viral crisis whose reality forced itself on our notice, there were reports of declines of life expectancy in America, rising rates of suicide, and other "deaths of despair." This is surely evidence of another crisis, though it was rarely described as such. The novel coronavirus has the potential for mitigation, treatment, and ultimately prevention. But a decline in hope and purpose is a crisis of civilization requiring reflection and generous care for the good of the whole society and its place in the world. We have been given the grounds and opportunity to do some very basic thinking. (Robinson 2020)

Just as Boccaccio does in the *Decameron,* Robinson reasserts the primacy of the Renaissance value of liberality—or "generous care"—which necessarily manifests in the way we relate to the bare fact of our obligation to the Other. Reflecting on this obligation, her analysis begins with a critique of the global economic system which focuses on the expansion of profit margins at the expense of human welfare in the realms of spiritual, intellectual, and physical wellbeing. She goes on to champion the virtues of a liberal education and decry the obsession with cost/benefit analysis, the idea of scarcity, and the general economic Darwinism that keeps many Americans in poverty in order to enrich a few. "Emergencies," Robinson (2020) writes, "remind us that people admire selflessness and enjoy demands on their generosity, and that the community as a whole is revivified by such demands." Ultimately, she says, there is a "need to recover and sharpen a functioning sense of justice based on a reverent appreciation of humankind, all together and one by one. The authenticity of our understanding must be demonstrated in our attempting to act justly even at steep cost to ourselves" (Robinson 2020). The tendency of Robinson's thinking is an indicator of the themes that will inform her post-pandemic literary production, which has—in her novels—always scrutinized the individual choice to act gracefully in response to the Other's particularity and fragility in spite of the overwhelming forces of history.

These contemporary authors forward the idea that the Other's face calls us to act amid, and through, the totalizing forces I've just mentioned. Indeed, like Camus' characters these authors will challenge their readers to an internal reckoning. However, this reckoning need not take place alone and in the shadows. Post-pandemic literature will tend to view this moment of force's apparent triumph as a moment to confront human suffering in all its forms both as artists—like the Florentine storytellers—and as agents of material and physical care—like Rieux, Tarrou, Grand, and Rambert. Whether, as with Enright, it comes with a preparatory recoiling from the incomprehensibility of current ineffectual leadership's self-serving rhetoric; or, like with Robinson, it comes from a return to basic thinking about how we should act to care for our fellow humans instead of endless economic growth and profit for a few; the themes that will drive post-pandemic literature will be concerned with acknowledging the responsibility that the face of the Other calls us to and, thereby, going to the limits of the *I* in order to apprehend the infinite nature of the individual human within the totalizing force we inhabit.

References

Boccaccio, G. (2008) *The Decameron*. Oxford: Oxford University Press.

Camus, A. (2001) *The Plague*. London: Penguin.

Enright, A. (2020) Anne Enright, Pandemic Journal, March 17–22. *The New York Review of Books*, 22 Mar [online]. Available at: https://www.nybooks.com/daily/2020/03/22/pandemic-journal/ (Accessed 17 August 2020).

Introduction to "The Illiad, or the Poem of Force," (1965) *Chicago Review*, 18(2), 5.

Hayat, Pierre. (1999) 'Preface.' *Alterity and Transcendence*. Trans. Michael B. Smith, pp. ix–xxiv.

Irvine, C. (2005) The other side of silence: Levinas, medicine, and literature. *Literature and Medicine*, 24(1), 8–18.

Judt, T. (2001) Introduction. *The Plague*. London: Penguin, pp. vii–xvii.

Levinas, E. (1991) *Totality and Infinity: An Essay on Exteriority*. Dordrecht: Kluwer.

Robinson, M. (2015) *The Givenness of Things: Essays*. Toronto: Harper Perennial.

Robinson, M. (2020) What kind of country do we want? *The New York Review of Books*, 11 Jun [online]. Available at: https://www.nybooks.com/articles/2020/06/11/what-kind-of-country-do-we-want/ (Accessed 17 August 2020).

Usher, J. (2008) Introduction. *The Decameron*. Oxford: Oxford University Press, pp. xv–xxxii.

Weil, S. (1965) The Illiad, or the poem of force. *Chicago Review*, 18(2), 5–30.

Wigand, M. E., Becker, T., and Steger, F. (2020) Psychosocial reactions to plagues in the cultural history of medicine: a medical humanities approach. *The Journal of Nervous and Mental Disease Volume*, 208(6), 443–44.

Embracing Digital Teaching and Learning: Innovation Upon COVID-19 in Higher Education

Edith M. Y. Yan

Abstract The sudden outbreak of COVID-19 forced most schools and universities around the world to abruptly change their instructional delivery from the traditional face-to-face to the fully online mode, which was an unprecedented experience for most teachers and students. This chapter surveys empirical studies that were conducted between January and July 2020 on university teaching and learning in order to provide a picture of how the new mode of teaching and learning has evolved in higher education settings. Twenty journal articles and five conference papers were reviewed for (1) new teaching and learning methods/strategies/technologies that are reported being used, (2) learning skills and practical knowledge that students gained when taking part in the teaching and learning activities, (3) aspects of teachers' professional development when implementing the teaching and learning activities. It was found that the empirical research of new teaching and learning methods/strategies/technologies used during the pandemic tended to focus on common e-learning applications/platforms/resources/devices (60%), preference for e-learning (32%), engaging e-learning techniques/strategies (24%), online adaptation to practice-based courses (20%), and specific e-learning applications/platforms (8%). This chapter ends with discussion of transformational and transcendent use of new technologies in teaching and learning for future higher education.

1 Introduction

The World Health Organization was first alerted to cases of atypical pneumonia in Wuhan, China, on 31 December 2019, and requested information on the reported cases from the Chinese authorities on 1 January 2020, which marked the beginning of the global outbreak of the COVID-19 pandemic. Based on a desktop analysis of direct university and government sources, news articles, and higher education outlets for 20 countries/territories collected in March 2020, Crawford et al. (2020)

E. M. Y. Yan (✉)
Beijing Normal University-Hong Kong Baptist University United International College, Zhuhai, China
e-mail: edithyan@uic.edu.cn

S.X.B. Zhao et al. (eds.), *COVID-19 Pandemic, Crisis Responses and the Changing World*, https://doi.org/10.1007/978-981-16-2430-8_19

reported the diverse responses of the universities across these countries/territories to the complex challenges of COVID-19 until March 2020. While only a few countries/territories (including mainland China, Hong Kong, India, South Korea, and South Africa) took the approach of extending the semester break in higher education, most countries/territories (such as Australia, Germany, Italy, the UK, mainland China, Hong Kong, Malaysia, South Korea, South Africa, etc.) had a country-wide/territory-wide policy on closing university campuses. These countries, except for Malaysia,[1] implemented an online mode of instruction to support students to continue with their studies (Crawford et al. 2020).

Such a sudden shift of instructional delivery from the traditional face-to-face to the fully online mode posed many challenges to students, teachers and educational institutions. Rasheed et al. (2020) reviewed previous studies, from 2014 to 2018, on the online component of blended learning instruction and identified challenges faced by the three types of stakeholder when employing online instruction. The key challenges faced by students involve self-regulation and using technology effectively for studying; teachers' challenges are mainly their unwillingness and negative perception of using technology for instruction; and educational institutions mainly find it difficult in providing suitable instructional technology and effective training support to teachers (Rasheed et al. 2020). The challenges from the perspectives of these three types of stakeholder indeed are interrelated. For example, students' ability to make proper use of learning technology and teachers' willingness to include technology in teaching largely depend on the technological infrastructure and support provided by their institutions.

On the other hand, the COVID-19 crisis may present an opportunity to mitigate the challenges of online teaching and learning. For example, during the pandemic period, most universities in countries, like China, Israel, the Philippines, and the U.S., provided academic staff with training on creating online courses and using a learning management system (LMS) through the institution's website or by direct online instructions (Cohen and Sabag 2020; Cuaton 2020; Kessler et al. 2020; Mulla et al. 2020; Ross and DiSalvo 2020; Zhu 2020). In China, the Ministry of Education also required providers of all LMSs offered in the country to provide technical support services to ensure online teaching could be run smoothly (Zhu 2020). It has been pointed out that faculty, including those who had been resistant to adopting e-learning tools for instruction before the crisis, had to implement online teaching and learning during the pandemic and realized the advantages and limitations of e-learning solutions; the experience may motivate them to couple e-learning with face-to-face instruction in the post-pandemic world (Mulla et al. 2020). Regarding the support offered to students during the pandemic, some universities had coaches reaching out to students proactively, suggesting techniques for time management and prompting them to connect with each other to reduce the challenges of learning

[1] The Ministry of Higher Education Malaysia declared that online mode of instruction may only be conducted if adequate preparation was done and students had satisfactory Internet connection (Kamal et al. 2020).

remotely (Kessler et al. 2020; Ross and DiSalvo 2020; Zhu 2020). Course instructors were also recommended to use the LMS analytics to track how often students view the material posted on the LMS as an indicator of how well they were involved in the course (Ross and DiSalvo 2020). As long as students' emotional and technical needs were addressed, the positive experience of online learning during the pandemic will be carried over and they may participate more actively in the online component of blended learning courses in the post-pandemic world. Indeed, scholars have considered the COVID-19 crisis a catalyst for the development and integration of novel technological resources to blended learning and distance learning in higher education (Cohen and Sabag 2020; Longhurst et al. 2020).

In view of the possible development and innovation in higher education during the pandemic, I carried out a systematic review of the empirical studies that were conducted between January and July 2020 on the positive experiences of university teaching and learning in order to provide a clearer picture of how teaching and learning has evolved in higher education settings. This study was guided by the following research questions:

RQ1: What empirical research was undertaken on the positive experiences of teaching and learning in higher education settings between January and July 2020? At what instructional levels (pre-university foundation, undergraduate, or postgraduate), with what target populations (students, teachers, or administrators) and their discipline areas, and in what countries/territories were these studies conducted?

RQ2: What new teaching and learning methods/strategies/technologies that are acceptable to teachers and students are reported as being used during the pandemic?

RQ3: What learning skills and practical knowledge are reported as having been gained by students who take part in teaching and learning activities online during the pandemic?

RQ4: What aspects of teachers' professional skills are reported as having been developed through the implementation of teaching and learning activities online during the pandemic?

2 Method

Literature published in English in 2020 was reviewed systematically to answer the research questions. Following the procedures outlined in Macaro et al. (2011) and Rasheed et al. (2020), the review process can be divided into three parts: literature search process, review with inclusion/exclusion criteria, and in-depth review.

2.1 Literature Search Process

First, two databases, Scopus and IEEE Xplore, were searched in early-mid August 2020. The two databases were selected because they contained both journal articles and conference papers related to education and technology. A search string, *(coronavirus OR COVID-19) AND ("higher education" OR university) AND (teaching OR learning)*, was keyed into the search option of the two databases. The published years were limited to 2020 and onwards, and the document types were confined to journal articles and conference papers. A total of 226 results were generated from Scopus and 54 results from IEEE Xplore. In addition, Google Scholar was queried to check for any missing suitable entries. Because too many results were generated, the search string for Google Scholar was refined as *(coronavirus OR COVID-19) AND ("higher education" OR university) AND (e-learning OR "distance learning" OR "online learning")*. The years of publication were also limited to 2020 and onwards, and books and patents were excluded. A total of 4680 results were generated, yet the search after the first 230 results was stopped when the relevancy of the results became lower.

2.2 Review with Inclusion/Exclusion Criteria

Inclusion and exclusion criteria were set to identify the studies to be included for in-depth review. The studies would be included if meeting all of the following criteria:

1. The paper reported empirical research with a clear data collection method;
2. The study is on teaching and learning in higher education settings;
3. The data were collected between January and July 2020 or during the pandemic in the country/territory; and
4. The paper was published in an English academic journal or conference proceedings.

Studies were excluded if falling into any of the following categories:

1. The paper is a commentary, book review or literature review;
2. The study is about pedagogy sharing, learning analytics, or e-learning tool/platform/system evaluation for the purpose of validating a theoretical model;
3. The study focuses on psychological aspects, socio-economic factors, or university/programme administration rather than aspects of teaching and learning in online class settings; and
4. The study reports only the challenges, difficulties or inadequacies of adopting certain e-learning tools/strategies/approaches.

First, the abstract and method sections of each paper selected from the databases were reviewed briefly according to the inclusion/exclusion criteria. This yielded a preliminary result of 53 studies. Then, the abstract, method, results and conclusion sections of these 53 papers were reviewed again carefully to ensure the studies to be included contain findings that reported positive teaching and learning experience in online class settings at university level. Twenty-eight studies were excluded after careful consideration according to the inclusion/exclusion criteria. This yielded a total of 25 studies (20 journal articles and 5 conference papers) for in-depth review.

2.3 In-Depth Review and Data Analysis

Each of the 25 papers was examined in detail to extract the relevant information to answer the defined research questions. All data were entered into an Excel spreadsheet, which included columns relevant to RQ1 (*Author & date*, *Research method*, *Instructional level [pre-university foundation/undergraduate/postgraduate]*, *Participants [students/teachers/administrators]*, *Discipline areas of participants*, *Country/Territory*, and *Sample size*), RQ2 (*New pedagogy*), RQ3 (*Student learning*), and RQ4 (*Teachers' professional development*). After that, data for RQ2 to RQ4 were duplicated into separate spreadsheets for further data analysis.

Thematic analysis was employed to analyze the data for RQ2 and RQ3. The extracted information for each of RQ2 and RQ3 was first read through for initial inductive coding. Then, the data was reviewed a second time to make adjustments to the initial codes and combine some similar codes. After that, the codes were considered for any emerging themes. Data were re-read to sort into these categories of themes and codes. Whenever the author had difficulties in assigning a code or theme to the extracted information, the original paper was reconsidered through again to determine the most appropriate code or theme.

3 Results and Discussion

Twenty-five empirical studies conducted between January and July 2020 were identified relating to the positive experiences of teaching and learning in higher education settings, which captured a wide range of research contexts. Among them, findings from 24 studies offered relevant information to answer RQ2, findings from six studies relevant to RQ3, and findings from three studies relevant to RQ4. Figure 1 summarizes the data extraction from the 25 studies for the four research questions. In this section, results related to each research question are presented and discussed one by one. After that, the future development of teaching and learning in higher education is discussed, followed by the comments on the limitations of the present study.

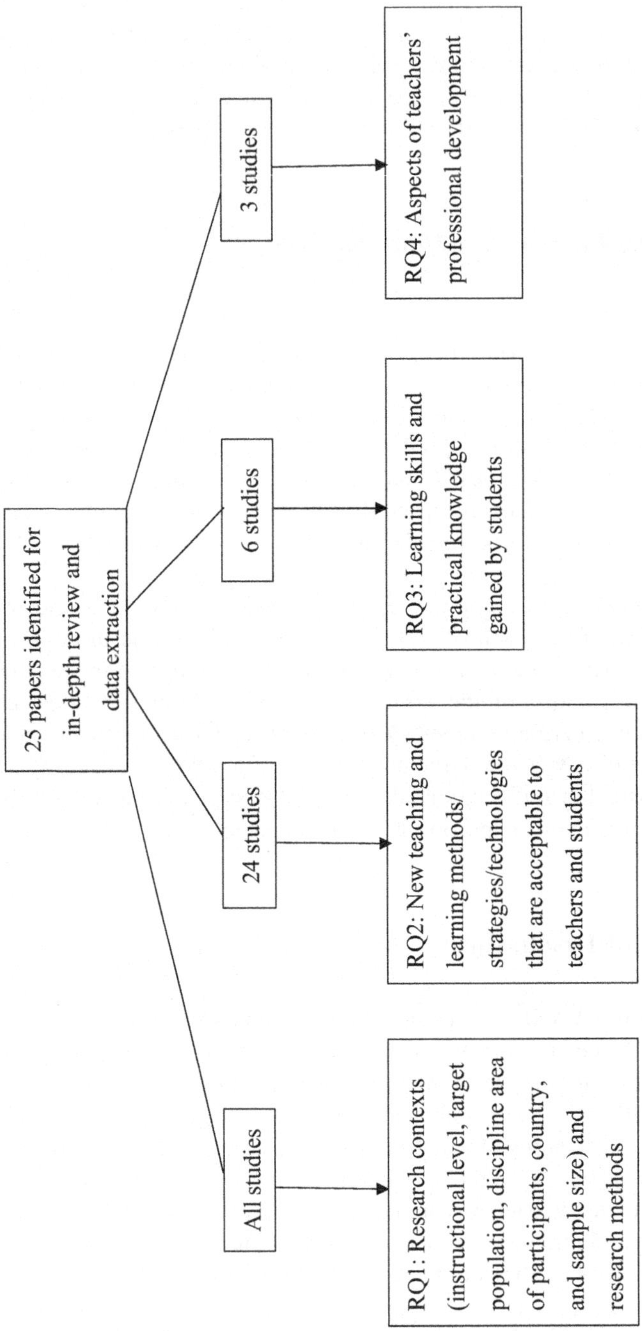

Fig. 1 A diagrammatic representation of data extraction from the papers under in-depth review for the research questions of the present study

3.1 RQ1: Research Contexts and Methods of the Empirical Research Identified Relating to the Positive Teaching and Learning Experience in Higher Education Settings During the Pandemic

Table 1 shows the research contexts and methods of the 25 studies identified for in-depth review. Most of the studies (60%) were quantitative research using questionnaire survey; 24% of the studies were qualitative, employing a range of qualitative research methods, such as interviews, focus groups, classroom observations, surveys with open-ended questions, and diaries and reflective journals; and 16% of the studies were mixed-methods research, which might be a combination of questionnaire surveys and interviews, or questionnaire surveys and evaluation of students performance through observations or grading essay assignments. The high percentage of studies employing only questionnaire surveys for investigation might be due to the urgency of collecting data and publishing the findings. The studies were primarily carried out between March and May 2020 when fully online teaching was implemented in the semester, and many of these studies were published online between May and early July so that the findings could be applied to the following new semester if there would still be a strong reliance on online teaching and learning. Questionnaire surveys, if constructed well, have the strengths of fast and relatively straightforward data processing, though the depth of investigation might be limited (Dörnyei 2007).

The sample of 25 studies captured a wide range of research contexts. Though as many as 40% of the studies did not indicate the instructional level they investigated, 32% of the studies focused on programmes/courses at undergraduate level and 24% of studies were on both undergraduate and postgraduate levels. There was also one study on programmes at pre-university foundation level. Regarding the target populations, 60% of the studies collected data from students, 20% of the studies from teachers and/or administrators, and 20% of the studies from both students and teachers and/or administrators. In terms of the participants' disciplinary areas, 24% of the studies dealt with health-related disciplines, 16% of the studies addressed disciplines related to science and technology, 12% of the studies addressed disciplines related to business and management, 4% of the studies were related to social science, and 16% of the studies covered a range of disciplinary areas. In addition, 28% of the studies did not indicate the disciplinary areas of the participants, who might be from a range of disciplinary areas. A high proportion of the studies was found relating to health-related disciplines and disciplines related to science and technology. These two discipline areas consisted of practice-based courses, which could be affected most during the pandemic. Thus, some studies focused on the impact of COVID-19 on the practice-based courses in these discipline areas and investigated their adaption to a fully online mode. Regarding the countries/territories where the studies were located, most of the studies were from Asian countries (64%), in particular South Asian countries (44%), and the rest of them (36%) were from North America, Europe, Africa and Oceania. According to the United Nations (2020), the Asian and African

Table 1 Research contexts and methods of the empirical research identified relating to the positive teaching and learning experience in higher education settings during the pandemic

Author and date	Research method	Instructional level (pre-university foundation/undergraduate/postgraduate)	Participants (students/teachers/administrators)	Discipline areas of participants	Country/Territory	Sample size
Abbasi et al. (2020)	Questionnaire survey	Undergraduate	Students	Medicine, Dentistry	Pakistan	377
Bahassoan et al. (2020)	Questionnaire survey	Undergraduate	Students	Management	Indonesia	115
Bordoloi et al. (2020)	Questionnaire survey	Not specified	Students, teachers, librarians	Not specified	India	120 (66% teachers, 21% students, 13% librarians)
Craig et al. (2020)	Questionnaire surveys and analysing essay assignments	Undergraduate	Students	Not specified	U.S.A.	49
Edelhauser and Lupu-Dima (2020)	Questionnaire survey	Undergraduate, postgraduate	Students	Mining, Mechanical & Electrical Engineering, Science	Romania	209
Gill et al. (2020)	Questionnaire surveys	Not specified	Students, teachers	Not specified	Mainland China	88 students, 16 teachers

(continued)

Table 1 (continued)

Author and date	Research method	Instructional level (pre-university foundation/undergraduate/postgraduate)	Participants (students/teachers/administrators)	Discipline areas of participants	Country/Territory	Sample size
Hoq (2020)	Questionnaire survey	Not specified	Teachers	Management & Information Technology	Saudi Arabia	28
Johnson et al. (2020)	Questionnaire survey	Not specified	Teachers, administrators	Not specified	U.S.A.	897
Kamal et al. (2020)	Questionnaire survey	Pre-university foundation	Students	Physical Science, Life Science, Science	Malaysia	557
Kapasia et al. (2020)	Questionnaire survey	Undergraduate, postgraduate	Students	Arts, Science, Commerce	India	232
Lall and Singh (2020)	Questionnaire survey	Not specified	Students	Pharmacy, Management, Computer Applications, Technology	India	200
Longhurst et al. (2020)	Questionnaire survey (with all open-ended questions)	Not specified	Administrators	Anatomy	U.K., Republic of Ireland	14 medical schools
Malan (2020)	Second cycle of action research (with student survey)	Undergraduate	Students, teacher	Accounting	South Africa	46 students, 1 teacher

(continued)

Table 1 (continued)

Author and date	Research method	Instructional level (pre-university foundation/undergraduate/postgraduate)	Participants (students/teachers/administrators)	Discipline areas of participants	Country/Territory	Sample size
Mukhtar et al. (2020)	Focus groups	Undergraduate	Students, teachers	Medicine, Dentistry	Pakistan	12 students, 12 teachers
Nadeak (2020)	Questionnaire survey	Not specified	Students	Not specified	Indonesia	250
Pather et al. (2020)	Written reflections	Undergraduate, postgraduate	Teachers	Anatomy, Histology, Embryology	Australia, New Zealand	18
Rahiem (2020)	Diaries, reflective essays, focus groups	Not specified	Students	Social Science	Indonesia	80
Rajhans et al. (2020)	Questionnaire survey	Undergraduate, postgraduate	Teachers	Optometry	India	78
Ramos-Morcillo et al. (2020)	Interviews	Undergraduate, postgraduate	Students	Nursing	Spain	32
Saif Almuraqab (2020)	Questionnaire survey	Undergraduate, postgraduate	Students	Business, Engineering & IT, Law	Saudi Arabia	133
Sobaih et al. (2020)	Questionnaire survey, interviews	Undergraduate	Students, teachers	Tourism & Hotel	Egypt	309 students, 304 teachers

(continued)

Table 1 (continued)

Author and date	Research method	Instructional level (pre-university foundation/undergraduate/postgraduate)	Participants (students/teachers/administrators)	Discipline areas of participants	Country/Territory	Sample size
Wang et al. (2020)	Questionnaire survey	Not specified	Students	Engineering	Hong Kong	496
Wargadinata et al. (2020)	Questionnaire survey, interviews	Not specified	Students	Not specified	Indonesia	225
Won et al. (2020)	Class observation, interviews	Undergraduate	Students	Business, Communication, Design & Environmental Analysis, Information Science, Computer Science	U.S.A.	24
Zheng et al. (2020)	Questionnaire survey	Undergraduate	Students	Not specified	Mainland China	513

countries/territories listed in Table 1 all belong to developing countries (72% of the studies), and the American, European, and Oceanian countries in the table are all developed countries (28% of the studies). Far more studies were from developing countries than developed countries. Institutions in many of the developing countries might not have sufficient IT infrastructure to support online teaching and learning. For example, Abbasi et al. (2020) reported that many institutions in Pakistan had never considered e-learning as a part of formal education until the outbreak of COVID-19. The greater challenges in delivering online classes in some of the developing countries might prompt more researchers to investigate how teaching and learning was shifted online during the pandemic.

In summary, the sample of 25 studies investigating the teaching and learning experiences during the pandemic reported mainly teaching and learning at undergraduate level (32% or higher), from student perspectives (60%), related to health-related disciplines and disciplines of science and technology (40%), and in Asian countries (64%).

3.2 RQ2: New Teaching and Learning Methods/Strategies/Technologies That Are Acceptable to Teachers and Students

The thematic analysis of the extracted information for RQ2 generated five themes: common e-learning applications/platforms/resources/devices (60% of the studies), preference for e-learning (32% of the studies), engaging e-learning techniques/strategies (28% of the studies), online adaptation to practice-based courses (20% of the studies), and specific e-learning applications/platforms (8% of the studies). These themes and sub-themes, and the relevant domain summaries and studies are given in Table 2.

3.2.1 Common e-Learning Applications/Platforms/Resources/Devices

Sixty percent of the reviewed studies (15 out of the 25 studies) investigated the common e-learning applications, platforms, resources or devices employed during the pandemic. Among them, 11 studies identified the most commonly used, suitable or effective e-learning applications, platforms, resources or devices as rated by the participants; six studies compared one type of e-learning applications, platforms or resources with another type for acceptance by the participants; seven studies addressed the strengths of the more popular, suitable or effective e-learning platforms, applications, resources or devices as identified by the participants; two studies pointed out the differentiated use of e-learning platforms, applications or resources by different groups of participants for teaching and learning; and one study highlighted

Table 2 New teaching and learning methods/strategies/technologies that are acceptable by teachers and students used during the pandemic

Theme (No. of studies, percent)[a]	Sub-theme or code	Domain summary	Studies (No. of studies, percent)[b]
Common e-learning applications/platforms/resources/devices (15, 60%)	Most popular/suitable/effective applications/platforms/resources/devices	Including WhatsApp (for delivering instruction and learning materials, carrying out discussions, and collecting assessments), Zoom (for delivering online classes), Panopto (for recorded presentations of lectures), institution's LMS (for hosting and distributing learning materials), Office 365 and Google Classroom (the participating university without a unitary e-learning platform), email (as an exam tool), e-books and e-journals (for studying), PPTs with audio (as a format of online classes), and mobile phones (for attending online courses)	Abbasi et al. (2020), Bahassoan et al. (2020), Bordoloi et al. (2020), Edelhauser and Lupu-Dima (2020), Gill et al. (2020), Kapasia et al. (2020), Johnson et al. (2020), Lall and Singh (2020), Longhurst et al. (2020), Rahiem (2020), and Wargadinata et al. (2020) (11, 44%)
	More popular/suitable/effective than another type of platforms/applications/resources	Including social media (over other videoconferencing and online collaboration tools) for academic communication, distribution of materials and collection of assignments; videoconferencing (over asynchronous pre-recorded videos) for delivering online lectures; electronic self-learning materials and e-textbooks (over printed learning materials) for studying	Bordoloi et al. (2020), Johnson et al. (2020), Nadeak (2020), Rajhans et al. (2020), Ramos-Morcillo et al. (2020), and Sobaih et al. (2020) (6, 24%)

(continued)

Table 2 (continued)

Theme (No. of studies, percent)[a]	Sub-theme or code	Domain summary	Studies (No. of studies, percent)[b]
	Strengths of the more popular/suitable/effective platforms/applications/resources/devices	WhatsApp for straightforward to access, low data usage, and allowing transmission of various types of files and resources; social media for accessible to all, easy to use, and interactivity that supports social learning and social presence; videoconferencing for most similar to the traditional face-to-face class, allowing interaction with the teacher, and being able to be recorded and watched later; LMS for the chat function that allows teachers easily communicate with students for assignment collection and task, the assignment function that allows teacher comments and reviews of the work done, and the quiz function that allows building question banks, automated grading, randomized presentation of questions and setting time constraint for quiz items; electronic learning materials for accessible anytime and anywhere; mobile phones for learning taking place anytime and anywhere	Abbasi et al. (2020), Bahassoan et al. (2020), Bordoloi et al. (2020), Longhurst et al. (2020), Ramos-Morcillo et al. (2020), Sobaih et al. (2020), and Wargadinata et al. (2020) (7, 28%)

(continued)

Table 2 (continued)

Theme (No. of studies, percent)[a]	Sub-theme or code	Domain summary	Studies (No. of studies, percent)[b]
	Differentiated use of applications/resources by different users	Including social media (sustaining formal teaching and learning by teachers, and engaging and supporting each other in the learning process by students) and lesson formats (Word, PPT and PDF documents provided by older teachers; and videoconferences and recorded classes delivered by younger teachers)	Ramos-Morcillo et al. (2020), Sobaih et al. (2020) (2, 8%)
	Combination of LMS and WhatsApp for optimal functions	Using WhatsApp for communicating the learning process and LMS for collecting assignments	Wargadinata et al. (2020) (1, 4%)
Preference for e-learning (8, 32%)	Most teachers/students satisfied with online teaching, or preferring the online mode to the face-to-face mode of teaching	–	Gill et al. (2020), Hoq (2020), Kamal et al. (2020), Lall and Singh (2020), Rajhans et al. (2020), and Saif Almuraqab (2020) (6, 24%)

(continued)

Table 2 (continued)

Theme (No. of studies, percent)[a]	Sub-theme or code	Domain summary	Studies (No. of studies, percent)[b]
	Reasons for supporting online learning	Including saving time and energy in editing and updating e-learning materials, interactive contents and sufficient technical support, accessible anytime and anywhere, re-usable lecture recordings saving teachers' time for handling other curriculum issues	Hoq (2020), Kamal et al. (2020), Lall and Singh (2020), Pather et al. (2020) and Mukhtar et al. (2020) (5, 20%)
Engaging e-learning techniques/strategies (7, 28%)	Blended strategies of e-learning and conventional learning techniques	Including pre-recorded videos from external sources as learning materials and a summary report as an assignment; sharing of notes, reading materials, or recorded lectures during or after online lectures; and construction of the whole-class network for a reading and individual reading responses to support personal engagement	Craig et al. (2020), Rahiem (2020), and Rajhans et al. (2020) (3, 12%)
	Strategies facilitating student-student interaction	Including breaking classes into smaller groups; minimal interactions of avatars in virtual worlds, such as nodding heads and hand tracking; and removing the requirement of having the group assignment submitted as a certain format for the groups to be creative in the division of labour	Malan (2020) and Won et al. (2020) (2, 8%)

(continued)

Table 2 (continued)

Theme (No. of studies, percent)[a]	Sub-theme or code	Domain summary	Studies (No. of studies, percent)[b]
	Strategies engaging students in synchronous and asynchronous online lectures	Including nominating students to answer questions; using interactive formative assessments, such as Kahoot! and Slido; using microlearning lessons or dividing the lesson content into several small modules to help students to focus and for them to consume the material in one go	Pather et al. (2020), Rahiem (2020), Rajhans et al. (2020), and Wang et al. (2020) (4, 16%)
	Multiple communication channels between the teacher and students	Including phone calls, social messaging, and discussion boards within the LMS for students to ask questions and teachers to make announcements	Malan (2020) and Rajhans et al. (2020) (2, 8%)
Online adaptation to practice-based courses (5, 20%)	Most common practices for practical sessions	Including asynchronous prerecorded lectures, synchronous lectures/tutorials, case discussion, demonstration using videos from external sources, (for anatomy) both digitized cadaveric resources and 3D virtual anatomy platforms	Gill et al. (2020), Longhurst et al. (2020), Pather et al. (2020), and Rajhans et al. (2020) (4, 16%)

(continued)

Table 2 (continued)

Theme (No. of studies, percent)[a]	Sub-theme or code	Domain summary	Studies (No. of studies, percent)[b]
	Specific practices for practical sessions	Including students repeatedly reviewing the procedures and techniques presented in microlearning lessons to improve the practical skills, teaching support staff creating videos of rotating models to give students a visual impression of the resources, and students working through previous clinical cases before accessing post-class videos on key subject knowledge	Pather et al. (2020) and Wang et al. (2020) (2, 8%)
	Strengths of particular online practices for practical sessions	Case discussions covering evidence-based practice, critical thinking and clinical decision-making skills, which was not taught in clinical skill teaching before; and online live sessions via Zoom offering opportunities for students to interact with experts in the field	Pather et al. (2020) and Rajhans et al. (2020) (2, 8%)
Specific e-learning applications/platforms (2, 8%)	Strengths of Net.Create	Including engaging peers socially when creating networks for subject content, allowing students to contribute meaningfully to the whole-class network, and encouraging students to think more explicitly about connections and causality in the network	Craig et al. (2020) (1, 4%)

(continued)

Table 2 (continued)

Theme (No. of studies, percent)[a]	Sub-theme or code	Domain summary	Studies (No. of studies, percent)[b]
	Strengths of Virtual Worlds	Including inherently interesting experience of visiting virtual worlds, students feeling closer to peers and the teacher when they see their avatars moving, and virtual field trips by guest lecturers connecting the class to anywhere of the world	Won et al. (2020) (1, 4%)

[a]The percentage was calculated by dividing the total number of studies covering at least one of sub-themes of that theme by the total number of studies reviewed (i.e., 25)
[b]The percentage was calculated by dividing the total number of studies covering that sub-theme by the total number of studies reviewed (i.e., 25)

the combination of the institution's LMS and a social media application (WhatsApp) for optimal functions in providing effective online learning for students.

A summary of findings is given as domain summary in Table 2. Depending on the populations that the studies investigated, conflicting findings might be obtained. For example, while Gill et al. (2020) and Johnson et al. (2020) found that the institution's LMS was the most popular platform for hosting and distributing online materials in the universities investigated in China and the U.S. respectively, Kapasia et al. (2020) pointed out that most participating students from Indian universities did not use much of the institution's learning platforms and obtained the learning materials from the teacher and their peers through WhatsApp groups. Nevertheless, some emerging trends about future teaching and learning practices can be found from the findings of the 15 studies. First, there may be an increasing use of social media, such as WhatsApp, for academic communication and distribution of learning materials when face-to-face classes are resumed. As both teachers and students are familiar with the features of certain social media applications and able to create and respond to messages quickly, the integration of social media communication into formal teaching could build an online learning community that supports social learning and social presence (Sobaih et al. 2020). This approach also echoed the findings from Wargadinata et al. (2020) about combining the institution's LMS and WhatsApp for optimal functions. Indeed, integrating social media with LMS has proved to enhance students' learning outcome and brought a higher level of satisfaction and engagement (Rasheed et al. 2020). Second, there may be a shift to mobile technology in classroom teaching and learning. Students' preference for electronic learning materials over printed materials for studying (Bordoloi et al. 2020) and mobile phones over other devices (such as laptops and desktops) for attending online courses (Abbasi et al. 2020; Edelhauser and Lupu-Dima 2020; Kapasia et al. 2020) suggested that they might continue their practices of using the mobile devices to view electronic materials and make annotations in the physical classroom. In this way, they could study the course materials anywhere and anytime. Third, for the universities with the institutions' own LMS, there might be an increasing proportion of online components in the face-to-face courses in the future. Before the pandemic, many course instructors would only use the LMS as "a repository for materials and information" (Cabero-Almenara et al. 2019, p. 31). During the pandemic, they had to explore the features other than uploading files and making announcements that were found on the institution's LMS in order to accommodate other teaching and learning activities for the online classes. Thus, while Longhurst et al. (2020) reported the features associated with quiz activities on the LMS, Wargadinata et al. (2020) specified the features of assignment activities. The accuracy and automation of running quizzes and grading assignments online on the LMS might prompt teachers to continue conducting the two types of activities online when face-to-face classes are resumed. Longhurst et al. (2020) have pointed out that the change might be more relevant to summative continuous assessments of practice-based courses, where a question bank of image-based quiz items could be built up for online exams in order to save the workload associated with designing and implementing station-based practical exams.

3.2.2 Preference for e-Learning

Thirty-two percent of the reviewed studies (8 out of the 25 studies) addressed the participants' preference for e-learning. Among them, six studies reported that most of their participants either were satisfied with online teaching or preferred the online mode to the face-to-face mode of teaching; and five studies provided reasons from the participants that supported online teaching and learning. As the online mode enabled greater versatility and flexibility in teaching and learning, Saif Almuraqab (2020) and Bordoloi et al. (2020) found that most participants, who were more used to the traditional classroom learning before the pandemic, indeed would like to study through blended learning (a combination of online and face-to-face modes) after the pandemic.

3.2.3 Engaging e-Learning Techniques/Strategies

Twenty-eight percent of the reviewed studies (7 out of the 25 studies) examined engaging e-learning techniques or strategies employed by teachers and students. Four sub-themes were identified from this category: blended strategies of e-learning and conventional learning techniques (3 studies), strategies facilitating student-student interaction (2 studies), strategies engaging students in synchronous and asynchronous online lectures (4 studies), and multiple communication channels between the teacher and students (2 studies).

The teaching and learning strategies identified under these four sub-themes might generate some guiding principles for effective delivery of online courses or the online components of blended learning courses. First, the sub-theme, *blended strategies of e-learning and conventional learning techniques*, suggested that online tasks or activities should be built in accordance with a format that students are familiar with, such as providing a printable version for students to take notes, or requiring a conventional written assignment so that students could follow easily. Rahiem (2020) found that students often studied the subject content using conventional media and methods even when an online mode of learning was used. Second, the two sub-themes, *strategies facilitating student-student interaction* and *strategies engaging students in synchronous and asynchronous online lectures*, highlighted the importance of establishing a collaborative and interactive online community, which essentially offers students a sense of ownership in the course (Rasheed et al. 2020). Finally, the sub-theme, *multiple communication channels between the teacher and students*, suggested setting up various channels, including social media, to enable students to raise questions easily when they encounter any problems in completing the online tasks or activities. This could also establish a safe learning environment for students as they can express their doubts and receive responses via these channels without disclosing their identity during the online class (Rajhans et al. 2020).

3.2.4 Online Adaptation to Practice-Based Courses

Twenty percent of the reviewed studies (5 out of the 25 studies) investigated how practice-based courses were adapted to the online mode during the pandemic, which generated three sub-themes: most common practices for practical sessions (4 studies), specific practices for practical sessions (2 studies), and strengths of particular online practices for practical sessions (2 studies). Most of the online adaption to the practice-based courses reported in the studies was about the use of various formats of digital representations (such as photos, videos, and 3D virtual anatomy images) of models, specimens, or demonstrations for students to watch and practise the procedures and techniques. Interestingly, no use of augmented or virtual reality (AR or VR) for the practical sessions was reported in these studies, which was commented on by Gill et al. (2020) as a missed opportunity. This indicated that the use of AR or VR for educational purposes in higher education was not common during the period. Besides that, the introduction of case discussions to practical sessions as reported in Pather et al. (2020) and Rajhans et al. (2020) enabled students to focus on evidence-based practice, critical thinking and clinical decision making in addition to practicing their psychomotor skills (Rajhans et al. 2020). Moreover, individual practitioners and researchers in the field were invited to the online practical sessions (Pather et al. 2020; Rajhans et al. 2020), which could bring in new knowledge and fresh perspectives to the course (Rajhans et al. 2020). Indeed, given the scale of change brought into many practice-based courses during the pandemic, some educators called into question traditional laboratory-based approaches to practice-based courses and were in favor of online approaches (Pather et al. 2020).

3.2.5 Specific e-Learning Applications/Platforms

Two reviewed studies reported the findings of implementing a particular e-learning application or platform in their online courses. One study was about using a network visualization tool to engage students socially and cognitively by building the whole-class network for assigned readings (Craig et al. 2020); the other was on students' experience of learning in virtual environments through virtual reality software (Won et al. 2020). Though the software employed was different in each study, authors of both studies highlighted the importance of the software in engaging students socially for learning (one by constructing a network collaboratively, and another by movements of avatars), which should be considered for future implementation for blended and online learning.

Table 3 Learning skills and practical knowledge that students gained when taking part in the teaching and learning activities during the pandemic

Theme	Domain summary	Studies
Independent learning	Students visiting YouTube, searching the Internet, or downloading free modules for answers when encountering difficulties in online course content	Bahassoan et al. (2020) and Zheng et al. (2020)
Self-directed learning	Students actively searching and bringing the relevant online content to the e-learning environment	Mukhtar et al. (2020) and Rajhans et al. (2020)
Technological knowledge	Developing ICT based knowledge and skills through accessing live online classes and using social media for a positive learning experience	Bordoloi et al. (2020) and Sobaih et al. (2020)

3.3 RQ3: Learning Skills and Practical Knowledge Gained by Students

Findings of six reviewed studies addressed the learning skills and practice knowledge that students gained through the online mode of teaching and learning, which can be categorized into three themes: independent learning[2] (2 studies), self-directed learning (2 studies) and technological knowledge (2 studies). Table 3 presents the three themes, their domain summaries and studies. Generally speaking, the shift from the face-to-face mode to an online mode of teaching and learning would also be accompanied with a shift of teaching approach from teacher-centered to student-centered. For example, Rajhans et al. (2020) compared the face-to-face mode of teaching and learning used for Optometry programmes in India in 2018 with the online mode used for the same type of programmes during the pandemic and found that the pedagogy for theoretical content had shifted from monotonous didactic lectures to interactive online lectures and learning assessments were switched from semester-end examinations to small and online unit assessments throughout the semester using various teaching and learning applications. The breaking down of subject content and assessments into smaller units for online delivery, the use of various online tools for teaching and learning, and the physical separation between the teacher and students in an online learning environment provided more room for students to find out their own answers in learning through the online resources (i.e.,

[2] According to Van Hout-Wolters et al. (2020), independent learning refers to the mental activity learners use when they figure out things on their own or together in a group without teacher supervision; whereas self-directed learning refers the decisions that learners take by themselves when they make their own time-planning, choose their own learning goals and activities, test their own progress, and reflect on their own errors and successes.

independent learning), set their learning goals and select their own learning materials (i.e., self-directed learning), and make use of various online tools to interact with each other and build rapport (gaining in technological knowledge).

3.4 RQ4: Aspects of Teachers' Professional Development

Three reviewed studies (Bordoloi et al. 2020; Rajhans et al. 2020; Won et al. 2020) attended to aspects of teachers' professional development when they implemented online teaching during the pandemic. All findings were related to the gain in technological pedagogical knowledge, "an understanding of how teaching and learning can change when particular technologies are used in particular ways" (Koehler and Mishra 2009, p. 65). While Bordoloi et al. (2020) reported generally that most participants (both teachers and students) agreed that accessing live online classes helped them to develop their ICT-based knowledge and skills, Rajhans et al. (2020) and Won et al. (2020) addressed specifically the technological pedagogical knowledge and techniques the teachers employed when delivering online teaching—such as using random questioning, chatbox, opinion polls, student-led summarization of the session to keep students active during synchronous online classes; giving longer wait time for student responses because the teacher could not rely on eye contact to elicit responses; and using a wide variety of online tools and applications to keep going with their teaching.

3.5 The Way Forward

The COVID-19 pandemic has provided a strong push to the adoption of new technologies in higher education. Most of the adoption in the reviewed studies was about translational use of technology, which introduces automation and efficiency without changing teaching and learning significantly (Magana 2017). For example, electronic self-learning materials replaced printed materials for flexible accessibility; live-streamed classes (recorded) and pre-recorded lectures substituted face-to-face lectures for flexible accessibility and repeated viewing; online quizzes on the LMS substituted pen and paper quizzes for randomization of quiz questions and automatic grading and feedback; and online assignment activities on the LMS replaced grading assignments in paper format for automatic compilation of scores and feedback. Yet, the e-learning resources and activities adopted during the pandemic could be re-organized in the post-pandemic era in such a way to help learners shift towards deeper phases of learning and higher orders of thinking. For example, the communication channels established via social media could be used as means for students to share their work among peers for peer feedback and peer assessments; and short videos of microlearning used for online classes before could also serve as examples or templates for students to produce their own microlearning lessons to demonstrate their understanding of certain concepts. These activities are what Magana (2017) refers to as transformational use of technology, during which learning is transformed into a process of knowledge development and production. In addition, video conferencing tools make it easier to invite practitioners or experts in a field to interact with students, and VR software enables guest lecturers to provide virtual field trips to connect the class to anywhere in the world. These guest lectures or virtual field trips could be set as the starting point for students to investigate a real-world problem beyond the confines of the classroom for a solution. This level of technology use is referred to as transcendent use of technology (Magana 2017), where newly acquired knowledge is applied toward solving real-life problems and improving their world. Such a shift in the use of new technologies for teaching and learning from translational to transformational and to transcendent will also be accompanied by an increase level of self-directed learning and independent work.

The reviewed studies (Bordoloi et al. 2020; Rajhans et al. 2020; Won et al. 2020) suggest a gain in technological pedagogical knowledge when teachers employed certain strategies to engage students in synchronous online lectures and used various video conferencing and social media applications for online classes. Indeed, the knowledge and skills that teachers need to select and integrate appropriate new technologies into their curriculum are more than the technological and pedagogical aspects. Koehler and Mishra (2009) conceptualize such knowledge and skills as technological pedagogical content knowledge (TPACK), which includes competence in content, pedagogy, technology and their interactions. TPACK offers a comprehensive approach for teachers to reflect on their current practices on technology integration and make changes in their instruction (Benson and Ward 2013; Herring et al. 2016). Therefore, if there is a shift in the use of new technologies in higher education settings from translational to transformational and to transcendent, more research has to be conducted regarding the development of faculty TPACK from both the teachers' and the students' perspectives in order to provide diagnostic feedback to teachers' practices.

3.6 Limitations

The most notable limitation of the present study is that it drew from papers published online only up to early-mid August of 2020, a time when the COVID-19 pandemic still impacted communities all over the world and traditional classroom teaching had not been resumed in many countries and territories. That means this systematic review only captured part of the studies which investigated teaching and learning experience during the early period of the pandemic. Studies conducted before or in July 2020 but published after mid-August 2020, or studies conducted after July 2020 were not included in the present study. If these two groups of studies had been included in the present study, the sample might have contained more qualitative and mixed-methods research and covered the teaching and learning practices in the fall semester of 2020, which might be different from those in the spring semester of 2020.

Another limitation is that the present study reviewed only the positive teaching and learning experience reported in the reviewed studies in order to address the research questions, and the challenges and difficulties encountered for online delivery were excluded. These challenges and difficulties might provide indirect evidence for future development of teaching and learning in higher education settings. A third limitation is that only studies written in English were included, which could have excluded any important studies produced in other languages. Nevertheless, the analysis conducted in the present study should be sufficient to portray a roadmap for developing digital teaching and learning in higher education in the post-pandemic era.

4 Conclusion

This chapter presents a systematic review of the positive teaching and learning experience in higher education settings based on 25 studies conducted during the COVID-19 pandemic up to July 2020. The studies reviewed encompassed a range of research methods, education levels, target populations, discipline areas of the participants, and countries or territories (as outlined in Table 1). Through thematic analysis of the literature, the present study found that the empirical research of new teaching and learning methods/strategies/technologies being used during the pandemic tended to focus on common e-learning applications/platforms/resources/devices (60%), preference for e-learning (32%), engaging e-learning techniques/strategies (24%), online adaptation to practice-based courses (20%), and specific e-learning applications/platforms (8%). In addition, a gain in the levels of independent learning, self-directed learning and technological knowledge by students and an increase in the level of technological pedagogical knowledge by teachers during the online teaching and learning were indicated in the empirical research. The surge of e-learning resources and activities during the pandemic provide the opportunities for educators and researchers of higher education to shift the translational use of new technologies to transformational and transcendent use for teaching and learning. Such a shift should also be coupled with research on the development of faculty TPACK so that the findings could provide diagnostic feedback to teachers' practices.

References

Abbasi, S., Ayoob, T., Malik, A. and Memon, S.I. (2020) Perception of students regarding learning during Covid-19 at a private medical college, *Pakistan Journal of Medical Sciences*, 36(COVID 19-S4), 57–61. Available at: https://doi.org/10.12669/pjms.36.COVID19-S4.2766. Accessed 10 August 2020.

Bahassoan, A., Ayuandiani, W., Mukhram, M. and Rahmat, A. (2020) Effectiveness of online learning in pandemic Covid-19, *International Journal of Science, Technology & Management*, 1(2), 100–106. Available at: https://ijstm.inarah.co.id/index.php/ijstm/article/view/30. Accessed 10 August 2020.

Benson, S.N.K. and Ward, C.L. (2013) Teaching with technology: Using TPACK to understand teaching expertise in online higher education, *Journal of Educational Computing Research*, 48(2), 153–172. Available at: https://doi.org/10.2190/EC.48.2.c. Accessed 30 December 2019).

Bordoloi, R., Das, P. and Das, K. (2020) Perception of online/blended learning at the time of the pandemic: An academic analytics in the Indian context, in E. Tsang, K.C. Li, P. Wang (eds.), *International Conference on Open and Innovative Education (ICOIE2020): Proceedings*, 2–4 July, The Open University of Hong Kong, Online, 335–354. Available at: http://icoie2020.ouhk.edu.hk/proceedings.html. Accessed 10 August 2020.

Cabero-Almenara, J., Arancibia, M.L. and Del Prete, A. (2019) Technical and didactic knowledge of the Moodle LMS in higher education: Beyond functional use, *Journal of New Approaches in Educational Research*, 8(1), 25–33. Available at: https://doi.org/10.7821/naer.2019.1.327. Accessed 30 December 2019.

Cohen, S. and Sabag, Z. (2020) The influence of the COVID-19 epidemic on teaching methods in higher education institutions in Israel, *Journal of Research in Higher Education*, 4(1), 44–71. Available at: https://doi.org/10.24193/JRHE.2020.1.4. Accessed 30 July 2020.

Craig, K., Humburg, M., Danish, J.A., Szostalo, M., Hmelo-Silver, C.E. and McCranie, A. (2020) Increasing students' social engagement during COVID-19 with Net.Create: Collaborative social network analysis to map historical pandemics during a pandemic, *Information and Learning Sciences*, 121(7/8), 533–547. Available at: https://doi.org/10.1108/ILS-04-2020-0105. Accessed 10 August 2020.

Crawford, J., Butler-Hendreson, K., Rudolph, J., Malkawi, B., Glowatz, M., Burton, R., Magni, P.A. and Lam, S. (2020) COVID-19: 20 countries' higher education intra-period digital pedagogy responses, *Journal of Applied Learning & Teaching*, 3(1) [online]. Available at: https://doi.org/10.37074/jalt.2020.3.1.7. Accessed 30 July 2020.

Cuaton, G.P. (2020) Philippines higher education institutions in the time of COVID-19 pandemic, *Revista Romaneasca pentru Educatie Multidimensionala*, 12(1Sup2), 61–70. Available at: https://doi.org/10.18662/rrem/12.1sup2/247. Accessed 30 July 2020.

Dörnyei, Z. (2007) *Research Methods in Applied Linguistics*. Oxford and New York: Oxford University Press.

Edelhauser, E. and Lupu-Dima, L. (2020) Is Romania prepared for e-learning during the COVID-19 pandemic?, *Sustainability*, 12 [online]. Available at: https://doi.org/10.3390/su12135438. Accessed 10 August 2020.

Gill, A., Irwin, D., Towey, D., Walker, J. and Zhang, Y. (2020) Reacting to the Coronavirus: A case study of science and engineering education switching to online learning in a Sino-foreign higher education institution, in E. Tsang, K.C. Li, P. Wang (eds.), *International Conference on Open and Innovative Education (ICOIE2020): Proceedings*, 2–4 July, The Open University of Hong Kong, Online, 385–404. Available at: http://icoie2020.ouhk.edu.hk/proceedings.html. Accessed 10 August 2020.

Herring, M.C., Meacham, S. and Mourlam, D. (2016) TPACK development in higher education, in M. C. Herring, M. J. Koehler and P. Mishra (eds.), *Handbook of technological pedagogical content knowledge (TPACK) for educators*. New York and London: Routledge, pp. 207–224.

Hoq, M.Z. (2020) E-learning during the period of pandemic (COVID-19) in the Kingdom of Saudi Arabia: An empirical study, *American Journal of Educational Research*, 8(7), 457–464. Available at: https://doi.org/10.12691/education-8-7-2. Accessed 10 August 2020.

Johnson, N., Veletsianos, G., and Seaman, J. (2020) U.S. faculty and administrators' experiences and approaches in the early weeks of the COVID-19 pandemic, *Online Learning*, 24(2), 6–21. Available at: https://doi.org/10.24059/olj.v24i2.2285. Accessed 10 August 2020.

Kamal, A.A., Shaipullah, N.M., Truna, L., Sabri, M. and Junaini, S.N. (2020) Transitioning to online learning during COVID-19 pandemic: Case study of a pre-university centre in Malaysia, *International Journal of Advanced Computer Science and Applications (IJACSA)*, 11(6), 217–223. Available at: https://doi.org/10.14569/IJACSA.2020.0110628. Accessed 10 August 2020.

Kapasia, N., Paul, P., Roy, A., Saha, J., Zaveri, A., Mallick, R., Barman, B., Das, P. and Chouhan, P. (2020) Impact of lockdown on learning status of undergraduate and postgraduate students during

COVID-19 pandemic in West Bengal, India, *Children and Youth Services Review*, 116 [online]. Available at: https://doi.org/10.1016/j.childyouth.2020.105194. Accessed 10 August 2020.

Kessler, A., Barnes, S., Rajagopal, K., Rankin, J., Pouchak, L., Silis, M. and Esser, W. (2020) Saving a semester of learning: MIT's emergency transition to online instruction, *Information and Learning Science*, 121(7/8), 587–597. Available at: https://doi.org/10.1108/ILS-04-2020-0097. Accessed 30 July 2020.

Koehler, M.J. and Mishra, P. (2009) What is technological pedagogical content knowledge?, *Contemporary Issues in Technology and Teacher Education*, 9 (1), 60–70.

Lall, S. and Singh, N. (2020) Covid-19: Unmasking the new face of education, *International Journal of Research in Pharmaceutical Sciences*, 11(1), 48–53. Available at: https://doi.org/10.26452/ijrps.v11iSPL1.2122. Accessed 10 August 2020.

Longhurst, G.J., Stone, D.M., Dulohery, K., Scully, D., Campbell, T. and Smith, C.F. (2020) Strength, weakness, opportunity, threat (SWOT) analysis of the adaptations to anatomical education in the United Kingdom and Republic of Ireland in response to the Covid-19 pandemic, *Anatomy Science Education*, 13, 298–308. Available at: https://doi.org/10.1002/ase.1967. Accessed 10 August 2020.

Macaro, E., Handley, Z. and Walter, C. (2011) A systematic review of CALL in English as a second language: Focus on primary and secondary education, *Language Teaching*, 45(1), 1–43. Available at: https://doi.org/10.1017/S0261444811000395. Accessed 30 December 2019.

Magana, S. (2017) *Disruptive classroom technologies: A framework for innovation in education*. Thousand Oaks: Corwin.

Malan, M. (2020) Engaging students in a fully online accounting degree: An action research study, *Accounting Education*, 29(4), 321–339. Available at: https://doi.org/10.1080/09639284.2020.1787855. Accessed 10 August 2020.

Mukhtar, K., Javed, K., Arooj, M. and Sethi, A. (2020) Advantages, limitations and recommendations for online learning during COVID-19 pandemic era, *Pakistan Journal of Medical Sciences*, 36(COVID19-S4), 27–31. Available at: https://doi.org/10.12669/pjms.36.COVID19-S4.2785. Accessed 10 August 2020.

Mulla, Z.D., Osland-Paton, V., Rodriguez, M.A, Vazquez, E. and Plavsic, S.K. (2020) Novel coronavirus, novel faculty development programs: Rapid transition to e-learning during the pandemic, *Journal of Perinatal Medicine*, 48(5), 446–449. Available at: https://doi.org/10.1515/jpm-2020-0197. Accessed 30 July 2020.

Nadeak, B. (2020) The effectiveness of distance learning using social media during the pandemic period of COVID-19: A case in *Universitas Kristen Indonesia, International Journal of Advance Science and Technology*, 29(7), 1764–1772.

Pather, N., Blyth, P., Chapman, J.A., Dayal, M.R., Flack, N.A.M.S., Fogg, Q.A., Green, R.A., Hulme, A.K., Johnson, I.P., Meyer, A.J., Morley, J.W., Shortland, P.J., Strkalj, G., Strkalj, M., Valter, K., Webb, A.L., Woodley, S.J. and Lazarus, M.D. (2020) Forced disruption of anatomy education in Australia and New Zealand: An acute response to the Covid-19 pandemic, *Anatomical Sciences Education*, 13, 284–297. Available at: https://doi.org/10.1002/ase.1968. Accessed 10 August 2020.

Rahiem, M.D.H. (2020) The emergency remote learning experience of university students in Indonesia amidst the COVID-19 crisis, *International Journal of Learning, Teaching and Educational Research*, 19(6), 1–26. Available at: https://doi.org/10.26803/ijlter.19.6.1. Accessed 10 August 2020.

Rajhans, V., Memon, U., Patil, V. and Goyal, A. (2020) Impact of COVID-19 on academic activities and way forward in Indian optometry, *Journal of Optometry* [online]. Available at: https://doi.org/10.1016/j.optom.2020.06.002. Accessed 10 August 2020.

Ramos-Morcillo, A.J., Leal-Costa, C., Moral-Garcia, J.E. and Ruzafa-Martinez, M. (2020) Experiences of nursing students during the abrupt change from face-to-face to e-learning education during the first month of confinement due to COVID-19 in Spain, *International Journal of Environmental Research and Public Health*, 17(15) [online]. Available at: https://doi.org/10.3390/ijerph17155519. Accessed 10 August 2020.

Rasheed, R.A., Kamsin, A. and Abdullah, N.A. (2020) Challenges in the online component of blended learning: A systematic review, *Computers & Education*, 144 [online]. Available at: https://doi.org/10.1016/j.compedu.2019.103701. Accessed 30 July 2020.

Ross, A.F. and DiSalvo, M.L. (2020) Negotiating displacement, regaining community: The Harvard Language Center's response to the COVID-19 crisis, *Foreign Language Annals*, 53, 371–379. Available at: https://doi.org/10.1111/flan.12463. Accessed 30 July 2020.

Saif Almuraqab, N.A. (2020) Shall universities at the UAE continue distance learning after the COVID-19 pandemic? Revealing students' perspective, *International Journal of Advanced Research in Engineering and Technology (IJARET)*, 11(5), 226–233. Available at: http://www.iaeme.com/IJARET/issues.asp?JType=IJARET&VType=11&IType=5. Accessed 10 August 2020.

Sobaih, A.E.E., Hasanein, A.M. and Abu Elnasr, A.E. (2020) Responses to COVID-19 in higher education: social media usage for sustaining formal academic communication in developing countries, *Sustainability*, 12 [online]. Available at: https://doi.org/10.3390/su12166520. Accessed 10 August 2020.

United Nations (2020) *World economic situation and prospects 2020* [online]. Available at: https://www.un.org/development/desa/dpad/publication/world-economic-situation-and-prospects-2020/. Accessed 30 August 2020.

Van Hout-Wolters, B., Simons, R.-J. and volet, Simone (2020) Active learning: Self-directed learning and independent work, in P.R.J. Simons, J.L. van der Linden and T. Duffy (eds.), *New learning*. Dordrecht: Kluwer Academic Publishers, pp. 21–37.

Wang, T., Towey, D. and Ng, R.Y.-K. (2020) Microlearning in technical and vocational education and training (TVET): A case study during the COVID-19 outbreak in Hong Kong, in E. Tsang, K.C. Li, P. Wang (eds.), *International Conference on Open and Innovative Education (ICOIE2020): Proceedings*, 2–4 July, The Open University of Hong Kong, Online, pp. 157–163. Available at: http://icoie2020.ouhk.edu.hk/proceedings.html. Accessed 10 August 2020.

Wargadinata, W., Maimunah, I., Dewi, E. and Rofiq, Z. (2020) Students responses on learning in the early COVID-19 pandemic, *Tadris: Journal of Education and Teacher Training*, 5(1), 141–153. Available at: https://doi.org/10.24042/tadris.v5i1.6153. Accessed 10 August 2020.

Won, A.S., Bailey, J.O. and Yi, S. (2020) Work-in-progress—Learning about virtual worlds in virtual worlds: How remote learning in a pandemic can inform future teaching, in D. Economou, A. Klippel, H. Dodds, A. Peña-Rios, M.J.W. Lee, D. Beck, J. Pirker, A. Dengel, T.M. Peres and J. Richter (eds.), *Immersive learning research network. Proceedings of 6th International Conference, iLRN 2020*, 21–25 June, Immersive Learning Research Network, Online, pp. 377–380. Available at: IEEE Xplore. Accessed 10 August 2020.

Zheng, J., Huang, Y., Li, S. Wang, C. and Zhong, K. (2020) Investigation of college students' online learning, in 2020 International Conference on Big Data and Information Education (ICBDIE), 23–25 April, IEEE, Zhangjiajie, China, pp. 139–142. Available at: IEEE Xplore. Accessed 10 August 2020.

Zhu, T. (2020) Empirical research on the application of online teaching in Chinese colleges and universities under the situation of novel coronavirus pneumonia prevention and control, *iJET*, 15(11), 119–136. Available at: https://doi.org/10.3991/ijet.v15i11.13935. Accessed 30 July 2020.

Navigating Public Relations in a Pandemic

Xiaomeng Lan

1 Introduction

The COVID-19 pandemic is not only a health crisis of immense proportions; it has also fundamentally impacted the landscape in which businesses operate. Companies have had to navigate the financial and operational challenges arising from the disruption in offshore supply chains, the movement restrictions imposed to stop or slow the spread of the disease, and an acute pullback in economic activity and demand (Craven et al. 2020b), while promptly addressing the changing needs and expectations of their employees, customers, and suppliers (Accenture 2020). Although much of the disturbance may be temporary, the COVID-19 crisis is understood to have accelerated and intensified some worrisome trends already underway, including the tendency toward less free and open global trade and investment flows (Amm and Prichard 2020), further challenging businesses to keep pace and refocus their strategies. Analysts and observers are murmuring about the "next normal" likely to emerge in the post-viral era, one divergent from the pre-2020 state of affairs (Sneader and Singhal 2020f). The question is: How can leaders across the public, private, and social sectors intervene positively in the current uncertainties and crises until we reach the other side of this pandemic? There is already agreement that the response of leaders and organisations to the pandemic will go a long way in determining the success of their institutions for years to come (Amm and Prichard 2020; PwC 2020). In this context, the present chapter attends to a particular facet of the corporate response to the COVID-19 crisis: the public relations efforts made by companies and business leaders during the pandemic.

Public relations is an important management function that helps establish and maintain relationships between an organisation and the stakeholders who have a

X. Lan (✉)
BNU-HKBU United International College,
Zhuhai, China
e-mail: maggiexmlan@uic.edu.cn

S.X.B. Zhao et al. (eds.), *COVID-19 Pandemic, Crisis Responses and the Changing World*, https://doi.org/10.1007/978-981-16-2430-8_20

vested interest in the success of the organisation and may represent a network of support during crises (Cutlip et al. 2000; Ulmer 2001). Public relations is of particular importance in times of uncertainty, as, at its best, it can inspire trust and solidarity, distil meaning from chaos, and act as a voice of reason (Mendy et al. 2020; Rattan 2020; Burke et al. 2020). Even before COVID-19, there was a growing sense that leaders of commerce needed to be weaned away from a strict focus on maximizing profits when conducting business, and companies were increasingly expected to bear wider social responsibilities and to embrace broad principles of stewardship, sustainability, employee wellbeing, and long-term value (Denning 2019; Sneader and Singhal 2020g; Amm and Prichard 2020). The COVID-19 pandemic has focused even more attention on individual and social needs and concerns, and at this pivotal time companies are poised to demonstrate their defining corporate purpose—what their core reason for being is, and where they can have a unique, positive impact on society (Amm and Prichard 2020; Gast et al. 2020e). They are expected not only to share resources to address genuine needs, but to provide timely and accurate information that helps people make sense of all that has happened (Mendy et al. 2020; Goldberg 2020; Boin et al. 2016).

Moreover, with the emerging postmodernist view on public relations that stresses the social construction of ethical values and meaning (Venkatesh 1992; Mickey 1997), there have been greater expectations that businesses and corporate leaders voice their opinions and take stances on socially and politically significant issues (Ulmer 2001; Lan et al. 2020; Dodd 2018). Companies' engagement in social advocacy and public discourse, however, may be overshadowed by the changes in public opinion triggered by the pandemic. The rising anti-globalisation and nationalist movements, for example, complicate the role of business in the public debate about globalisation (Altman 2020c). These developments form the larger context for the subsequent discussion and also point to the need for an axiological reflection on public relations during and after the pandemic.

2 Challenging Information Environment and Public Relations as Meaning-Making

COVID-19 has put public relations in a tricky spot. The good news, as Jill Avery and Richard Edelman observe, is that people want to hear from businesses during the crisis (Avery and Edelman 2020). But there is a serious potential downside for companies in speaking to the public: the overwhelming and complex information environment they are facing can actually hurt the effectiveness of their public relations efforts. This is an environment already complicated by an overabundance of information, competing values, and spurious or slanted content (Anderson and Rainie 2017). Ideologically divergent social groups, motivated to defend their own identities and value systems, draw on radically different combinations of values and facts to sustain their worldviews (Scheufele et al. 2020). The strong instinct people have to find and believe information that aligns with their understanding or views grants advantages to unreliable information wherever it reinforces biases. That makes it harder for them to agree on the "common knowledge" necessary for communication and coordination of behaviours within a society (Anderson and Rainie 2017; Vanderschraaf and Sillari 2014).

The ubiquity of new media platforms has made it easier for more groups to construct and distribute their own narratives or "alternative realities," heightening people's vulnerability to falsehoods (Schmidt et al. 2017). This, together with the increased reliance on social media as a main source of news and information, biased algorithms replacing human judgment, economic incentives for producing misinformation for online advertising markets and popular social networks, as well as the undermining of society's trust in traditional journalism's ability to accurately and fairly report the news, have all given rise to the so-called "fake news" phenomenon (Allcott and Gentzkow 2017; Berthon and Pitt 2018; Wendling 2018). A "new shape of truth" has come into being; as Kevin Kelly, co-founder of *Wired* magazine, put it, "Truth is no longer dictated by authorities, but is networked by peers. For every fact there is a counterfact and all these counterfacts and facts look identical online, which is confusing to most people" (as cited in Anderson and Rainie 2017). We are said to have entered a "post-truth" era, where "objective facts are less influential in shaping public opinion than appeals to emotion and personal belief" (Oxford Languages 2016).

The sudden onset of the new, highly contagious coronavirus seems only to have accelerated these troublesome trends. This is the first time in history when technology and social media are being used on such an immense scale in a pandemic situation (World Health Organization 2020). The greater dependence on social media and digital platforms during the crisis is enabling and amplifying what U.N. Secretary-General António Guterres called a "pandemic of misinformation," a phenomenon that describes COVID-19's severe strain on the discourse of the public sphere, in which trustworthy information is difficult to distinguish from the overwhelming noise of competing, and in some cases conflicting, messages (World Health Organization 2020; Pazzanese 2020). This COVID-19 "infodemic," as the WHO calls it, includes deliberate attempts to disseminate incorrect information to undermine the public health response and advance alternative agendas of groups or individuals (World Health Organization 2020).

In the meantime, those politicians, scientists, journalists, and communication practitioners making well-intentioned communication efforts face an uphill battle: the use of evidence in policy-making and public debate around COVID-19 is complicated and jeopardized by the "epistemic uncertainty" and ambiguity surrounding the scientific facts and knowledge about the disease (Roberts 2020). As Scheufele et al. (2020) have said, accuracy of information "is a tenuous notion during a crisis such as this, in which uncertainty reigns." Something that was considered correct at the outset may turn out to be incorrect or incomplete, making it even harder to draw a clear line between fact and fabrication.

These transformations of the public arena have so impacted contemporary public discourse that rational and meaningful communication is giving way to emotionality and distraction (Thompson 2020). Some public relations scholars (Heath 1992; Heath and Frandsen 2008) would argue all this requires public relations to engage in and foster dialogue that helps create and enact meaning for the good of society. One belief underlying this view on public relations is that of the "marketplace of ideas," which refers to the faith that "the test of the truth or acceptance of ideas depends on their competition with one another" (Schultz 2017). As Cutlip (1994) reasoned, "...only through the expertise of public relations can causes, industries, individuals, and institutions make their voice heard in the public forum where thousands of shrill, competing voices daily re-create the Tower of Babel" (p. ix). Within this process, public relations perhaps "cannot escape the virtue and pitfalls of advocacy, argument, persuasion, and the co-creation or mutual shaping of shared meaning," but it can add value to society through ethical practice of meaning-making (Heath and Frandsen 2008, 349). The meaning-making virtue of public relations is further explicated by M. Taylor (2009):

> The role of public relations in civil society is quite clear. When we focus on meaning making, language, rhetorical argument, and persuasion, then we have enormous potential to see how public relations theory can serve civil society interests. The focus on meaning making also ensures that if one group, through money, access, or media ownership, tries to dominate the civil sphere, then other actors or organizations may be able to moderate the self-serving interests. (p. 89)

3 Corporate Public Relations Responses During COVID-19

The COVID-19 crisis has created an urgent and unprecedented demand for companies to practice purpose-driven leadership and corporate social responsibility. Companies have faced extraordinary financial and operational challenges, and as every industry and business is tested in unique ways, the best response may be different for each (Just Capital 2020). While the evolving COVID-19 pandemic has in many ways limited the resources and tools available for public relations, companies have been actively engaging in the following public relations activities during the pandemic.

Educating the public. Many companies have used their brand power and media presence to spread reliable, factual information that instructed people about the crisis, how to protect themselves during it, and the progress being made against it (Avery and Edelman 2020). For example, Jeep encouraged consumers to stay home by passing along the message #StayOffTheRoad (Buss 2020), and Dove released a video on social media that illustrated proper hand-washing techniques to help stop the spread of the virus (Avery and Edelman 2020). Some media and advertising companies are using public service announcements (PSAs) as a creative alternative to amplify the message from authoritative sources, and calling for industry involvement to ensure that the public is directed to official, factual information from health experts (Lin 2020; Graham 2020b). In addition, individual agencies and companies are utilizing their specific tools and resources to connect their audiences with the PSA campaign message (Faw 2020).

Fighting COVID-19 misinformation. Tech and communications companies have been at the forefront of battling misinformation and disinformation around COVID-19. WhatsApp, for example, has limited message forwarding to slow distribution of coronavirus misinformation (Paul 2020). Facebook has been removing content about the virus that may contribute to "imminent physical harm" or that makes "false claims about cures, treatments, the availability of essential services or the location and severity of the outbreak" (Clegg 2020). This included a post by U.S. President Trump playing down the deadliness of COVID-19 (Horwitz 2020). Twitter also responded to a similar claim by the president on its own platform by appending a notice that his tweet violated its rules on spreading harmful information related to the virus. YouTube has taken the approach of pairing misleading COVID-19 content with a link to an alternative expert source, such as the Centers for Disease Control and Prevention or World Health Organization (Chakravorti 2020). Google has pledged $6.5 million in funding to fact-checkers and nonprofit groups fighting against coronavirus information. This includes support for the creation of data resources for reporters working on COVID-19, thus helping journalists tell data-driven stories that have impacted their communities (Mantzarlis 2020).

Supporting employees. A study by McKinsey & Company found that many companies have done a solid job of addressing their employees' basic needs for safety, stability, and security (Emmett et al. 2020a). Some companies are boosting pay for front-line workers or offering paid leave for those who are unable to work because of COVID-19. PepsiCo, for example, announced it would provide enhanced benefits to employees who produce, transport, or deliver its products. It would also pay the salary of employees diagnosed with COVID-19 or caring for a family member with the virus (PepsiCo 2020). Some companies took measures to help offset financial pressures caused by the pandemic. Citigoup, for example, said the bank will send $1,000 awards to some employees to compensate them for the financial burden of working during the coronavirus pandemic (Son 2020a). Some companies have prioritized virtual wellness programmes and initiatives to help ease the stress and anxiety of working from home. The Bank of Ireland, for example, launched a new wellbeing app that offers employees online seminars, live feeds, and interactive sessions on mental, physical, and financial wellbeing (Churchill 2020).

Helping combat coronavirus. Companies across the world are helping in the fight against COVID-19. As documented by the World Economic Forum (Fleming 2020), some companies have been augmenting the work of public bodies, while others have been filling gaps that might otherwise have been neglected. For example, Alibaba has made massive donations of testing kits, masks, and protective suits and face shields to African countries. Microsoft, Amazon, and Starbucks donated to Seattle-area public–private COVID-19 Response Fund to support coronavirus relief efforts in local communities. Manufacturers like Ford, GE, and 3 M started producing life-saving ventilators. Luxury brands like LVMH and Prada used their production lines to produce large quantities of sanitizers, hospital gowns, and masks for healthcare professionals. Ride-sharing company Uber said it would provide 10 million free rides and food deliveries to "health care workers, seniors, and people in need" across the world. It would also use its Uber Eats delivery service to provide 300,000 free meals to first responders and health care workers (Stebbins and Suneson 2020).

While this list of public relations efforts is by no means exhaustive—and focuses only on the earlier phase of the COVID-19 crisis—it sheds some light on the way companies and business leaders approached public relations when the pandemic hit. However, new challenges are emerging, calling for a more sophisticated approach as companies enter the next phase of the crisis.

4 Public Relations in a Post-Pandemic Future

Changes that the pandemic has engendered—and will continue to engender in the years ahead—require business leaders to plot their future approach to public relations to help the companies adapt to the post-COVID-19 era. In the unprecedented new reality, as predicted by the analysts from McKinsey & Company (Sneader and Singhal 2020f), there will be "a dramatic restructuring of the economic and social order in which business and society have traditionally operated." In the scenarios envisioned in that white paper, there may be adjustment to international business and localisation or regionalisation of supply chains that would represent a setback for globalisation. For large companies, particularly multinational corporations, it is imperative to prepare for a world where both globalisation and anti-globalisation pressures remain enduring features of the business environment (Altman 2020c). Superpower frictions and reinforced nationalism have added new layers of complexity (Altman 2020c; Rachman 2020). This would complicate the management and public communications of multinational firms that need to carefully navigate amid globalisation's turbulence.

Meanwhile, COVID-19 is changing the relations between government and business, and between business and society. The pandemic's economic consequences demand urgent policy responses to keep the economy afloat and enable people to retain their jobs and incomes (OECD 2020). This may result in an expansion of state power, and stricter regulation of the private sector, especially with many businesses operating to some extent with public money (Sneader and Singhal 2020g; Altman 2020c). Governments may feel obliged or emboldened to take a much more active role in shaping economic activity. As McKinsey analysts wrote, "The implications for the role of the state will materially affect the way business is conducted; business leaders in many more sectors will have to adjust to the next normal of greater government intervention" (Sneader and Singhal 2020g). This could also make government relations a more important aspect of public relations than ever in the post-COVID-19 period, for large and small companies alike, as they put increased resources into lobbying and advocacy in hopes of shaping policy agendas and bailout decisions.

The relations between business and society, on the other hand, may also undergo a series of tests and scrutiny from the public. The pandemic has drawn more attention to how business and society intersect, revealing the heightened expectations for societal engagement and corporate citizenship (Paine 2020b). As the coronavirus reveals or highlights social fractures and systemic concerns such as increasing income and wealth inequality, climate change, racial and ethnic discrimination, and declining public health and education, business will likely face increased public pressure to help in finding long-term solutions (Sneader and Singhal 2020g). In a time of extreme uncertainty, people look to governments and large companies for leadership. Boin et al. (2016) argued that effective crisis leadership consists of more than "doing the right thing"; leaders from different sectors must also manage the meaning-making process. COVID-19 started as a public health crisis and quickly evolved into a contest of meanings, ideologies, and values. Companies, therefore, need to be more strategic about their public communications.

For the leaders of companies, all this should underscore the importance of employee relationships and alliances. The pandemic has made all too clear that society depends on well-functioning companies to meet its basic needs, and that companies cannot fulfil those needs without prioritizing the health and safety of employees. Coming out of the crisis, businesses must make sure their employees have a shared understanding of the company's purpose and strategy. Building a common sense of purpose gives employees a sense of direction while fuelling and guiding collaboration within organisations (Andriotis 2017). To this end, companies need to not only engage employees regarding their purpose, mission, and values through structured internal communication (Hannum 2020), but also to involve employees in the solutions and view them as co-creators (Schaninger et al. 2020c). It has been pointed out that employees are now a company's most powerful interest group, as well as one of the major forces behind CEO activism, the growing trend among top executives to speak out on sensitive social and political issues (A. Taylor 2018). As more and more companies take a shared value approach to corporate responsibility, it would be beneficial to build a corporate culture that incorporates employees' values and provides continuous alignment with the vision, purpose, and goals of the organisation (Baumgartner 2020).

The pandemic has caused a still-unfolding crisis for the economy and financial system. As Sneader and Singhal (2020f) summarized, for some organisations, near-term survival is the only agenda item. Others are trying to peer further into the uncertain future while bearing great financial stresses. The new environment is characterized by an increasingly complex set of pressures and demands from various stakeholder groups—including greater government influence on economic activity and heightened public expectations of corporate responsibilities (Paine 2020b). To confront the crisis, leaders of companies should foster collaboration. As some analysts point out, forming alliances can help reboot businesses, industries, as well as the larger economy (Kearney 2020). Together, companies would gain an increased bargaining power and voice that could help balance government interventions and economic and social welfare, and drive the business-government-society dynamic.

References

Allcott, H., & Gentzkow, M. (2017) Social media and fake news in the 2016 election. *Journal of Economic Perspectives, 31*(2), 211–236, https://doi.org/10.3386/w23089.

Amobee. (2020) COVID-19 PSA campaign goes global with the World Health Organization (WHO). Accessed 25 March 2020.

Andriotis, N. (2017) What embracing shared purpose can do to benefit your organization. *eFront.*

Bain & Company. (2020) Leading during times of uncertainty. May 1.

BBC Trending. (2018) The (almost) complete history of 'fake news'. January 22.

Beehive Strategic Communication. (2020) Engaging employees in purpose, mission and values through strategic communication. Accessed 11 April 2020.

Berthon, P. R., & Pitt, L. F. (2018) Brands, truthiness and post-fact: Managing brands in a post-rational world. *Journal of Macromarketing*, 1–10, https://doi.org/10.1177/0276146718755869.

Boin, A., t Hart, P., Stern, E., & Sundelius, B (2016). *The Politics of Crisis Management: Public Leadership Under Pressure* (2nd ed.). Cambridge, UK: Cambridge University Press.

Cision. (2020) Leading digital and tech platforms join Ad Council, White House, HHS and CDC to address COVID-19 crisis.

CNBC. (2020a) Citigroup is giving some employees a $1,000 bonus for working through the coronavirus pandemic.

CNBC. (2020b) NBCU, ViacomCBS, Walt Disney Television and other media companies will run new coronavirus PSAs. March 17.

Corporate Knights. (2020) How to craft your business strategy for a post-pandemic world.

Cutlip, S. M. (1994) *The Unseen Power: Public Relations. A History.* Hillsdale, NJ: Lawrence Erlbaum Associates.

Cutlip, S. M., Center, A. H., & Broom, G. M. (2000) *Effective Public Relations* (8th ed.). Upper Saddle River, NJ: Prentice Hall.

Dodd, M. D. (2018) Globalization, pluralization, and erosion: The impact of shifting societal expectations for advocacy and public good. *The Journal of Public Interest Communications, 2*(2), 221–238.

Facebook. (2020) Combating COVID-19 misinformation across our apps.

Financial Times. (2020) Nationalism is a side effect of coronavirus. March 23.

Forbes. (2019) Why maximizing shareholder value is finally dying. August 19.

Forbes. (2020) FCA combines inspiration, deals In 1st Jeep, Ram ads during COVID-19.

Google. (2020) COVID-19: $6.5 million to help fight coronavirus misinformation.

Harvard Business Review. (2018) When CEOs should speak up on polarizing issues. October 31.

Harvard Business Review. (2020a) Build a culture that aligns with people's values.

Harvard Business Review. (2020b) Covid-19 is rewriting the rules of corporate governance.

Harvard Business Review. (2020c) Will Covid-19 have a lasting impact on globalization? May 20.

Harvard Business School Working Knowledge. (2020) What customers need to hear from you during the COVID crisis. April 7.

Heath, R. L. (1992) The Wrangle in the Marketplace: A rhetorical perspective of public relations. In E. L. Toth, & R. L. Heath (Eds.), *Rhetorical and critical approaches to public relations* (pp. 17–36). Hillsdale, NJ: Lawrence Erlbaum Associates.

Heath, R. L., & Frandsen, F. (2008) Rhetorical perspective and public relations: Meaning matters. In A. Zerfass, B. van Ruler, & K. Sriramesh (Eds.), *Public relations research: European and international perspectives and innovations* (pp. 349–364). Wiesbaden, Germany: VS Verlag für Sozialwissenschaften.

Issues in Science and Technology. (2020) How not to lose the COVID-19 communication war. April 17.

Just Capital. (2020). The COVID-19 corporate response tracker: How America's largest employers are treating stakeholders amid the coronavirus crisis.

Kearney. (2020) Rebooting value chains in the wake of an international crisis.

Lan, X., Tarasevich, S., Proverbs, P., Myslik, B., & Kiousis, S. (2020) President Trump vs. CEOs: A comparison of presidential and corporate agenda building. *Journal of Public Relations Research, 32*(1–2), 30–46, https://doi.org/10.1080/1062726X.2020.1719494.

McKinsey & Company. (2020a) COVID-19 and the employee experience: How leaders can seize the moment.

McKinsey & Company. (2020b) COVID-19: Implications for business.

McKinsey & Company. (2020c) Demonstrating corporate purpose in the time of coronavirus.

McKinsey & Company. (2020d) How to communicate effectively in times of uncertainty.

McKinsey & Company. (2020e) Purpose: Shifting from why to how. April 22.

McKinsey & Company. (2020f) Beyond coronavirus: The path to the next normal.

McKinsey & Company. (2020g) The future is not what it used to be: Thoughts on the shape of the next normal. April 14.

Media Post. (2020) More companies join Ad Council, White House COVID-19 PSA initiative. March 25.

Mickey, T. J. (1997) A postmodern view of public relations: Sign and reality. *Public Relations Review, 23*(3), 271–284, https://doi.org/10.1016/S0363-8111(97)90036-9.

OECD. (2020) Government support and the COVID-19 pandemic.

Outmaneuver uncertainty: Navigating the human and business impact of Covid-19. (2020) Available at: https://www.accenture.com/us-en/about/company/coronavirus-business-economic-impact.

Oxford Languages. (2016) Oxford Word of the Year 2016.

People Management. (2020) How are people teams responding to coronavirus? ...Bank of Ireland. April 24.

Pew Research Center. (2017) The future of truth and misinformation online. October 19.

PR Newswire. (2020) PepsiCo to provide enhanced benefits to all U.S. employees and additional compensation to U.S. frontline during unprecedented health pandemic. March 20.

PRSA. (2020) COVID-19: Lessons of past pandemics are more timely than ever for crisis management.

PwC. (2020) COVID 19: Confidently navigate through the coronavirus crisis.

Rattan, T. (2020) The role of public relations in a pandemic. Impact.

Reuters. (2020) WhatsApp limits message forwarding to slow spread of coronavirus misinformation. April 7.

Schmidt, A. L., Zollo, F., Del Vicario, M., Bessi, A., Scala, A., Caldarelli, G., et al. (2017) Anatomy of news consumption on Facebook. *Proceedings of the National Academy of Sciences, 114*(12), 3035–3039, https://doi.org/10.1073/pnas.1617052114.

Schultz, D. (2017) Marketplace of ideas. *The First Amendment encyclopedia*.

Taylor, M. (2009) Civil society as a rhetorical process. In R. L. Heath, E. L. Toth, & D. Waymer (Eds.), *Rhetorical and critical approaches to public relations II* (pp. 76–91). New York, NY: Routledge.

The Conversation. (2020) Social media companies are taking steps to tamp down coronavirus misinformation—But they can do more.

The Harvard Gazette. (2020) Battling the 'pandemic of misinformation'.

The New York Times. (2020) Embracing the uncertainties. Accessed 7 April 2020.

The Wall Street Journal. (2020) Facebook removes Trump's post about Covid-19, citing misinformation rules. Accessed 6 October 2020.

Thompson, G. (2020) *Post-truth public relations: Communication in an era of digital disinformation*. London: Routledge.

Ulmer, R. R. (2001) Effective crisis management through established stakeholder relationships: Malden Mills as a case study. *Management Communication Quarterly, 14*(4), 590–615, https://doi.org/10.1177/0893318901144003.

USA Today. (2020) Amazon, Apple among the companies that are helping Americans fight COVID-19.

Vanderschraaf, P., & Sillari, G. (2014) Common knowledge. In E. N. Zalta (Ed.), *The Stanford Encyclopedia of Philosophy* (Spring 2014 ed.).

Venkatesh, A. (1992) Postmodernism, consumer culture and the society of the spectacle. *NA—Advances in Consumer Research, 19*, 199–202.

World Economic Forum. (2020) How big business is joining the fight against COVID-19. March 20.

World Health Organization. (2020) Managing the COVID-19 infodemic: Promoting healthy behaviours and mitigating the harm from misinformation and disinformation.

The Pandemic and Advertising: Be (AD)Normal

Chai Lee Lim

Abstract The coronavirus (COVID-19) has severely impacted numerous industries through country lockdowns and border closures, affecting daily routines and leading to an era of 'remote everything'. These are challenging times for brands as consumer behaviour, purchasing patterns, and media habits are quickly changing. However, not everything will adhere to the new norm. While brands can benefit from this situation and finding opportunities to engage with consumers, the heart of the matter is, should brands advertise? Do consumers wish to hear from brands? If yes, what do consumers need during the pandemic? Accordingly, this chapter aims to discuss key trends in media consumption during the COVID-19 pandemic and its implications on brand strategy and advertising. Moreover, given the growth in digital traffic during this time, *quarantainment* came to dominate all types of screen and redefined the uses and gratifications afforded by media. In this context, brands needed to practise empathy, embrace purpose-led communications, accelerate digital capabilities and amplify brand community to improve brand resonance. In particular they needed to adapt to four types of pandemic-induced consumer type, which can be identified as worrywart, unflappable, hard-headed and unbothered. The pandemic has proven that the value of media is growing, and brands should stay in the conversation for contribution, not just conversion.

Keywords Advertising · Brand strategy · COVID-19 · Consumer behaviour

1 Introduction: An Unprecedented Crisis

The coronavirus (COVID-19) pandemic has disrupted industry and countries on an unprecedented scale, resulting in significant restrictions with more than one-third of the world's population under lockdown in mid-April 2020. Stay-at-home orders and *cordons sanitaire* have also been implemented worldwide in response to

C. L. Lim (✉)
Beijing Normal University Hong Kong Baptist University United International College (BNU-HKBU UIC), Zhuhai, China
e-mail: chaileelim@uic.edu.cn

S.X.B. Zhao et al. (eds.), *COVID-19 Pandemic, Crisis Responses and the Changing World*, https://doi.org/10.1007/978-981-16-2430-8_21

the pandemic, such as the movement control order (MCO) in Malaysia, shelter-in-place restrictions in the United Kingdom (UK) and Singapore's circuit breaker (CB) measures.

However, this pandemic is more than a global health crisis and has turned into a significant economic crisis. The scale and magnitude of quarantine measures have brought economic activity to a halt which triggered an unfavourable impact on gross domestic product (GDP), an immediate drop in advertising spending worldwide as well as a change in our way of living (Hoekstra and Leeflang 2020). It is likely that the COVID-19 crisis will have substantial consequences on people's livelihoods, changing our daily routines, social interaction, and how businesses serve communities. This is an unexplored territory for many, affecting commodities, services, brands, businesses, marketing on a global scale. A survey conducted in March 2020, revealed that 9 in 10 advertisers in the United States (US) revisited their budgets in response to COVID-19 (Fromm et al. 2020a), in which 49% of advertisers said they were holding back campaign launching, and 45% stopped or pulled a campaign in mid-flight. The same survey conducted in June forecast a 60% decrease in total advertising spend in 2020 compared to 2019, but with spending improving each quarter; from a 72% reduction in the second quarter to 54% in the third quarter and 40% in the fourth quarter (Fromm et al. 2020b).

Advertising in a recession drives companies to reduce their advertising budget (Verma and Kumar 2017). This scenario comes to pass when companies treat marketing as a cost and advertising as an expense rather than an investment (Drucker 2017). Moreover, it is seen as a perspicuous practice, especially in financially difficult times. Advertising budgets are always vulnerable, given they are not committed until spent and can be held back and cut without having any immediate or visible impact on the ongoing productivity of the business. Given the prevailing tension in perceiving the role of advertising, brands become indecisive in adjusting their advertising budgets.

2 No One Is Immune from COVID-19

There is no doubt that the world has changed given the harm and stress resulting from COVID-19. For instance, the present economic downturn in Europe and the US in a single quarter is likely to be far greater than the economic loss experienced during the great depression of the 1930s (Sneader and Singhal 2020). A vast amount of statistics has shown the extent of the economic pain from staff layoffs, salary cuts, unemployment, and reductions in consumer spending, retail sales and production.

In the "What Worries the World" global survey, more than half the respondents ranked COVID-19 as most concerning, followed by unemployment in February, March, and April 2020. However, in the same survey, the change since May 2020, has replaced COVID-19 with unemployment as the top issue; an increase of 11% compared to April 2020 (IPSOS 2020). The fear and anxiety are not without substance, given that 16 million jobs were lost in just two weeks in the US in March as the pandemic brought the economy to a near standstill (*The Guardian* 2020).

Other major shortfalls can be seen in media revenue, as cited by Twitter, *#CancelEverything* especially regarding changes to flagship global events like the European Football Championship 2020 and the Tokyo Olympics. The postponement or cancellation of these mega sporting events will no doubt be a major blow not only to scheduled broadcast coverage but advertising, such as sponsorship and promotional programmes (Graham 2020). The lower spending on out-of-home media under the "shelter-in-place" policy, enforced across most of the nation, has resulted in media revenue facing a turbulent rollercoaster ride to an unknown destination.

Moreover, at a time when the COVID-19 infections are increasing, further unpredictable turmoil in our lives and livelihoods and the unknown new normal (or "norm") remain unsolved. This pandemic is impacting our lives in many ways, and will no doubt lead to the economic restructuring and social order where businesses and society have traditionally operated. People are being challenged to re-evaluate their needs and priorities in life which will then lead to changes in buying behaviour. There is a rule of thumb in the advertising industry that when consumer behaviour shifts, advertising effort has to be adjusted in response. However, to advertisers, while walking a tightrope at this trying time; the question is, should brand advertise?

3 Learning from Past Recessions

Tellis and Tellis (2009) conducted a review on advertising in a recession, discovering that companies that advertise less during a decline in the economy not only experience falling sales during the slowdown but also after the economy begins to recover. In contrast, companies that maintain their marketing strategy during low market periods are more likely to boost short and long-term sales. In another study of recessions in the US, Tellis and Tellis (2009) highlighted that McGraw-Hill Research analysed 600 companies covering 16 different industries between 1980 and 1985, echoing a similar outcome concerning advertising. Also, firms that maintained or increased their advertising expenses during the 1981–1982 recessions averaged significantly higher sales growth, both during the recession and in the following three years. By 1985, sales of those companies that were aggressive advertisers during the recession had risen by 256% compared to those not continuing to advertise.

Overall, most of the research reviewed has revealed that advertising has positive outcomes even during economic contractions. It is well documented that brands that neglect to advertise during a recession, believing that everyone else is also cutting back, end up weakening the brand, making it less profitable after the recession (Consterdine 2009). However, the impact and duration of the present COVID-19 pandemic-induced recession remain to be seen. Slashing advertising budgets will decrease brand visibility and leave a space in the consumer's mind, especially for aggressive marketers to make strong inroads in the long run (Fader 2008).

Aside from the research mentioned and evidence about the importance of advertising in a recession, it may be useful to explore the most recent disease-related outbreak, the Severe Acute Respiratory Syndrome (SARS) that occurred in 2003. This will enable learning on how a virus-induced recession provides a window of opportunity for the development of new and innovative business models. Many suggest that the SARS pandemic boosted China's e-commerce economy and was a significant turning point for two online retail players, Alibaba and JD.com. However, others suggest the SARS outbreak was not the reason why e-commerce boomed in China. Alibaba was already an established business-to-business (B2B) e-commerce platform, and eBay had equally been performing strongly; the 2003 SARS epidemic was merely an inspiration rather than a driving force.

Nevertheless, both pandemics, SARS and COVID-19, have comparable conditions regarding travel restrictions and shop closures. Many foreign businesses turned to Alibaba to source Chinese goods given travel warnings at the time, while local Chinese suppliers, facing fewer alternatives, joined Alibaba's platform, venturing into online marketing. Being the only bridge between wholesaler and retailer at that time, Alibaba foresaw strong sales growth which led to the birth of Taobao, as a consumer-to-consumer (C2C) marketplace. Meanwhile, the owner of JD.com, who previously owned 12 offline stores in Beijing, was forced to close all but one store to conserve resources. He then discovered new ways of reaching consumers by posting in online forums. This further aroused his interest in conducting business online. JD.com later grew to become a top player in online retail of electronics consumables in China.

It may be overly simplistic to consider making a direct comparison between what occurred in decades past to the situation today, especially when digital marketing was only a portion of the entire marketing mix back in 2008 while the current delivery and logistic services are considerably well-developed. However, the past lessons highlight how retailers can navigate through a crisis in identifying business or marketing gaps that need to be filled. It serves as a useful baseline for brands to recognise there are always opportunities that emerge from a crisis and knowing that adjustments to consumer demands need to be made even during a recession.

4 Advertiser, Do Not Go Dark

During this worrisome time of uncertainty, the act of going dark may seem tempting since it has little impact on the brand or business metrics in the short term. However, seeing a COVID-19 related Tweet every 45 ms at the beginning of the outbreak (Josephson and Eimear 2020), it signals to brands that people are hunger for information.

According to Kantar's COVID-19 Barometer, a global survey of 35,000 consumers showed that in April 2020, only 5% of consumers thought that brands should not advertise. This was a decline from 8% in March 2020 (Chen 2020). Twitter Marketing (2020) research on brand communication guidelines also indicated that the majority of respondents (68%) said that brands should continue to advertise, with 77% agreeing that they felt positive about the need for brands to support society and 51% expressing the view that seeing or hearing advertisements gave them a sense of normality.

Undoubtedly, communication is at the very core of our society, and people wish to hear from brands amid the uncertainty brought about by the virus. Doyle Dane Bernbach (DDB), as cited in Marketing Interactive (2020), conducted a consumer survey in Hong Kong, asking respondents what they expected to hear from brands at the time of the survey compared to the coming months. The survey revealed a shift in expectations on what consumers wanted to hear and a transition from a state of panic and frustration to a more forward-looking condition. According to the results, concrete actions to help society and provide information about the virus were most desired before the containment of the virus. In contrast, it is interesting to observe that people tend to be more open to promotional communications and expected brands to provide them with positive distraction during the latter stage of the outbreak or after the outbreak is contained.

Apart from the shift in expectations on what to hear at different stages, there is also a shift in expectations across generations. In another COVID-19 tracker survey conducted by Dentsu Aegis Network, some diversity in content preference across different generations is again noticeable (Lundstrom 2020). In particular, generation Z (age 16–25) and millennials (age 26–39) were concerned about their mental health at the beginning, but later expressed a desire to become involved in the crisis and wanted brands to show how to accomplish this and help them to ease anxiety. This is consistent with the earlier DDB Hong Kong survey. On the other hand, baby boomers (age 60–74) were concerned about their health and the economy at the beginning of the pandemic and later moved to view brands as supporting their employees. Overall, the reactions and expectations of brands varied between generations and changed as the pandemic progressed.

During the initial stage of shock and uncertainty fueled by the pandemic, brands were expected to react and respond by providing accurate information, primarily aimed at offering a feeling of relief and a sense of psychological comfort. However, as the pandemic progressed, the wave of bad economic news eroded consumer confidence and buying power. This stage presented an opportunity for brands to persevere with uncertainty instead of being overpowered and engulfed. In determining an economically viable and socially acceptable path to the next norm, and to connect with existing and potential consumers, brands must make better judgement and act on insights based on consumer patterns. It is also essential for brands that wish to survive and remain relevant to know not just what consumers wish to hear at various stages of a crisis, but also where and how to get their message across.

To consumer-facing companies, adopting a brand strategy towards emerging consumer needs and behaviour is key to survival. Consumer insight is critical for brands in anticipating and meeting the evolving needs, attitudes, and trends of consumers. However, nothing is certain; focusing attention on consumer media habits could help brands to identify opportunities and gaps in fulfilling consumer's needs. Once a pattern is known, decisions can be made to survive a crisis and build future capabilities. For brands to adjust according to consumer demand, brands should first identify the current media consumption pattern of consumers. With the restriction of movement and social distancing measures fast becoming the new norm, consumers needed to redefine and re-adapt along with a drastic change in media habits. There are three key trends in media consumption in the COVID-19 era, namely, the surge in digital traffic, the awareness that all eyes on the screen and new uses and gratifications.

5 Key Trends in Media Consumption

5.1 The Surge in Digital Traffic

In this new era of "remote everything" with the population of most countries sheltering from COVID-19 and practising social distancing, there has been a notable spike in internet usage and the consumption of digital media. From a survey conducted by Nielsen of 9,100 people across six countries, including China and the US, concerning media consumption and preferences during COVID-19, between 80 and 90% of people consumed news and entertainment online for an average of 23.6 h a week, while 60% of consumers of global service were willing to register for free or pay to use and engage with online media content (Hall and Li 2020).

Another study investigating consumer behaviour by country highlighted some remarkable statistics revealing a massive increase in digital traffic (Agarwal 2020). Among the countries experiencing notable upsurges, Australia witnessed a 925% growth in educational gaming apps, and a 473% growth in news apps. In South Korea, a country with a popular eSports culture, there was a 191% rise in board games and an increase of 334% in card game apps. After the CB measures announced in early April 2020, Singapore saw a 3700% growth in the use of communication apps. All these figures suggest more than merely increased usage, but a growing preference and inclination of consumers towards digital activity and content.

The usage of super apps is particularly unique and quickly growing in Asia, driven by COVID-19 (Aakerlund and Dias 2020). WeChat, the all-in social media app, also known as the "king of super apps" in China, has around 1.165 billion monthly active users (MAUs) and offers more than 100 Chinese municipal services, using a mini programme in the apps to share information and statistics on COVID-19. Another short-video platform, Tik Tok, known as Douyin in China, has managed to connect 500 million users among which more than 12 million were unique visitors from the US who had registered between January and March 2020. With its broad coverage, Tik Tok announced a new content partnership programme with the World Health Organisation (WHO), launching the *#StayAtHome Live!* initiative to promote public service announcements (PSA). In India, Paytm, the largest domestic mobile payment and commerce platform has streamlined almost all types of payments for utilities in their 'go contactless' programme.

Other initiatives have also been witnessed aside from utility-based super apps, such as business apps, online education tools and digital health platforms, which strengthen and streamline the way the community and business interacts. One of the must-go-to platforms developed during this time has been 'Zoom', a video conferencing cloud-based platform. At the end of February 2020, Zoom was reported to have helped over 90,000 schools across 20 countries to continue education remotely, with an influx of daily users surging to 200 million users in March from a base of approximately 10 million users in December 2019 (Yuan 2020).

Indeed, the statistics just mentioned, contribute to the year-on-year global digital growth reported in April 2020 by Hootsuite (2020a), in which global digital growth and adoption increased across all digital platforms, accounting for an increase of 7.1% (301 million) of global internet users and 8.7% (304 million) growth in global active social media users. Digital platforms have become an integral part of our lives, providing new lifeblood for businesses, motivating the development of innovative digitally enabled business models and facilitating a global digital economy in the post-COVID 'new norm'.

The current pandemic has also inspired a new format in creating and distributing content, namely, live streaming and user-generated content (UGC). With multitudes of people forced to remain at home to help prevent the spread of COVID-19, live streaming traffic has spiked across media platforms such as Twiter, YouTube and Facebook with different content creators streaming a variety of topics. In China, there were more than 41 million watching live stream events at its peak, particularly the construction of the Leishenshan hospital, a temporary hospital in Wuhan. Likewise, the Weibo lockdown diary, a type of UGC which encourages Weibo users to journal and record their daily lives also received a high response rate. With the majority of major sporting events either cancelled, suspended or postponed, ESPN embraced UGC to remain relevant by inviting sports fans themselves to substitute for missing sports content.

As such, the new norm of "remote everything" has brought everyone online in some way or form for socialising, learning, working, entertainment and leisure across social, education, business, government, and healthcare platforms (Spataro 2020).

6 All Eyes on the Screen

Since COVID-19 has placed the majority of the world's population into unprecedented confinement, many are turning to or are almost entirely reliant on digital screens. Networks and electronic devices have provided vital help to people in coping with everyday life as part of the new norm. The home has become the new hub for our daily lives and a multiverse for news, *hometainment* and *quarantainment* through a myriad of different screen sizes.

Referring to Hootsuite's (2020b) July Global Statshot Report on how people globally are using the internet and mobile devices, there has been a consistent rise in the use of connected devices since April 2020, despite many countries temporarily, at least, easing restrictions. The majority of internet users aged between 16 and 64 years are spending the most time using smartphone devices or mobile phones (70%), followed by laptops (47%), desktop computers (33%) and tablet devices (23%). When it comes to reporting their screen time leisure activities, more than half were found to be watching shows and films on streaming services. Other top activities included spending extended time using social media, messenger services and mobile apps, listening to music through streaming services and for gaming. Comparing Hootsuite's (2020b) July report and Ericsson's Mobility Report (2020) in June 2020, it is evident that not only are people accessing and using information and communication technology for entertainment and utility purposes, but they are also using them to relieve anxiety during lockdowns and restrictions. For example, technology helps users cope by enabling parents to support their children's education (76%), keeping children entertained at home and engaged (65%), improving mental health and wellbeing (43%) and keeping fit and exercising (40%).

Overall, the time spent viewing digital media via multiple screens has recorded steady growth, including time watching television. However, other screens have contributed to this phenomenal growth. According to Media Partners Asia's (2020) report on the growing depth of the streaming economy in Southeast Asia between January and April 2020 in Indonesia, Singapore, Thailand and the Philippines, the total minutes per week recorded, for online video on mobile devices, rose sharply by 60% following the onset of COVID-19.

Furthermore, most of the over-the-top (OTT) media, a streaming media service offered directly to viewers via the internet, reported a significant uptake in consumption in these four countries: in China iQIYI grew by 500%, in Hong Kong Viu increased by 274% with a significant jump of 115% for Netflix. In Malaysia, iflix recorded a growth of 118% in consumption. Similarly, PS4 devices and games in Singapore also showed a growing interest during the first two weeks in March, as high as 713% and according to GIPHY's online database, video game searches worldwide are also up 928% in March (Stein 2020).

7 New Uses and Gratifications

People are not only turning to familiar ways of using media to manage their anxiety as COVID-19 wreaks havoc globally; under curfew and facing the same environment day in and day out, they are also finding new uses and gratifications in their attempts to keep physically and mentally active. During this time of uncertainty and instability, most consumers focus on achieving optimal health, especially mental wellness and emotional health. As such, having hobbies and self-care are crucial as this results in positive experiences and therapeutic benefits (Alfonso 2020).

Since people are using social media to search, share and discuss home experiences, 'Brandwatch' (a research institution) conducted a study in the Asia Pacific region in the context of the online phenomena in April 2020 on how people are spending their time. The findings showed that home workouts were top, followed by baking/cooking, reading, spring cleaning and learning a skill (Lee 2020). As people are actively seeking new ways to enrich their life under quarantine by informing brands what they want, brands could also help to explore new hobbies as well.

As reported in some news articles, dumbbells were added to the list of panic buying items (Koren 2020) to staying fits while exercising at home. By observing this demand for exercise equipment and weights and the broad social embrace of fitness, marketers can respond by developing brand strategies and creating content. The upsurge in stay-at-home fitness has not only created massive online traffic for digitally guided stay-at-home workouts via sports apps and short videos but has inspired a variety of streaming services and virtual trainers. For example, there has been a rise in hosting free yoga classes via YouTube, live stream meditation, and live fitness classes through apps and websites. Consequently, home and digital fitness have proven to be an invaluable outlet during the COVID-19 pandemic and may emerge as the new norm or 'hybrid' approach for post-virus wellbeing.

Besides home workouts, people are also registering for courses on self-enrichment and personal development during self-quarantine, resulting in exponential growth for massive online open courses (MOOCs). Several online learning platforms such as Coursera, Udacity, and Udemy provide a wide range of free programmes and training to meet the needs of quarantined adult learners. In contrast, prestigious schools like Harvard University and the Massachusetts Institute of Technology also offer a variety of open learning opportunities free-of-charge to the public, including online courses and modules to expand their knowledge. As much as the course completion rate, learning experience and effectiveness is subject to debate, at least, it brings new trends in media uses and gratifications in light. Knowing consumers of today have become active, and conscious in their selection, interest and media usage is of paramount importance in developing brand positioning. Brands that gratify the needs of people during this difficult time constitute the brands' that people will remember when the economy begins to reopen.

The desire for novel gratification is evident in trends such as the Dalgona coffee challenge. As cited in Kirkwood (2020), "Dalgona coffee" garnered a surge in searches worldwide by 1,800% in mid-March 2020, becoming the most searched coffee recipe worldwide via Google search. Moreover, the hashtag *#dalgonacoffee* garnered 423.8 million views on Tik Tok (2020). Such online challenges inform companies and brands about the new forms of gratification people are searching for. In particular, for social media food trends, it is rarely about the food itself, but the social capital one can relate to; experience sharing, staying current with the trend or, at least, in this case, showing that one can rustle up a foamy café-inspired coffee while stuck at home.

Covid-19 has imposed a challenge for us all. However, people need an anchor in familiarity for their comfort and to remain positive. Staying close to consumers, navigating and recognising these new behaviours and desires can help brands to create stability for housebound consumers. Unquestionably, there is a call for brands to be agile in fulfilling new gratifications and helping people to explore new hobbies, such as the online craze for the 'lockdown's got talent' show over the social media platforms.

8 Adapting Brand Strategies for COVID-19

The coronavirus pandemic has significantly changed media and the consumption of content. Media habits, as discussed, provide clarity on how consumer behaviour and media preferences are changing. However, these changes are equivocal, and it is difficult to postulate whether changes in behaviour will continue post-COVID-19. Though the redefined patterns of media consumption serve as a catalyst for brands in the immediate future, advertisers need to be alert to further changes in order to remain relevant. Brands that continue to be resilient in adapting to the new reality will have a better chance of remaining viable in the time coming. It is salient in this respect to observe that a study in social psychology has found that, on average, it takes 66 days for a behaviour to become a habit (Lally et al. 2010). Given the period of time that it will take to return to 'normality', even with the availability of vaccines, it is likely that some new trends will continue post-COVID.

Managing brand strategy is critical and needs to stress relevancy, authenticity and contextual needs. Given the new trends in media consumption, four implications are evident in relation to brand strategy, namely, being empathetic, not opportunistic; staying true through purpose-led communication; enhancing the brand's digital capabilities; and amplifying brand community.

9 Key Implications for Brand Strategy

9.1 Not Being Opportunistic, Being Empathetic with a Strong Social Presence

The fear and anxiety associated with self-isolation and enforced quarantine can be quite overwhelming and cause strong psycho-emotionally driven behaviour in people. During this trying time, the priority relative to people is essential in creating brand strategies that reflect empathy and the needs of people. However, brands need to be prudent as well as balancing empathy and opportunism. "Going dark" and doing nothing tends to signal indifference and sends out situation-insensitive and impractical messages can also fall into the 'do nothing' category.

Furthermore, in an atmosphere of distress, society will expect consumer-facing companies to address and respond to this issue in addition to being part of the solution. Therefore, the social presence of brands plays a pivotal role during a pandemic, such as COVID-19. Also, maintaining a social presence across different type of media, especially earned, shared, and owned, offers brands an opportunity to gain publicity and exposure under pressurised budgets. Especially at a time when there is an obvious temptation to cut marketing budgets; a social presence can lessen advertising clutter and stimulate a better brand recall and resonance for consumers.

Acknowledging the disruption caused by COVID-19 can be best reflected in the brand's intention in addressing and combating this virus. Brand strategy should focus on the aspects relevant to how they can contribute to helping resolve the threat of COVID-19. For instance, Google cancelled its popular April Fools' jokes programme, a tradition practised since the year 2000, as a sign of respect to those fighting the spread of COVID-19. Google's move helped to direct other forms of resources in helping communities stay well-informed and connected via exposure to notifications systems and a widening range of distance learning apps and tools.

Similarly, telecommunication providers are offering free mobile data services to help those in need and housebound to remain connected. Likewise, fashion labels such as John Lewis, Burberry and Mango have repurposed their factories to address the global shortage of personal protective equipment (PPE), that include face masks and hospital gowns. However, not all effort expended has been received positively, as brands must also ensure they present the best capability and proficiency in this endeavour for the right intentions otherwise the effort and sincerity go to waste. For instance, the first batch of Brewdog, a brewery brand that sold beer and cider and instead turned to produce hand sanitiser, was rejected by a local hospital since the company did not meet the medical standards required.

Overall, maintaining a brand's social presence is truly important, and brand strategy must be well-aligned to address existing threats by remaining relevant to the brand's core values and competency.

10 Staying True through Purpose-led Communication

Amid the chaos brought about by COVID-19, brand strategies must cut through the noise and build a creative environment to interact with consumers in a meaningful way. Without having a sense of purpose, a brand will fail to accomplish its full potential. Further, a brand strategy that revolves around purpose-led communication will ensure that the brand survives, and the brand name is reinforced, thanks to growing consumer loyalty cementing its position in the market-place in the long term (Wilson 2020). There are two principles in translating brand purpose into communication and practices, namely, purposeful stakeholder engagement and strategic brand equity.

Purpose-driven communication must not only be directed to consumers but other stakeholders as well, especially employees. In a brand strategy that prioritizes people, consumer and talent should be given equal consideration. Consumers continue to relate to companies who are caring and looking after the wellbeing of their employees in times of crisis, leading to a better reputation and trustworthiness (Kohll 2020). For example, the French high fashion luxury-goods company, Hermès, announced that they would maintain the basic salary of its employees worldwide in addition to the company's donation of EUR20 million to public hospitals in the Paris region. During this time, when many people are worried about unemployment, not only did Domino commit to feeding people with pizza, they also made sure the company was providing job opportunities to those in need by offering 10,000 job openings in the US. In these uncertain times, the inclusion of different stakeholders in providing purposeful communication and engagement tells a unique story about the brand.

A purpose-driven speech was delivered by the CEO of Marriott International, Arne Sorenson, who released a 6-min video to all Marriott associates addressing the company's challenges in the face of COVID-19. The CEO displayed compassionate leadership in managing stakeholder expectations by having the courage to deliver the bad news 'face-to-face' and shared in the sacrifices by forgoing his salary for the remainder of 2020 and cutting the salary of his executive team by half. This demonstrated the CEO's vulnerability and humility in dealing with this unprecedented crisis and the address ended with an emotional yet optimistic note assuring that together, they would survive.

Secondly, brands should leverage media channels to communicate with consumers for better brand equity. Communicating about charitable relief, medical assistance, and public health messages is a purpose-led communication. However, brands are reminded not to adopt humorous messages during PSAs as it is better to convey practical and relevant messages. On the other hand, a strategic communications plan will help to keep messages aligned with evolving market needs and demands and highlight important attributes of brands in creating a meaningful differentiation of the brand and accentuate its desirability. For instance, Nike launched a campaign encouraging people to practise social distancing and to stay indoors during COVID-19. The text-based advertisement read: "*If you ever dreamed of playing for millions around the world, now is your chance. Play inside, play for the world*". The campaign also featured Nike's high-profile endorsers, including renowned footballer Cristiano Ronaldo, who shared posts of himself 'playing inside'. Nike was also offering free studio-style streaming workouts and tips on remaining in shape while at home.

Another strategic brand equity communication was that of Dove's 'Courage is Beautiful' campaign celebrating the strength and beauty of frontline workers by showing the faces of healthcare workers, their skin marked by masks and PPE equipment. This campaign very much resonated with Dove's award-winning and worldwide Real Beauty campaign and its central notion of real beauty. Brand positioning and highlighting brand core values help to create a purposeful brand strategy for greater brand recall and recognition.

11 Accelerating Digital Commerce and Digital Experience Capabilities

'Go digital' is perhaps the new catchphrase nowadays, given the movement in digital adoption rates (Fabius et al. 2020). Undeniably, technology orientated commerce and experience offer a safer option, greater flexibility and convenience to consumers. COVID-19 continues to serve as a super accelerant in solidifying digital consumer behaviour. Moreover, in remaining ahead of competitors, brand strategies must focus on digital-first initiatives, particularly in e-commerce and omnichannel communication platforms by providing seamless customer experience from a physical store to virtual world.

The surge in online shopping and 'click-and-collect' options during the pandemic has forced brands, and companies to accelerate e-commerce in order to remain competitive in the new norm. Shoppers worldwide have adopted e-commerce at an unprecedented rate, especially in grocery and food shopping, changing one of the last footholds if not strongholds of retailers. For instance, in China, Alibaba reported a four-fold increase in online grocery orders placed by people born in the 1960s during the Spring Festival when the country was still experiencing new COVID-19 cases each day (Fan 2020). The number of e-commerce users in ASEAN in September 2020 reached 340 million, surpassing the 2025 forecast (Bernama 2020). Seeing this growth in e-commerce, there is no excuse for brands not to move to digital platforms.

Furthermore, exploring the feasibility of e-commerce infrastructure, marketers need to rethink their omnichannel digital experience and capability in line with new consumer behaviour. In catering to the rising demand of online shopping experiences, Forest Cabin, a Shanghai-based cosmetics brand saw a 90% decline in sales after temporarily closing half of its 337 stores across China and instead developed a live streaming strategy as its core marketing channel, gaining a 45% uptake in sales in just 15 days. The company trained a total of 1,600 shop attendants on how to host a live stream session on Taobao Live and witnessed a significant jump in viewers and new loyalty members; the proportion of online sales was boosted from 25 to 90%. Also, as consumer media habits are changing, brands that anchor omnichannel strategies in connecting with consumers will gain a competitive advantage.

Omnichannel communication is providing more options and flexibility for consumers to engage with brands. The rapid movement of digital experience through different channels and screens has also been made possible through offline-online migration. The rise of virtual museum and gallery tours, and the streaming of live music concerts and opera performances have driven the need to digitise cultural experiences and strengthened the demand for online experiences. By analogy, the snack brand Emily Crisps found a digital solution to the problem of launching its first outdoor advertising campaign during the lockdown, by bringing the offline online. The brand shared photos of the outdoor advertisements online on social media, along with self-deprecating and humourous light copy. This migration provided confidence for other brands to accelerate their digital transformation, catering for the user experience via their marketing.

12 Amplifying Brand Community: Prepare for the Rebound

During the COVID-19 pandemic, there is no doubt that shopping consumption will continue to decline, given the focus of people has changed from only buying necessities such as food. As a result, many brands are struggling to adapt to meet the changing market needs of consumers. At a time when people are turning to local news, and travel restrictions are imposed, brands need to re-adjust their strategies in connecting locally with consumers.

Indeed, business operations and supply chains are not excluded from this disruption. As such, consumers have begun to support small businesses locally, seeking locally produced consumables. It also allows brands to become much closer to local markets, especially with small businesses. When brands are capable of maintaining sufficient social presence, awareness and bridging the gap to the new norm, it will undoubtedly strengthen engagement going forward with the local community and brand preparedness for post-COVID-19 recovery.

Another possible brand strategy in amplifying brand community is by bringing people together, albeit virtually but *#alonetogether* (a popular hashtag during COVID times which illustrates how people stay interconnected while practising social distancing). Some initiatives sought to focus on the quintessential social activity, namely sharing food. For example, IKEA released the secret recipe for its signature Swedish meatball dish online for stay-at-home foodies, while DoubleTree by Hilton for the first time, shared its official bake-at-home recipe for chocolate chip cookie, famous for being the world's first cookie baked in space. These brands have thus created a warm and comforting experience for people with engaging content that seeks to maintain a sense of community.

Aside from recipe sharing, there has also been an online challenge inspired by the Rijksmuseum in Amsterdam, asking fans and followers to recreate iconic artworks using household items. The initiative received thousands of re-creations online with the tagline "*Don't just look at an artwork, be the artwork and make it yourself!*". The rationale behind amplifying the notion of community is primarily to stimulate people's emotional response to brands. Without being cynical, the promotion of shared minds, shared voices and shared hearts, can also translate into market share.

13 Adapting to Changes in Consumer Behaviour and Spending Patterns

COVID-19 has no doubt been a transformative event creating many unprecedented changes on a global scale. The period of contagion, self-isolation and economic uncertainty has over a relatively short period transformed the way we live and has marked a profound change in human behaviour. Similarly, the pandemic-related public health and economic crises have virtually reshaped consumer behaviour and spending patterns. However, the broad shifts to new behaviour hide significant variation since people have different personality characteristics (Amalia et al. 2012).

During times of crisis, according to Mehta et al. (2020), there are two important factors in studying consumer behavioural change: risk attitude and risk perception. Risk attitude refers to the interpretation by consumers of the risk content, and how much he or she is worried about the content of that risk. In contrast, risk perception refers to the interpretation by the consumer of the chance of being exposed to the risk

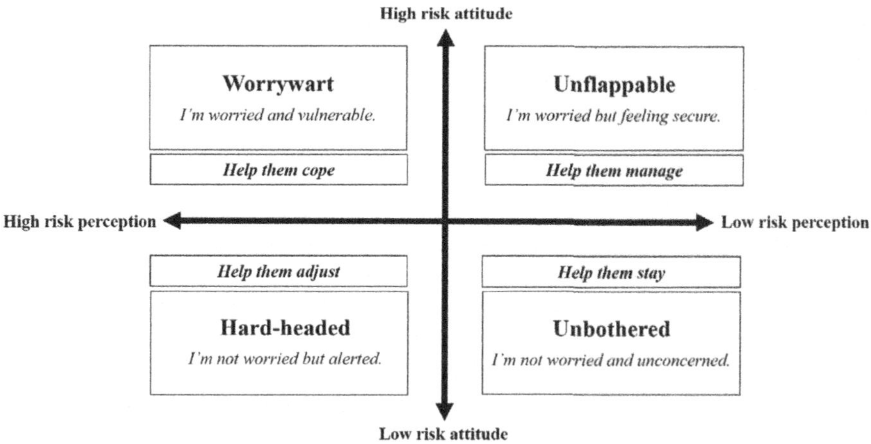

Fig. 1 Four types of consumer segment

content. These factors allow us to review consumer behaviour from a psychological perspective, instead of by demographics, since people think, feel, and make decisions differently. Figure 1 shows four types of consumer segment by their level of risk attitude and risk perception.

The **Worrywart** represents the hardest hit segment, and also the most pessimistic and vulnerable. Worrywarts tend to spend less across all product categories and prioritise essential goods. This segment is not only exclusive to the lower-income group, it can be from the higher-income class as well. Brands should provide a solution to help them cope through tough times; be it financially or psychologically. For instance, brands may attract worrywarts by offering a discount and smaller pack sizes at a lower price.

The **Unflappable** segment of consumers is not directly impacted by the crisis. Unflappable consumers are resilient and resolutely optimistic. As time passes, they may start spending on affordable indulgence. This segment consists of the under-affected realists, who, though feeling anxious, remain calm and positive. Brands can address this segment by initiating a cause-related campaign and providing accurate and reliable information to foster a sense of security. They may also prioritise customer care, helping the unflappables to manage change.

The **Hard-headed** consumer represents a segment that is less concerned but pessimistic about the long-term effect of the crisis. Here, spending tends to be less across all product categories but in a less aggressive way than the Worrywarts. This segment is prepared and aware, and also acts cautiously and vigilantly. Brands may offer options to help the hard-headed consumers to adjust to living in the new norm. Health-minded buying, preparation in quarantine living and affordable alternatives are appropriate for this segment.

The **Unbothered** category is the least concerned segment and can be perceived as overly-optimistic. Unbothered consumers will probably not be changing their spending habits and continue to buy favoured brands and products across all categories. This segment is close to indifferent as they retain their habits, but they are still open to living under the new norm. Brands can seize their openness by offering good deals, extra benefits and added convenience to help them stay positive during the crisis.

Notably, the COVID-crisis has fundamentally shifted consumer behaviour towards more utilitarian-based demands for essential needs. This global phenomenon has implicated brands in rethinking how and when to connect with consumers, re-examine messages, persona and strategies to engage with consumers and re-adjust operations to match the new shopping patterns. These four segments just described are constructed based on one's risk perception and attitude. By understanding consumer psychology, advertisers should achieve better persuasion, influence, and marketing efforts. However, there will be frequent starts, stops and resets in consumer behaviour driven by factors such as the changing conditions of the crisis, new values, new consumer experiences, disparities in the effects of the crisis in different geographical areas and more.

The changes in global consumer behaviour are evident. However, the cornerstone of the deviation is about what the next norm may entail and how sharply its contours will diverge from those with which we are familiar. This is because not all trends will survive post-COVID, some trends will be advanced, slowed or arrested by the recession. Knowing what to communicate to a different market segment of consumers via SMART—using storytelling, medium-based, authentic, relevant and trustworthy content—should help to protect brand resonance during and post times of crisis. New trends are likely to waver, and for a brand to sustain its profile amid this uncertainty, it must employ SMART content to drive the connection with consumers and maintain growth.

14 Key Implications in Advertising

Based on the above discussion of new trends in media consumption, brand strategy and emerging consumer behaviour, there are four implications with respect to advertising strategies, which offer new insights to advertisers on how advertising strategies affect brand resilience during economic adversity.

Relevance over reach: The COVID-19 pandemic has demonstrated how interconnected we all are to the extent that no one is safe until everyone is safe. The nature of interdependence echoes the need for realignment coupled with evolving consumer needs and exploiting the new consumer segments described above. While maintaining a social presence is critical, being online is not a prerogative; the crux is staying relevant to the shifting market demands.

Conversation over conversion: These unprecedented COVID times have brought about huge challenges and collective anxiety in the marketplace. People are searching for reliable information to stay safe, looking for distraction and levity while staying at home and seeking ways to remain positive. At times like this, brands should stay in the conversation for contribution, engagement and encouragement rather than conversion.

Solving over selling: Consumers expect brands to be part of the community and part of the solution in helping the less fortunate and disadvantaged during times of crisis. Brands should leverage their owned and shared media in responsible marketing and to build trust. Publicity gained from earned media, too, contributes to brand awareness and its social presence, particularly through customer reviews, mentions, shares and retweets in social media platforms or printed media. It is certainly not a marketing opportunity to capitalise upon but rather, maintaining media investment for brand building, promoting new advantages and digital reinvention as a means of addressing the immediate challenges.

Value over visibility: Making a brand's social presence felt in the marketplace via advertising efforts is critical for brand visibility, recognition and awareness. However, in times of crisis, brands should value quality over quantity for business resilience and continuity. A good impression and positive word-of-mouth are more effective and influential with regards to brand acceptance. Additionally, message personalisation and association with locality and current needs generate support at a much deeper emotional level.

15 Conclusion

The effects of COVID-19 are far-reaching, causing unprecedented disruptions worldwide. During an economic slowdown like this, advertisers, though, are reluctant to spend even though past recessions have demonstrated how continued advertising provides reassurance about the brand during periods of uncertainty. Nonetheless, times of crisis also demonstrate that the value of media is growing, if it is aligned with changes in media consumption. Remaining contextually relevant is the key for brand survival, while adapting to recent trends and understanding new consumer behaviour is the key in moving forward, especially post-COVID-19.

Even though lockdowns and restrictions have separated millions of people, there is a tendency for communities to band together and help each other. Given that we hope to learn from these unprecedented times, there is a fine balance between identifying opportunities and remaining opportunistic about the future. Also, being purpose-driven in communication and providing solutions to assist and embrace communities should be a high priority. Brands should do more than merely communicate but instead connect with consumers, continue to advertise, and above all, accommodate and adjust to remain relevant and true to the brand's core value. An advertising mantra summed it up best. "When times are good you should advertise; when times are bad you must advertise".

References

Aakerlund, K., Dias, N. (2020) The new abnormal—media habits in cathartic times. MMA Webinar Series. Available at: https://www.mmaglobal.com/webinars/apac-webinar-new-abnormal-media-habits-cathartic-times. (Accessed 16 April 2020).

Agarwal, V. (2020) Navigating the shift in consumer behaviour in Asia during COVID-19. Mobile Marketing Association. Available at: https://www.mmaglobal.com/files/webinars/inmobi_mma_covid19_webinar.pdf. (Accessed 29 April 2020).

Alfonso, F. (2020) The long lost hobbies people around the world are revisiting during the coronavirus pandemic. CNN International. Available at: https://edition.cnn.com/2020/04/05/world/old-hobbies-quarantine-coronavirus-wellness-trnd/index.html. (Accessed 4 May 2020).

Amalia, P., Mihaela, D., Ionut, P. (2012) From market orientation to the community orientation for an open public administration: A conceptual framework. *Procedia: Social & Behavioral Sciences*, 62:871–875.

Bernama. (2020) E-commerce users in ASEAN surpasses 2025 forecast. The Edge Markets. Available at: https://www.theedgemarkets.com/article/ecommerce-users-asean-surpasses-2025-forecast. (Accessed 27 September 2020).

Chen, E. (2020) Advertising in the time of COVID: Perspectives from consumers and the automotive, QSR and retail sectors. KANTAR Media. Available at: https://www.kantarmedia.com/us/thinking-and-resources/blog/advertising-in-the-time-of-covid-perspectives-from-consumers-and-the-automotive-qsr-retail-sectors. (Accessed 8 September 2020).

Consterdine, G. (2009) *Advertising in a recession: It pays to maintain marketing pressure.* Dublin: Periodical Publishers Association of Ireland.

Drucker, P. (2017) View marketing as an investment—not an expense. Tribal Vision. Available at: https://tribalvision.com/tips-to-market-smarter/view-marketing-investment-not-expense/. (Accessed 20 August 2020).

Ericsson Mobility Report. (2020) Available at: https://www.ericsson.com/49da93/assets/local/mobility-report/documents/2020/june2020-ericsson-mobility-report.pdf. (Accessed 22 September 2020).

Fabius, V., Kohli, S., Veranen, S. M., Timelin, B. (2020) Meet the next-normal consumer. McKinsey & Company. Available at: https://www.mckinsey.com/business-functions/marketing-and-sales/our-insights/meet-the-next-normal-consumer. (Accessed 18 September 2020).

Fader, P. (2008) When the going gets tough, the tough don't skimp on their ad budgets. Knowledge@Wharton, University of Pennsylvania. Available at: https://knowledge.wharton.upenn.edu/article/when-the-going-gets-tough-the-tough-dont-skimp-on-their-ad-budgets/. (Accessed 18 September 2020).

Fan, Y. Y. (2020) How COVID-19 sparked a silver tech revolution in China. Sixth Tone. Available at: https://www.sixthtone.com/news/1005303/how-covid-19-sparked-a-silver-tech-revolution-in-china. (Accessed 18 September 2020).

Fromm, J., Bolton, S., Fisher, L. (2020a) Coronavirus effect on advertising report: A new series of studies based on the effect of the Coronavirus on ad spending. Advertiser Perceptions. Available at https://www.advertiserperceptions.com/wp-content/uploads/2020/03/03.25.2020-Coronavirus-Effect-on-Advertising-WEBINAR-PDF-1.pdf. (Accessed 19 August 2020).

Fromm, J., Bolton, S., Fisher, L. (2020b) Coronavirus effect on advertising report: a new series of studies based on the effect of the Coronavirus on ad spending (Wave 6). Advertiser Perceptions. Available at: https://s3.amazonaws.com/media.mediapost.com/uploads/CoronavirusWave6.pdf. (Accessed 19 August 2020).

Graham, M. (2020) Global ad spending will likely fall if spread of coronavirus continues. CNBC TECH. Available at https://www.cnbc.com/2020/03/03/how-coronavirus-could-impact-advertising-spending.html. (Accessed 29 August 2020).

Hall, S. Li, C. (2020) COVID-19 proves that media's value is growing—but we need to find better ways to measure it. World Economic Forum. Available at: https://www.weforum.org/agenda/2020/04/covid-19-media-value/. (Accessed 17 August 2020).

Hoekstra, J. C., Leeflang, P. S. H. (2020) Marketing in the era of COVID-19. *Italian Journal of Marketing*, 249–260.
Hootsuite. (2020a) Digital 2020 April global statshot report. Available at: https://hootsuite.com/pages/digital-2020. (Accessed 27 September 2020).
Hootsuite. (2020b) Digital 2020 July global statshot report. Available at: https://hootsuite.com/pages/digital-2020. (Accessed 27 September 2020).
IPSOS. (2020) What worries the world—May 2020. IPSOS. Available at: https://www.ipsos.com/en/what-worries-world-may-2020. (Accessed 30 August 2020).
Josephson, A., Lambe, E. (2020) Brand communications in time of crisis. Twitter company. Available at: https://blog.twitter.com/en_us/topics/company/2020/Brand-communications-in-time-of-crisis.html. (Accessed 30 August 2020).
Kirkwood, K. (2020) What is Dalgona coffee? The whipped coffee trend taking over the internet during coronavirus isolation. The Conversation. Available at: https://theconversation.com/what-is-dalgona-coffee-the-whipped-coffee-trend-taking-over-the-internet-during-coronavirus-isolation-137068. (Accessed 24 September 2020).
Kohll, A. (2020) How one company is taking care of employees during COVID-19. *Forbes*. Available at: https://www.forbes.com/sites/alankohll/2020/04/06/how-one-company-is-taking-care-of-employees-during-covid-19/#34f58226488d. (Accessed 7 September 2020).
Koren, M. (2020) The healthiest way to sweat out a pandemic. *The Atlantic*. Available at: https://www.theatlantic.com/health/archive/2020/03/coronavirus-gyms-exercise-social-distancing/608278/. (Accessed 12 September 2020).
Lally, P., Van Jaarsveld, C. H., Potts, H. W., Wardle, J. (2010) How are habits formed: Modelling habit formation in the real world. *European Journal of Social Psychology*, 40(6):998–1009.
Lee, S. (2020) Covid-19 and APAC: hobbies and creating positive experiences at home. Available at: https://www.brandwatch.com/blog/covid-19-apac-hobbies/. (Accessed 10 September 2020).
Lundstrom, K. (2020) Millennials, gen z want distraction—and action—from brands during crisis. Available at: https://www.adweek.com/brand-marketing/millennials-gen-z-want-distraction-action-from-brands-coronavirus/. (Accessed 20 September 2020).
Marketing Interactive. (2020) Five lessons from lockdown: COVID-19, Hong Kong consumer sentiment, and brand implications. Available at: https://marketing-interactive.com/five-lessons-from-lockdown-covid-19,-hong-kong-consumer-sentiment,-and-brand-implications. (Accessed 20 September 2020).
Media Partners Asia. (2020) Online video streaming minutes in Southeast Asia skyrocket after COVID-19 impact according to new MPA study. Available at: https://www.media-partners-asia.com/article.php?id=2325. (Accessed 27 August 2020).
Mehta, S., Saxena, T., Purohit, N. (2020) The new consumer behaviour paradigm amid COVID-19: Permanent or transient? *Journal of Health Management* , 22(2):291–301.
Sneader, K., Singhal, S. (2020) Beyond coronavirus: The path to the next normal. Available at: https://www.mckinsey.com/industries/healthcare-systems-and-services/our-insights/beyond-coronavirus-the-path-to-the-next-normal. (Accessed 10 September 2020).
Spataro, J. (2020) 2 years of digital transformation in 2 months. Microsoft. Available at: https://www.microsoft.com/en-us/microsoft-365/blog/2020/04/30/2-years-digital-transformation-2-months/. (Accessed 17 August 2020).
Stein, L. (2020) Here's how people are using GIFs during social distancing. Campaign US. Available at: https://www.campaignlive.com/article/heres-people-using-gifs-during-social-distancing/1679829. (Accessed 5 January 2021.
Tellis, G. J., Tellis, K. (2009) A critical review and synthesis of research on advertising in a recession. *Journal of Advertising Research,* 49(3):304–327.
The Guardian. (2020) US unemployment rises 6.6m in a week as coronavirus takes its toll. Available at: https://www.theguardian.com/business/2020/apr/09/us-unemployment-filings-coronavirus. (Accessed 24 September 2020).
Tik Tok. (2020) Tik Tok tag. Available at: https://www.tiktok.com/tag/dalgonacoffee. (Accessed 20 September 2020).

Twitter Marketing. (2020) Advertising during COVID-19. Available at: https://marketing.twitter.com/en_gb/insights/twitter-covid19-advertising-policy. (Accessed 4 January 2021).
Verma, S., Kumar, V. (2017) Advertising in recession: a competitive strategy to crush small players. *The Catalyst—Journal of Management*, 2(2): 28–35.
Wilson, J. (2020) Sustainable brands can pivot with purpose to help address COVID-19. Nielsen. Available at: https://www.nielsen.com/my/en/insights/article/2020/sustainable-brands-can-pivot-with-purpose-to-help-address-covid-19/. (Accessed 6 September 2020).
Yuan, E. S. (2020) A message to our users. Zoom Company News. Available at: https://blog.zoom.us/a-message-to-our-users/. (Accessed 17 August 2020).

University Image Building via WeChat During the Covid-19 Pandemic: A Case Study of a Chinese Higher Education Institution

Hong Qian and Jia Zhang

Abstract The contagious nature of the Covid-19 coronavirus has seriously challenged universities all over the world, as millions of students have been unable to attend classes on campus. For universities such as BNU-HKBU United International College (UIC), given the loss of face-to-face communication channels, social media such as UIC WeChat Account have been playing an important role in connecting students, parents and the university, and in displaying the university's image. The shift toward the use of social media during the Covid-19 pandemic has drawn our attention to the fact that most scholarly discussion of university image building has been from the perspective of tertiary institution management, while little attention has been given to the multimodal resources employed in WeChat posts during the image building process. This study thus focuses on an investigation, from a multimodal perspective, of image building of UIC, a higher education institution with English as the medium of instruction in China, during the Covid-19 pandemic. The study was conducted by drawing on the theoretical framework of the Corporate Identity system (CIS) which includes the Mind Identity System (MIS), Behavior Identity System (BIS) and Visual Identity System (VIS). From a bottom-up approach, in the first place, posts published by UIC from the outbreak of the pandemic were collected to build a small corpus. Then texts and pictures were categorized and analyzed to find out how different components and modes work together to form the BIS and VIS, and what MIS of UIC has been demonstrated. The study shows how multimodal resources on social media have supported the development of a university image in a time of crisis and social distancing.

1 Introduction

Kotler and Fox (1995) define 'image' broadly as one's general impression of a certain object; it refers to people's perceptions of reality (Gotsi and Wilson 2001). Often

H. Qian · J. Zhang (✉)
Beijing Normal University - Hong Kong Baptist University United International College (BNU-HKBU UIC), Zhuhai, China
e-mail: jiazhang@uic.edu.cn

S.X.B. Zhao et al. (eds.), *COVID-19 Pandemic, Crisis Responses and the Changing World*, https://doi.org/10.1007/978-981-16-2430-8_22

discussed in the commercial world, especially in marketing and advertising, this concept might still seem to many to have little relation to higher education. However, several decades ago universities had been analyzed as examples of marketization by academics (e.g., Fairclough 1993; Osman 2008). Kwong (2000: 89) defines the marketizing process in higher education as the "adoption of free market practices in running school" via strategies such as "cutting production cost, abandoning goods not in demand, producing only popular products and advertising products to increase sales and the profit margin". With the growth of intense competition among universities to attract higher quality students, universities have been operating more like private businesses, and university management have begun to view university image as a marketing tool in enhancing the reputation of the institution. From that moment on, traditional universities have changed into so-called corporate universities (Jarvis 2001), and they had taken up more of a corporate form and functioned more like a corporation. Consequently, scholarly attention has also been paid to university image as it has been found that a university's image plays a crucial part in its development (e.g., Chandra et al. 2019).

The outbreak of the Covid19 pandemic in 2020 brought unprecedented challenges to university image building that demand scholarly attention. When teaching had to be conducted online, to avoid possible infection, how could a university present itself to its students, and to the outside world? It is evident that with the loss of face-to-face communication, almost all universities relied even more than they had done hitherto on digital means such as websites, emails or social media tools to stay in touch with their students. On the Chinese mainland, with the popularity of the social media app, WeChat, WeChat Official Accounts (hereinafter WOAs) have become a vital platform for universities to interact with the subscribers and to present their corporate image. As corporate culture (Treadwell and Treadwell 2000) is a kind of new university culture, most of those universities have established departments responsible for corporate communications (Osman 2005) to handle corporate matters. Those departments would undertake corporate information management and publication, and would project a positive image of their universities, all of which belong to corporate advertising.

In this chapter, drawing on the Corporate Identity System (hereinafter CIS) as a theoretical framework, the authors investigate the image building of Beijing Normal University-Hong Kong Baptist University United International College (hereinafter UIC) via a multimodal approach. The WOAs published by the Media and Public Relations Office of UIC are the research objects. According to Osman (2008: 61), "any publications from universities, particularly those produced by the Corporate or Public Relations Office, are referred to as corporate genre". We are interested in what image of UIC has been projected through the WOAs.

UIC was selected as our study object because of its representativeness considering the corporate nature. UIC is a university jointly founded by Hong Kong Baptist University and Beijing Normal University, one of the very first cooperation between Mainland China and Hong Kong. As a self-financed university, UIC receives not much funding from governments, and mainly relies on income from students' tuition fees to survive and expand. Therefore, unlike most universities in mainland China with government funding, UIC operates more like a general business. It also has more urgent needs than other universities to increase its reputation and attract more quality students. Therefore, we deem it a good example for the analysis of image building.

A multimodal approach takes into consideration a range of multimodal semiotic resources, such as verbal texts and visual images, instead of a narrow analysis of language alone, as, without the broader context, analysts "may lose essential aspects of meaning, and subsequent interpretations of communicative effects, cultural values and ideology may be partial or incorrect" (Feng 2019: 65). The multimodal dimension to the study on the image building of UIC during the pandemic period is hoped to deepen our understanding on this kind of corporate genre.

2 University Image

Images are reflected in the positive or negative opinions formed in people's mind after interacting with the elements of a system or an organization for a period of time (Dichter 1985). They can only be formed on the basis of one's experience. They might also be perceived differently by different people owing to variations in the information received (Dowling 1988). Likewise, a brand image, a concept much studied in the commercial world, represents the beliefs, associations, attitudes, and impressions held by customers when interacting with any given brand. Two further related terms, corporate image and organizational image, have also been thoroughly investigated by researchers. Those terms in recent years have been applied to the study of image in a university setting, a topic that hitherto has been relatively neglected. Researchers are now using the terms 'university image' or 'higher education institution (HEI) image'. For example, Alcaide-Pulido et al. (2017) defines university image as a set of students' mental perceptions which will impact on their opinions about the university. In our research, the term 'university image' is also used, and it refers to the perceived perception of a university by students and parents on the basis of information and experience. Parents are also included in our definition, because unlike many other universities, UIC involves extensively parents in students' whole person education, which has been written into its education philosophy. Parents are also the targets of university promotions, either parents of current students or those of future students.

Universities, for a long time, were regarded as non-profit organizations, and thus image, which is assumed to affect consumers' purchase decision-making and thus companies' profitability, seemed irrelevant to universities. As the difficulty of accessing higher education has declined, the competition among universities to attract higher quality students has intensified. People began to view a university's image as a marketing tool to enhance the university's attractiveness to applicants and private funders. In addition, measuring a university's image also might provide universities with a better understanding of their own strengths and weaknesses.

Universities, during the pandemic, have been faced with a situation where many face-to-face channels of information dissemination become impossible. Popular social media platforms among young people, such as WeChat, were thus increasingly relied upon as effective means to spread information and enhance experience. It is worth studying how it helps to shape a positive image among students and parents.

The few scholars of marketing who have addressed university image building mainly probe into three aspects: the importance and impact of a university image, key factors in building a university image, and the means of enhancing a university image.

Most of these studies find that university image now plays a crucial part in the development of the university. Various research instruments have been used that demonstrate its positive impact on many aspects including student satisfaction, student loyalty and student Behavior. For instance, Chandra et al. (2019) employs a set of survey instruments to confirm that a university image positively and significantly influences student satisfaction and student loyalty. In another study, Polat (2011) measures students' perceived university image and finds out that the more accurately students perceive the image of the university, the higher their academic achievement is.

Other research identifies factors that might affect university image, by measuring it from different perspectives such as those of current students, graduates, and parents of prospective students. Aghaz et al. (2015) examined factors contributing to university image on the basis of postgraduate students' opinions and finds that those factors consist of internal and international reputation, university members, academic planning and university environment. Wilkins and Huisman (2013) designed a questionnaire of 25 items to identify factors which prospective international students use to assess university image.

A small number of researchers have also explored various means to improve and enhance university image, especially marketing models. Foroudi et al. (2019) explored customer value co-creation behavior in higher education institutions, which refers to customer (student in the case of higher education) participation in creating and delivering customer experiences. He confirmed in a quantitative study that there is a positive link between website features and customer value co-creation behavior and thus this helps to create university image.

The few studies of university image building have hitherto attended largely to websites, service quality, and student satisfaction. During the Covid-19 pandemic social media became the pre-eminent means by which universities sought to communicate with and maintain their image amongst students. Their popularity amongst most students, their ease of use and their interactivity make social media a powerful means of establishing and sustaining a university image in higher education. This chapter therefore focuses on WeChat, currently the most popular social media platform in China, to explore how a Chinese institution sustained its image during the pandemic.

3 WeChat Official Accounts

WeChat currently offers three different types of accounts: a service account, a subscription account, and an enterprise account, each with an emphasis on different functions. In most cases, individuals and organizations choose to open up subscription accounts, for the purpose of "posting stories and information, innovating author-reader interaction and content management" (WeChat Official Account Platform 2020).

Compared with an official university website, WeChat official subscription accounts can facilitate more active interaction: once an article is sent, subscribers are notified immediately, and can easily access the article via mobile phones and other devices.

WeChat official accounts have only become popular in recent years. Owing to its popularity amongst students, universities have also been opening up official accounts to post information and interact with students and parents. However, research on the impact of university WeChat official accounts is still scarce.

Among those who have explored the use of WOA in academic settings, Xu et al. (2015) in their investigation of the use of WOA of 39 academic libraries in China, found that one third of the universities sampled used WeChat explicitly as a marketing tool. In addition, most of the universities at that time adopted only the most basic functions of the app, but failed to use more advanced functions. Wei (2016) discusses the use of WOA in the management of universities, analyzing problems in student management and attempting to apply the functions of WeChat to solving those problems.

Several other studies probe various ways in which academic institutions might increase reader views and likes of their pages. Zhou and Lu (2017) collected articles from the WOA of university libraries, analyzed the features and writing rules of those articles, and proposed ways of increasing reader views. Li et al. (2018) took the WOA of Communist Youth League of Guangxi University as an example to assess the factors that help increase the number of followers. They note that to enhance the attractiveness of the institution, official accounts have to provide useful services or be entertaining.

Thus far, studies of the impact of university WeChat public accounts are still limited in number. Most focus on the various functions of WeChat and suggest ideas for the better utilization of those functions. Though the attractiveness of the university is sometimes discussed, university image as such is rarely mentioned. In addition, when WeChat articles are analyzed, the purpose is usually to identify the writing patterns and features. Not much attention is given to image building or multimodal aspects beyond the verbal elements.

4 Corporate Identity System

The concept of the Corporate Identity System (hereafter CIS) can be traced back as far as the nineteenth century (Feng and Li 2004). It is a system that is intended to aid corporate image recognition (Zhang and Chen 2016). This system aims at creating a unified, simple, and distinctive image that helps a corporation stand out from others. CIS these days is not only applied in the image building of corporations, but also in the image building of cities, colleges, and other collectives.

CIS includes the Mind Identity System, Visual Identity System and Behavior Identity System. At the core is Mind Identity System (hereafter MIS) which includes corporate culture and management philosophy. MIS comprises the highest principles that a corporation upholds in operation. It will determine the management and operation strategies of a corporation and the internal rules and regulations.

The Behavior Identity System (hereafter BIS) refers to various activities carried out by corporations with the guidance of MIS, which in turn reflects the management philosophy and culture of corporations. Those activities might be internal, such as employee training and staff welfare, or external, such as marketing and public relations. The public can directly feel the image of a corporation, and thus recognition is formed.

Visual Identity System (hereafter VIS) is a set of visual elements designed to leave a profound impression on people and increase the recognition of the brand. Information about a corporation and its management philosophy is also delivered via those elements, such as logos, trademarks, and packages. At the end of the twentieth century, universities have also changed their roles played in society. Originally, universities were to serve the state in managing society, while now they will serve the industry and businesses so as to guarantee the employment of people in society (Jarvis 2001).

Universities, especially private-funded universities, are faced with more and more pressure in student enrollment, image of a university plays an important role in attracting prospective students. CIS is a proven effective system in building up image of corporations and has been borrowed and tested in the image building of cities and organizations. In this paper, it will be applied to the analysis of university image by analyzing WeChat articles.

5 Integrating CIS with UIC Image Analysis

This study combines a qualitative and quantitative approach to the exploration of university image in UIC. Qualitatively, The CIS system works as the theoretical framework which enables us to explore the university image via the BIS and VIS subsystems. The verbal resources employed in the published WeChat articles are analyzed so as to find out the behavior of UIC during the pandemic period. The visual elements are investigated to reveal the VIS system of UIC. With the understanding of the UIC's BIS and VIS systems in the Covid-19 pandemic period, we can account for the MIS so as to have a clear understanding of the focus in image building against the backdrop of Covid-19. The quantitative data, all WOA articles published by UIC during the pandemic, act as a supplement to further reveal the MIS. As noted above, both visual and verbal codes are analyzed and discussed, as this is a study that involves intersemiotic resources and multimodal analysis.

The research design aims to address the following questions: What BIS is constructed via the WOA articles of UIC during the pandemic? What VIS has been constructed via the WOA during the pandemic? What image of UIC has been shaped via the BIS and VIS? Is this image consistent with the announced mission and does it serve the purpose of university promotion well? If not, what are the possible reasons?

WOA articles, were collected from the official WeChat account of UIC. The duration is from January 22, 2020–May 15, 2020, approximately four months altogether. The rationale is that the first article on Covid-19 to be published in the UIC WeChat account, appeared on January 22, 2020. On April 8th, in the meeting of the Standing Committee of the Political Bureau of the CPC Central Committee Chinese President Xi Jinping analyzed the COVID-19 situation and mentioned that "regular prevention and control measures" should be adhered to (Regular Epidemic Prevention and Control 2020), which indicates that China had just gone through the most serious phase of the pandemic. By mid-May 2020, for China, the most serious period had already passed and the country had entered a new phase of regular epidemic prevention and control. Therefore, we deemed it reasonable to collect and analyze the articles published during this period to determine how the college presented itself via social media at the height of the crisis in China.

During the four months, January to May 2020, 115 articles in total were published in UIC WOA, among which 14 were quoted from other sources. The other 101 were originally composed by UIC. We will mainly focus on the 101 articles. The 115 articles are firstly categorized based on the themes. The purpose is to understand the BIS: what has been done and what was prioritized or emphasized during this phase of the pandemic. The categorization processes were conducted by the current two authors independently. The articles were coded in an excel sheet. There was not much disagreement over the coding, but when disagreement arose, it was resolved through discussion.

6 BIS of UIC Constructed via the WOA Articles

6.1 Summarizing the Data on BIS

Table 1 is a summary of the coded themes. It is evident that university-related articles are the most frequent, totaling 62 articles. When we coded the articles as university-related, we meant that the university provided information to students about how to take classes, how to prevent the pandemic, and about the improvement of UIC. When

Table 1 A summary of the BIS of UIC

Code	Category	Sub-category	Number of articles (sub-category)	Number of articles (category)	Percentage (category) (%)
1	University	1.1 Teaching	12	62	54
		1.2 Measures and actions related to the pandemic	13		
		1.3 University improvement	4		
		1.4 Admission	21		
		1.5 Graduation	2		
		1.6 Pandemic prevention knowledge	10		
2	Students	2.1 Study	5	42	36
		2.2 Student activities	17		
		2.3 Contribution to pandemic prevention	11		
		2.4 Life back at campus	1		
		2.5 Alumni	8		
3	Teachers	3.1 Staff	5	11	10
		3.2 President	6		
		Total		115	100

focusing on the pandemic related topics, it is clear that articles in the subcategories 1.1 *teaching,* 1.2 *measures and actions related to the pandemic* and 1.6 *pandemic prevention knowledge* are actually most directly related to the pandemic. The total number is 35, accounting for over 50% of the total number of articles in this category. The number of *admission related* articles is also impressive, taking up one third of the total number. Comparatively, the articles on *graduation* and *university improvement* are relatively few.

Articles related to students themselves number 42. It can be seen that articles about student activities are the most frequent. Then students' contribution to pandemic prevention is the second highest occurrence. Stories about alumni regularly appear during the four months, so there are eight such articles. Study, which might be considered one of the most important topics for students, was not explicitly discussed very often.

The number of articles about teachers is only 11, much fewer than articles about university and students, taking up only 10% of the total number. The number of articles related to teachers is six. The total number relating Professor Tang, the

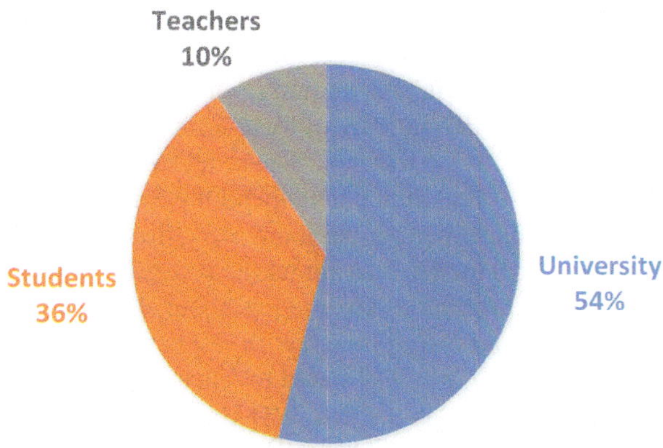

Fig. 1 The visual display of the themes of the articles

President of UIC is five, including articles written by him introducing historic sites in Zhuhai, letters written to students during the pandemic, etc. (Fig. 1).

7 Decoding the BIS

The figures shown above indicate that articles related to the university are the most frequent, then the students and the teachers. The university, therefore, has been highlighted in the published WOA articles during the pandemic period. As the categories demonstrate, the articles are mainly about how to address the pandemic.

The college showed its students and other readers that it was a responsible and caring higher education institution by publishing the most articles on pandemic-related issues including how to prevent the pandemic, how to take classes during the pandemic, how to relieve the mental stress which was brought about by the pandemic, etc.

In the following part, cases will be analyzed to demonstrate how the BIS is reflected via the WOA articles. Overall, the BIS of UIC in the studied period is constructed from four aspects via the verbal resources. Three of them are concerned with university management and one is related to students.

7.1 Pandemic Prevention and Teaching Adjustment: A Quick and Responsible Response

On January 20, Prof. Zhong Nanshan, China's top epidemiologist, who has also made the greatest contribution to defeat SARS in 2003, announced that the virus could be spread by infection from one human being to another (*Chinanews* 2020). The situation across the whole of China immediately became severe. Very quickly, on January 22, 2020, UIC's first WOA article about the pandemic was published, reminding students to protect themselves properly. Most of the content was not originally written by UIC, but quoted from the WHO, telling people how to properly wear masks, wash hands etc. The title, however, was original to UIC, conveying messages to both students and teachers. The article asked them to take proper actions to protect themselves so that they could spend the Spring Festival vacation without too much worry. At that time, people knew very little about the pandemic, neither knowing how to protect themselves nor taking it very seriously. UIC's prompt response, which provided authoritative knowledge about the Covid-19 virus, began establishing a responsible and caring image with respect to the imminent crisis.

There are 12 articles related to teaching arrangement or adjustment. The one on February 3, 2020, is the first WOA article to inform students about adjustments to teaching during the pandemic. It includes information about how to add and drop courses, the use of the Panopto video platform for online teaching and the implications for assuring teaching quality. Published only 13 days after the announcement of the virus, this article covered most of the teaching issues that students were likely to be concerned with, explaining how the college would conduct its courses online.

The two articles (January 22 and February 3) clearly showed the reader that the college was fair, responsible and caring about the wellbeing of its students. Furthermore, when affected by the sudden attack of the pandemic, the college could, almost without delay, provide information about self-protection and systematic teaching rearrangements. The image created was of an institution that was prepared for the upcoming emergency, and put student welfare first.

7.2 Admission: Tough and Challenging

As Table 1 shows, there are 21 articles on university admission, which account for the most items in percentage terms. Admission is one of the most important factors to boost the development of the college. Every year's admission process is tough and competitive, since it is a challenge to attract the best students to the college. Considering the contagious nature of the Covid-19 virus, promotion trips were suddenly impossible. From the number of articles on the topic of admission, it can be seen that the college was trying every means to shift the promotion online, and to ensure the quality of incoming students. The potential readers, most of whom were current students/parents, prospective students/parents thus could be reassured of the quality of the intake and their confidence in UIC would be strengthened. In a sense, these articles can be regarded as a kind of transformed prospectus, which has become a 'genre of consumer advertising colonizing professional and public service orders of discourse on a massive scale, generating many new hybrid partly promotional genres' (Fairclough 1993: 139).

The image built here is a tough team who were responding valiantly under pressure to ensure the continuing growth of the college, and played a role.

7.3 *President: Low Profile*

Another feature observed by the current authors, is the number of WOA articles related to the President of UIC, Prof. Tang Tao. No fewer than six articles are related to Prof. Tang. Among them, there are letters written by him to UIC students about the semester adjustments during the pandemic as well as articles written by President Tang about some renowned historic sites in Zhuhai, near the UIC campus. The number of articles related to the president is relatively fewer compared with that in the same period of the previous year (Nine out of 60 articles were related with the President). The likely functions of the relatively low ratio of the articles related with President Tang are twofold. Firstly, in such an unprecedented pandemic period, the letters written by the President of UIC might comfort students and parents so that they would not worry too much about studies. Secondly, the articles about the Zhuhai historic sites series show students the optimistic attitude of the President towards the pandemic, as the writing style is informal and friendly, and the articles were attractively illustrated with photographs of the historic sites. The words from senior management can work well to encourage students and build confidence in their minds, along with the belief that their study and life will soon resume as normal. The aura of the office of the President cannot be replaced by that of other people, especially during a crisis. And on the other hand, as it can be seen, the President was not foregrounded in this period. Instead, the articles related to university especially the management in the pandemic arear were frequently presented to the readers. By doing so, the image of a well-managed higher institution was framed, which could work well to inform and promote.

7.4 *Students: Positive, Courageous and Confident*

There are altogether 42 WOA articles about students, discussing their studies, activities, contribution to pandemic prevention and alumni stories, etc. The percentage is a little lower than that of articles categorized in the University topic (see Table 1). 17 articles are about student activities such as cooking and keeping fit. and 11 articles are about their contribution to the pandemic prevention. The first WOA article about home-stay study was published on February 19, 2020, two days after the spring semester started. As mentioned above, at this point in the pandemic, students had to stay at home to take courses online. This experience was quite new to many of them and probably a considerable number had some difficulty in adjusting quickly to this teaching style. Entitled "Which way of home-stay study is better? Find the one that suits you" (translated by the current authors), the first article provided various tips on home-stay study that were shared by experienced, peer students. This article was published quite in time, and in consideration of the real needs of students.

Starting from February 5, 2020, the UIC WOA published a series of articles about students' contributions to the community in the pandemic. The one published on February 10 is one of the most impressive when several stories about how UIC students fought the pandemic and contributed to Wuhan and their hometowns were reported. In late January and early February, people still knew very little about Covid-19, and the whole country was in a lockdown. Almost no one dared to go out as the virus was rampantly infectious. The article, therefore, presented to readers an image of their fellow students as being very positive, active, courageous and responsible. They were shown to have a strong sense of social responsibility, which motivated them to be actively engaged in the fight against the pandemic.

On the whole, the image of the students in this category of articles has been framed as valiant, having high sense of social responsibility and having great passion for life as well. The image of UIC thus has been conveyed to the reader as a cradle for nurturing such talents.

As mentioned above, the MIS is jointly constructed by the BIS and VIS. In the next section, The VIS of UIC will be analyzed in hoping to unfold a more comprehensive image built via the WOA articles.

8 The VIS of UIC Constructed via the WOA Articles

8.1 A Summary of the Data on VIS

Most of the WOA articles are a hybrid of different semiotic modes such as the verbal mode, visual mode, audio mode etc. The verbal mode and visual mode are most often seen. The BIS of the WOA of UIC are mainly reflected via the verbal mode. The visual modes, which indicate the Visual Identity System of UIC, are presented via different channels such as photos, screenshots, posters, illustrations etc. As shown in Table 2, there are in total 759 pictures. Based on the theme, they are categorized respectively as *students, teachers, campus landscape, college management* and *others*. Among these subcategories, the pictures of students are the most frequent, accounting for 37% of the total. The pictures of college management rank the second, taking up 23%. There are 62 pictures about teachers, which is 8% of the total. From these

Table 2 Figures indicating the VIS of UIC

Category		Number of pictures	Percentage (%)
Students		278	37
Teachers		62	8
Campus landscape		74	10
College management	Routine	33	4
	Pandemic-related	143	19
Others		169	22
Total		759	100

statistics, we can see that pictures of students are the most prominent during this phase of the pandemic. In this section, we will systematically examine the VIS of the WOA.

9 Decoding the VIS

With reference to examples from our collected data, we will discuss several prominent features constructed by the VIS. Firstly, there is a sharp contrast between WOA articles without pictures and the first article with abundant pictures. We found that the appearance of these articles basically coincides with the timeline of the outbreak of the pandemic. When most of the people knew little about Covid-19, they felt lost. The only thing people could do was to well protect themselves by staying at home and wear gloves and masks when going out. The WOA articles published at that time were mainly concerned with this kind of topic as well as teaching arrangement to cope with the unexpected pandemic. In terms of style, they tended to be formal. In terms of the content, it was mainly informative. Pictures could be hardly seen in those articles. With time passing by, the whole country as well as UIC gradually returned to the track. The WOA articles, whose functions are informative and promotional, started to feature pictures instead of merely providing plain information.

Besides, the scenery of the campus, which very often appears in ordinary WOA articles to align student readers as they are familiar with them, was presented in a particular way. In the pictures of the campus landscape, there are not only campus scenery, but also the presence of people who safeguard the scenes. These people include students, the university President and many collegiate staff. In the following part, several such pictures will be examined in turn.

9.1 WOA Articles without Pictures

An interesting phenomenon to be noticed when attending to the visual mode of the WOA articles is their frequent lack of visual content. The first article on Covid-19, as we said, was published on January 22. Starting from January 22 to February 4, there are altogether eight articles published. Six of them have no pictures. Considering that over 700 pictures that have been observed by us, and the intersemiotic nature of WOA articles, it is relatively unusual. When analyzing the topics of the six articles, we found that the first pictureless one was published shortly after the declaration of the outbreak of the pandemic on January 20, which meant that the whole nation had entered a state of emergency. Everyone kept a close eye on the development of the pandemic. So, the period from January 20 to early February 2020 was the hardest to go through, as people still knew little about it and the infection cases have happened seriously especially in Wuhan. As a higher education institution, UIC WOA published timely instructions to suggest students on how to protect themselves against the Covid-19 virus. And in the other five articles without pictures, the topics are respectively about postponing the starting time of the spring semester, a letter from the President acknowledging the severity of the situation and advising how to react to it as college students, notices about teaching rearrangements, etc. The appearance of the "pictureless" articles coincide exactly with the time of the outbreak of the pandemic. In the first a couple of days of the outbreak, when people knew almost nothing about the Covid-19 virus, a cautious attitude was adopted. Everyone was serious about the prevention measures. A formal style thus can best reflect the attitude of the university towards the pandemic as well as the students. Visual devices, however, such as pictures, photos, illustrations, screenshots can well facilitate people's understanding of WOA articles and make them more interesting. However, with the increase of the appealing function, the degree of the formal style is usually decreased. For formal documents such as government, legal or scientific documents, few pictures could be found in them.

In addition, we have also studied the WOA articles published in a different time. It was found that when it came to some serious topics, the articles usually were not illustrated. For instance, there are no photos in articles introducing the *Guangdong School Safety Regulations* (July 2, 2020) or regulations on UIC's recruiting the students passing National Entrance Examinations (June 26, 2020). We can safely say that the non-adoption of the visual modes is a kind of practice for the Media and Public Relations Office when touching upon serious topics. And it may also serve as a way to construct the college image in a special period of time, demonstrating to the putative readers the serious attitudes held by UIC.

9.2 The First Illustrated Article

Photo illustrations began to appear in the third article published on February 5, 2020. The first two articles are both still advising about teaching arrangements during the pandemic. The third article, however, which is one of a category mentioned in the previous section, reports on students' activities to protect the community from infection. In this article, various visual means are employed to produce strong visual effects. In total, 16 pictures illustrate this article, which includes a photo of a UIC student, who was in Wuhan, the most severely stricken city in China, and possibly even in the world at that time. In one of the pictures, he was studying with his laptop and in the other, wearing a mask, he was voluntarily sterilizing the panel of the lift in his apartment building. The two pictures are designed to demonstrate the resilient and socially engaged character of UIC students. From one aspect, as students, they still prioritize their studies, even in an emergency. From another, they help to do whatever they can, despite any risks to themselves (Fig. 2).

Besides the two pictures in the article, there are three screenshots. One is the WeChat group set up by UIC to get in touch with students in Hubei, the most affected area in China at that time. The other two are the screenshots of the social media Weibo, a Chinese version of Twitter. As another platform to communicate with students and

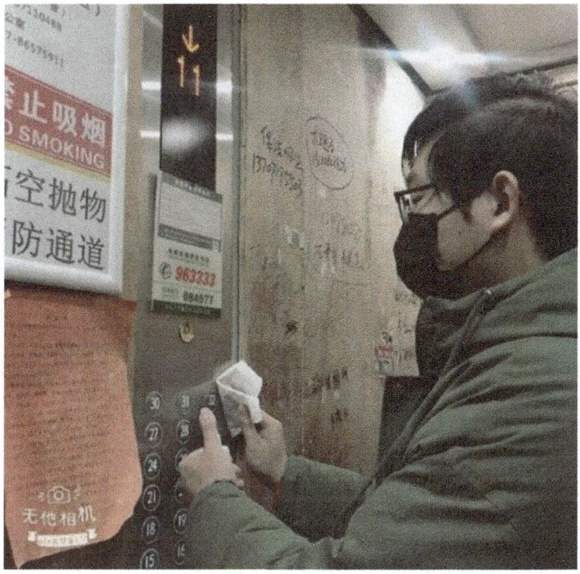

Fig. 2 A student cleaning an elevator panel

parents, UIC Weibo showed readers how much the college had donated to Hubei, which was in great need of help. And the Weibo of President Tang showed his interaction with students. In addition, 11 of the pictures were photos of students' handwritten messages of good will to the doctors working in the affected province. Various semiotic modes such as screenshots and photos diversify the visual content of the article.

As the first WOA article illustrated with as many as 16 colorful pictures ever since January 20, 2020, it has formed a sharp contrast with the previously mentioned pictureless articles. The illustrated stories and messages are no longer about informing and reminding. Instead, they are more appealing, visualizing the actions taken by UIC students, demonstrating the social responsibility taken by UIC and the students.

9.3 Student Wellbeing is Always the Concern of the College

From the very outbreak of the pandemic, as mentioned above, the college has published articles to stabilize the mental state of students, informing them the teaching arrangement in the pandemic period. The texts are more formal and most of them are notices, letters related with teaching adjustments. And we also have discussed some possible reasons for "pictureless" articles. As normality began to return, students started their online study at home. The articles no longer centered around notices or adjustments. They were more related to student life and study,

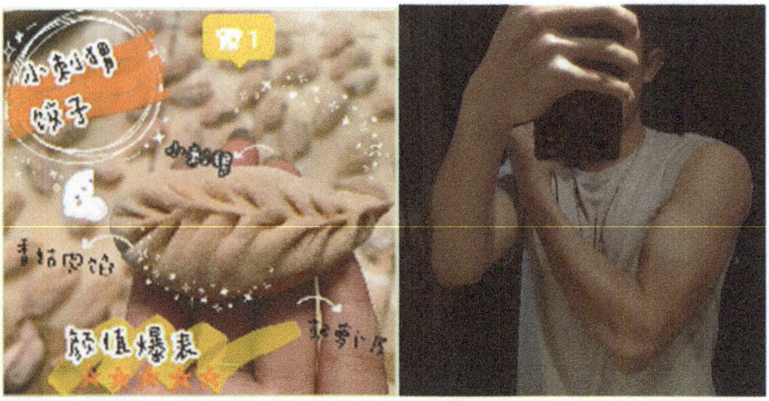

Fig. 3 Colorful homestay life

which can be more often read in the normal period. Pictures have also become an important part of those articles as they can be frequently seen in non-pandemic period.

The WOA articles published on February 24 and 27, showed the colorful homestay life of students. Altogether, more than 30 pictures are used in the two articles. There are drawings of UIC campus made by students, of food prepared by students, of books with notes, and of the muscles after hard work-out (Fig. 3).

In the first picture, a cutely shaped Jiaozi was in the center, which was held in the hand of the "chef". And there are more in the background. Some funny comments were added around the Jiaozi, saying "hedgehog Jiaozi" and "stunningly beautiful" etc. Those images can reflect the relatively relived mood of the student though he/she was still at home. The article accompanied also mentioned that by motivating students to show their cooking skills and prepare food for family members, it was hoped that love could always be felt by them.

The second picture simply consists of a boy student "showing off" the muscles of his arms. It was after days of work-out according to the article. The purpose, however, was to raise money for a hospital in Wuhan, Hubei. The muscles in the picture clearly showed the determination of the student to contribute. And at the same time, the homestay life was enriched by the workout.

These activities were intended to lessen students' stress of home-stay study, and relieve their worry about the pandemic. More importantly, they aimed to nurture students into loving persons by organizing such activities even when they were at home. The UIC image thus constructed is student-centered and responsible.

9.4 Foregrounding the President

President Tang appears in 25 of the 759 pictures in our data. The number is not a small one that can be ignored as pictures of teachers are 62. The high exposure rate compared with common teachers has interested us. As mentioned above (see Table 1) there are 6 texts related to President Tang. It seems that the rate of the visual mode is not in accordance with the verbal mode. On February 7, in his second letter to UIC students, explaining about the teaching arrangement in the pandemic period, his picture appeared. It is a group photo. President Tang was standing in the center; other colleagues were around him. Smiles were worn on their faces. In early February, the situation of the pandemic was still serious, and the college has postponed the opening of the spring semester. When this picture was provided to students along with the letter, the positive attitudes and their smiles were hoped to be received by the reader so that they would feel less worried about the future study. Actually, all through the four months, the smiling face of President Tang could be seen from time to time in the WOA articles. In addition, compared with the similar period of previous year, there are more photos of the President in the pandemic period (Fig. 4).

What has been constructed vis this VIS is care and support for the senior management. As a matter of fact, if scrutinizing the mission of UIC declared on the website, this high exposure of the senior management seems to go against with the "student-centered" philosophy. However, from our perspective, it is more meaningful to be against the philosophy in the pandemic context. With the strong support from the senior management and the President, who is the representative of the management as well as all the staff.

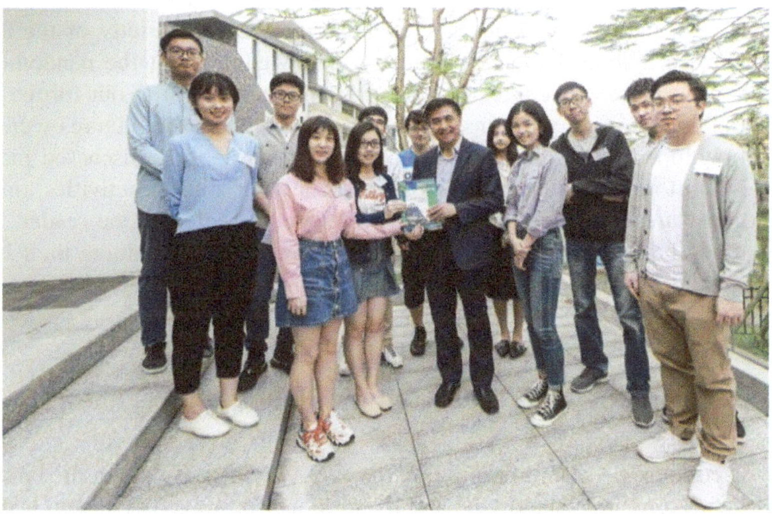

Fig. 4 President Tang and UIC colleagues

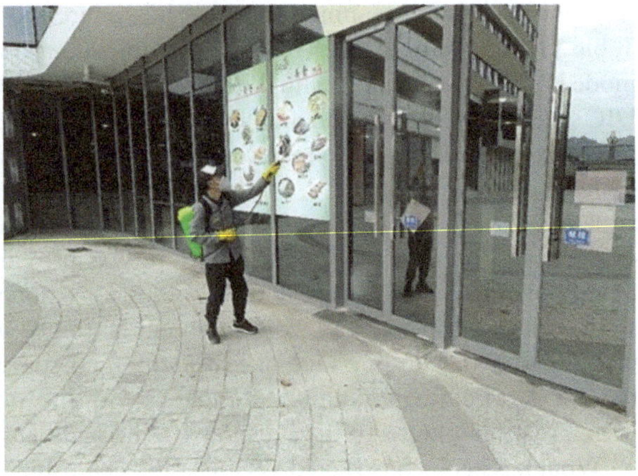

Fig. 5 Sterilizing the school canteen

9.5 We Do Everything to Safeguard Our Campus

The pictures about college management, especially the management against the pandemic are also abundant. An article published on April 7 can work as an example. The major components of the article are pictures, which are as many as 27. They clearly show every measure that have been taken to safeguard the campus. These pictures are all photos taken on campus, ensuring the authenticity of the article. These photos are about banners publicizing knowledge about the pandemic, the pandemic prevention procedures like taking temperature, filling out forms, sterilizing dorms, classrooms, canteens and library. The staff in the pictures were fully and well equipped with sterilizing devices. Unlike previously discussed pictures, there were no foregrounding of the campus scenery, or student activities, only the concrete measures fighting against the virus were presented to the reader. In the photos, it can be seen that everyone is fairly serious. They are doing their best to safeguard the campus which is waiting students to come back (Fig. 5).

10 Exploring the MIS of UIC in the Pandemic Period

Before discussing the MIS presented by the WOA articles of UIC in the pandemic period, we need to understand UIC and its mission. As previously mentioned, UIC was jointly founded by Beijing Normal University and Hong Kong Baptist University (HKBU). It is the first full-scale cooperation in higher education between the Mainland and Hong Kong. It is also the first college in Chinese Mainland embracing whole person education and takes the lead in implementing liberal arts education. This was also clearly stated in the WeChat Account. The education philosophy which could be found from the website is "A **Liberal Arts Education** is student-centered and cultivates open-minded, well-rounded talents" and "The College is committed to advancing the internationalization of Chinese higher education and takes the lead in implementing Whole Person Education and Four-Point Education" (Educational Philosophy 2020). The education philosophy here can be regarded as the Mind Identity System, which determines the general direction of the college in its teaching, administration as well as promotion. With students positioned as the center in the mission statement, the WOA, as a social media platform, is expected to show students and parents their study and lives in a panoramic way. However, the BIS analysis has shown us that during the pandemic period, the articles about the college are much more than those about students. The articles about the university takes up 54% of the overall 101 articles. Why do we see the deviation here? Then how about VIS? In Table 2, https://doi/org/10.1007/978-981-16-2430-8_5, the pictures of students take up 37%. The pictures about UIC is 41%, which is a little bit higher than that of students and also seemingly a deviation from the stated MIS in the website.

We argue that it is the impact brought about by the unprecedented pandemic. When struck by the pandemic, a college caring about their students would like to show them and other readers such as parents and prospective students their care, support and to build up confidence in them. The WOA articles analyzed in Sect. 7 also show this. The college reacted to the warning of the pandemic very quickly, providing students pandemic related knowledge to protect themselves. Besides, students were informed of the teaching adjustments and other administrative measures. Probably that's why the BIS and VIS couldn't reflect the education philosophy on the surface. But when giving it a second thought, it could be found that all these arrangements aim at facilitating the home-stay study and help to reduce their stress and pressure under such a circumstance. As a result, the ultimate focus conveyed via the foregrounded BIS and VIS on UIC and the senior management in the WeChat articles is still students. The WOA articles published in the pandemic period contribute to build the image of UIC as responsible and caring, serving for the consolidation of MIS.

In addition, we argue that the whole person education is also a component of the MIS. Besides helping students to achieve academic excellence, an interdisciplinary understanding, in the special circumstance of the pandemic, increasing students' awareness of taking the social responsibility is also fairly vital. The analysis of the BIS could well reflect this point as every measure taken by UIC and teachers is for the well-being and healthy growth of the students. And more importantly, this responsible image has been presented to students and become their role model. The students therefore were also actively involved in the anti-pandemic campaign.

11 Conclusion

In the backdrop of the Covid-19 pandemic, many face-to-face communication channels became impossible; thus, many activities, including teaching and students' events, were all moved online. Universities, under such situations, had also relied more on online social media to interact with students. In China, WeChat, a very popular social media app, became an essential tool.

This study focused on an investigation of image building of UIC via WeChat from a multimodal perspective. By drawing on the theoretical framework of the Corporate Identity system, WeChat articles published by UIC during the pandemic were collected, and the texts and pictures in those articles were categorized and analyzed. We intend to find out how the college maintained and built its image via social media during the crisis.

WOA published had displayed student activities, online learning, and students' contribution to pandemic prevention. In a time of online teaching and a closed campus, students were also innovative and moved many events online.

UIC has claimed in its educational philosophy that a liberal arts education is student-centered and this was echoed with the stories chosen to be reported in WOA. In addition to articles displaying students' online learning or extra-curriculum activities, there were many articles about the university. However, it can be noted that those articles were still closely related to students. UIC chose to publish articles on pandemic control and teaching adjustment, which demonstrated that the college cared for students' wellbeing and study. Articles about mental health were also chosen to help students handle the stress during the lock-down. When the campus was mentioned in those articles, the focus was still on providing a safe environment for students.

The pictures in those articles were also chosen to reflect the "student-centered" philosophy. Pictures of students in many different occasions were posted. For instance, there were pictures of students taking online lectures, participating online events, and helping with pandemic prevention. Even in articles about the universities, pictures of students were still included.

With its emphasis on whole person education, UIC also foregrounded students' responsibility to the community. Stories about students' contribution to the pandemic prevention were included, not only to show that students were tough and courageous, but also to set good examples for other students, in the hope of conveying ideological value and changing students' behaviour.

Sometimes the university had to act quickly to maintain its image. In the time of a pandemic, when situation changed, articles had to be published immediately to show that the college put students' need and safety first. Therefore, we saw some text-heavy articles, with no pictures included. This kind of article, formal to a certain degree, showed the urgency of the situation.

The pandemic has certainly posited great challenges to students, teachers, and senior management of the university, but the changes made during this special time can be an opportunity for the university to rethink its strategies of image building.

Acknowledgements 1. This work is supported by the UIC Research Grant Project (R201925) of BNU-HKBU United International College; Zhuhai Philosophy and Social Sciences Foundation and UIC Research Grant Project (R202042) of BNU—HKBU United International College.

2. Special thanks to the Media and Public Relations Office of BNU-HKBU United International College for allowing us to use the articles and reproduce the images in UIC WeChat Official Account as research data.

References

Aghaz, A., Hashemi, A., & Sharifi Atashgah, M. S. (2015) Factors contributing to university image: The postgraduate students' points of view. *Journal of Marketing for Higher Education*, 25(1), pp. 104–126.

Alcaide-Pulido, P., Alves, H., & Gutiérrez-Villar, B. (2017) Development of a model to analyze HEI image: A case based on a private and a public university. *Journal of Marketing for Higher Education*, 27(2), pp. 162–187.

Chandra, T., Hafni, L., Chandra, S., Purwati, A. A., & Chandra, J. (2019) The influence of service quality, university image on student satisfaction and student loyalty. *Benchmarking: An International Journal*, 26(5), pp. 1533–1549.

Chinanews [online]. Available at: http://www.chinanews.com/gn/2020/02-01/9075387.shtml. (Accessed: 20 September 2020).

Dichter, E. (1985) What's in an image. *Journal of Consumer Marketing*, 2, pp. 75–81.

Dowling, G. R. (1988) Measuring corporate images: A review of alternative approaches. *Journal of Business Research*, 17(1), pp. 27–34.

Educational Philosophy [online]. Available at: https://www.uic.edu.hk/en/about-us/educational-philosophy. (Accessed 15 September 2020).

Fairclough, N. (1993) Critical discourse analysis and the marketization of public discourse: The universities. *Discourse & Society*, 4(2), pp. 133–168.

Feng, D. W. (2019) Analyzing multimodal Chinese discourse: Integrating social semiotic and conceptual metaphor theories, in Shei C. (ed.) *The Routledge Handbook of Chinese Discourse Analysis*, Routledge, pp. 65–81.

Feng, Y., & Li, H. (2004) *Xian Dai Ying Xiao Guan Li Jiao Cheng (A textbook on modern marketing management)*. Dalian: Dongbei University of Finance and Economics Press.

Foroudi, P., Yu, Q., Gupta, S., & Foroudi, M. (2019) Enhancing university brand image and reputation through customer value co-creation behaviour. *Technological Forecasting and Social Change*, 138, pp. 218–227.

Gotsi, M., & Wilson, A. M. (2001) Corporate reputation: Seeking a definition. *Corporate Communications: An International Journal*, 6(1), pp. 24–30.

Jarvis, P. (2001) *Universities and Corporate Universities*. London: Kogan Page.

Kotler, P., & Fox, K. F. A. (1995). *Strategic Marketing for Educational Institutions*. (2nd ed.) Prentice Hall.

Kwong, J. (2000) Introduction: Marketization and privatization in education. *International Journal of Educational Development*, 20(2), pp. 87–92.

Li, K., Huang, X., & He, X. Y. (2018) Research on the construction of the attractiveness of universities WeChat public accounts—Taking Communist Youth league public platform of Guangxi University as an example. In *2018 International Joint Conference on Information, Media and Engineering (ICIME)*. IEEE, pp. 183–186.

Osman, H. (2005) 'Structural organization and socio-cognitive strategies in University Brochures: Implications for ESP', unpublished PhD thesis, University of Malaya.

Osman, H. (2008) Re-branding academic institutions with corporate advertising: A genre perspective. *Discourse & Communication*, 2(1), pp. 57–77.

Polat, S. (2011). The Relationship between University Students' Academic Achievement and Perceived Organizational Image. *Educational sciences: Theory and practice, 11*(1), 257–262.

Regular epidemic prevention and control [online]. Available at: https://english.koolearn.com/20200410/828860.html. (Accessed 18 September 2020)

Treadwell, D., & Treadwell, J. B. (2000) *Public Relations Writing: Principles and Practice*. Boston, MA: Allyn & Bacon.

WeChat Offcial Account Platform [online]. Available at: https://mp.weixin.qq.com/?lang=en_US&token=. (Accessed 12 September 2020).

Wei, M. (2016) Discussion on the application of "WeChat public platform" in the fine management of universities. In *2016 6th International Conference on Mechatronics, Computer and Education Informationization (MCEI 2016)*. Atlantis Press, pp. 842–845.
Wilkins, S., & Huisman, J. (2013) Student evaluation of university image attractiveness and its impact on student attachment to international branch campuses. *Journal of Studies in International Education*, 17(5), pp. 607–623.
Xu, J., Kang, Q., Song, Z., & Clarke, C. P. (2015) Applications of mobile social media: WeChat among academic libraries in China. *The Journal of Academic Librarianship*, 41(1), pp. 21–30.
Zhang, J., & Chen, X. (2016) City CIS in shaping the role of urban cultural characteristics. In *2016 International Conference on Economy, Management and Education Technology*. Atlantis Press, pp. 1912–1915.
Zhou, H., & Lu, H. (2017). Research on WeChat Official Account of "985 Project" university libraries. *Journal of Academic Libraries*, 01.

Native Advertising Discourse During the COVID-19 Pandemic: The Case of WeChat Official Accounts

Jiaqi Liang and Xiaying Xu

Abstract Social distancing policies during the COVID-19 pandemic impacted offline and outdoor advertising significantly, forcing many advertising activities to move online. Native advertising, a new form of advertising, is regarded as complementary to traditional advertising. The term native advertising refers to a relationship between an advertiser and a publisher whereby the advertiser pays to distribute content on the publisher's platform, thereby taking advantage of the format and substance of the publisher's content. Most of the previous research on native advertising is based on western media platforms. In China, Tencent's WeChat is the largest social media platform. This chapter focuses on native advertising on Tencent's WeChat official accounts (WOAs). It employs qualitative discourse analysis to understand how native ads on WOAs address the pandemic while seeking to persuade consumers. Referencing Burke's theory of identification and Green's theory of narrative transportation, we argue that native ads enjoy the advantage of generating emotional resonance with consumers by talking about pandemic-related topics. However, they risk being perceived as deceptive and manipulative.

Keywords Native advertising · Advertising discourse · WeChat advertising

1 Introduction

The COVID-19 pandemic has changed the advertising industry dramatically. Nearly 90% of advertisers postponed advertising plans, and 60% of major companies reduced their advertising budgets as an immediate response to the crisis, according to the World Federation of Advertisers (McCall 2020). Various degrees of lockdown and social distancing practices have caused the suspension of many businesses. Hence, there is a surging need for online advertising. Offline advertising, compared

This chapter is supported by UIC Research Grant. Project code: R202037.

J. Liang · X. Xu (✉)
Beijing Normal University Hong Kong Baptist University United International College (BNU-HKBU UIC), Zhuhai, China
e-mail: richardxu@uic.edu.cn

S.X.B. Zhao et al. (eds.), *COVID-19 Pandemic, Crisis Responses and the Changing World*, https://doi.org/10.1007/978-981-16-2430-8_23

to online advertising, has been deeply affected, as has advertising production that requires offline production, such as traditional advertising photography and videography. Cinemas are shut, so there is no demand for ads to accompany movies. Pop-up stores, roadshows, and conferences are restricted, also reducing possible advertising outlets.

During the pandemic, the expanding needs of online advertising risked prompting a backlash from the public, which had already shown concern about ads that use big data to target specific groups of consumers. According to a Statista survey, 51% of American adults thought that online targeted advertising made inappropriate use of personal data (Guttmann 2019). The two major tasks of advertising, to attract and to persuade, became even more challenging during the pandemic. Public attention was directed to pandemic-related information, especially during the initial outbreak in early January 2020. Recent research indicates that the pandemic has changed individuals' media habits, thereby changing the economic environment, making this a potential topic for ongoing investigation. For example, Taylor (2020, p. 588) called for further research into the effectiveness of digital formats and consumer targeting in a context in which customers are spending more hours at home. He also floated the idea that ads with an emotional appeal are more likely to be successful during a pandemic. Therefore, he urges researchers to explore the role of emotion in the processing of ads by consumers, the effectiveness of appeals to the emotions, and how word-of-mouth recommendations have been disseminated digitally during the COVID-19 crisis (Taylor 2020, p. 588).

Accordingly, we address how to advertise effectively during a pandemic. This chapter examines the discourse of native ads on WeChat official accounts (WOAs) during the initial stage of the COVID-19 pandemic in China. It looks at how these ads deal with the pandemic in relation to adverting messages and how audiences are persuaded and affected by the ads. Native advertising refers to the advertiser–publisher relationship, whereby an advertiser pays to distribute content on the publisher's platform, taking advantage of the publisher's form and content (Sweetser et al. 2016, p. 1). Wojdynski and Evans (2016) define native ads as "any paid advertising that takes the specific form and appearance of editorial content of the publisher itself" (p. 157).

Our approach to discourse analysis combines text and context, interacting in a way that is perceived as meaningful and unified by the participants (who are both part of the context and observers of it.). The task of discourse analysis is to describe the phenomenon of native advertising in general and in particular, and to account for how participants distinguish one type of discourse from another (Cook, 2001, p. 4).

The WOA is a platform affiliated with the Chinese social app WeChat. It allows WeChat users to publish multimedia content, and it feeds the content to its subscribers. According to Tencent, the owner of WeChat, by 5 July, 2020, there were over 20 million WOAs (Tencent 2020a). The presence of WOAs is pervasive, as domestic and international government organizations, traditional media and new media, businesses, and the general public can set up accounts on this platform. Users can access various forms of news and other content on WOAs, according to their reading interests. WeChat is the largest social media platform in China, its user scale and commercial functions giving it unparalleled advantages (Xiao 2019; Tencent 2020b). Official accounts on WeChat have become an important carrier of native advertising, for which they provide an optimized context (Tencent 2020b).

In China, native advertising, a new type of advertising with special characteristics, is becoming increasingly popular (Yang 2018, p. 6; Li and Liu 2017, p. 22; Ji 2016, p. 8). Yang (2018) argues that, as a new form of production, native advertising offsets the disadvantages of traditional advertising by being less intrusive and more acceptable. Native ads on WOA are becoming a popular channel for advertising, and this study will focus on "native ads."

The objective of this study is to examine how native advertising works to attract and persuade consumers during the outbreak of the pandemic. We conducted a discourse analysis of native ads on WOAs, with Burke's theory of identification and Green's theory of narrative transportation as our main theoretical reference points. Our central argument is that the native ads on WOAs during the pandemic generally attract attention by starting with a title and topic highly relevant to the pandemic. The discourse of the ad thus generates identification, and its internal textual logic brings people seamlessly to the advertised product. Such ads have the advantage of presenting useful information to readers during the pandemic, but they run the risk of deception and improper manipulation.

2 Theory of Identification and Narrative Transportation

"Identification" and "narrative transportation" are two important terms in media research. The concept of identification has been applied to account for connections between the media characters (including newscasters, sports personalities, cartoon characters, etc.) and the audience; it is a process of understanding and accepting the narrative (Cohen 2001, p. 247). Yan and Yang (2013) suggest that before identification is generated, individuals need to attend to the time, places, and characters to comprehend the narrative world. Therefore, they argue that identification results from narrative transportation (p. 1126). Burke saw identification as a key mechanism underlying persuasion, and he further explained that "identification occurs when one individual shares the interests of another individual or believes that he or she shares the interests of another" (1969, p. 180). From a Burkean perspective, later commentators assert that media consumers adopt the attitudes, values, beliefs, and behaviors of the media personae that are already similar to their own (cf. Brown 2015, p. 264). Identification is defined as a deliberative device, as when the speaker or writer seeks to identify themself with the audience, and as an end in itself, as when individuals are eager to identify themselves with one group or another (Zhong 2017, p. 68). According to Cohen (2001), identification focuses on sharing feelings with others (p. 251).

In 1972, Burke proposed three strategies for achieving content identification: identification by sympathy, identification by antithesis, and identification by inaccuracy (Zhong 2017, p. 69; Connaughton and Jarvis 2004, p. 40). Identification by sympathy involves taking advantage of a similarity in the emotional background and perception of different groups (Zhong 2017, p. 69). Advertisements promote identification with individuals by promising to satisfy needs, by sharing similar values and similar emotions. These means enable advertisers to achieve their goal of persuasion (Chen 2009, p. 135). Yan (2015) explains that in ads, the producer presents a similar goal-realization pattern and an opportunity-taking pattern to attain identification and to persuade the audience (p. 236).

Identification by antithesis is the generation of identification by setting up a common enemy, an urgent problem, or a hazardous status (Zhong 2017, p. 73; Connaughton and Jarvis 2004, p. 40). In ads, identification by antithesis can be introduced as a problem–solution structure, whereby a joint effort is needed to solve the problems or challenges (Yan 2015, p. 237; Chen 2009, p. 136). Chen (2009) proposed an advertising discourse mode concerning identification by antithesis: the producer raises a problem or challenge in daily life, attracts the attention of the audience, and provides a solution to the problem (p. 136). In this problem–solution structure, the advertised product is seen as a solution (Chen 2009, p. 136).

Identification inaccuracy refers to the attainment of identification by inaccurate cognition, unconsciously or subconsciously, which may lead individuals to mistakenly assume that what happens to others will also happen to them (Zhong 2017, p. 73; Chen 2009, p. 136; Connaughton and Jarvis 2004, p. 40). The advertising image will generate familiar emotions in the audience. Consequently, when exposed to the ad, the audience may inaccurately regard themselves as the characters in the ads, and they will share the product experience (Chen 2009, p. 136). In the same vein as Yan (2015) explained that, by immersing themselves in ads, members of the audience think that using the same product is a way to be as beautiful or happy as the characters in the ads (p. 237). In addition to these points, in 2014, Connaughton and Jarvis proposed that the use of "we" can help the audience associate themselves with the content (p. 41). Zhong (2017) observed the same phenomenon. By responding to particular personal pronouns, readers unconsciously align themselves with the writer and accept the views presented (Zhong 2017, p. 73). Similarly, Chen (2009) found that ads featuring celebrities use the first-personpronouns, such as "I" and "we", to highlight the assertion that a celebrity's experience of a product was wonderful. Through identification, the audience aligns with the celebrity and shares a sense of status as well as the emotions and values presented (p. 136). During the pandemic, what kinds of content work to generate identification?

3 Narrative Transportation in Advertising Studies

Narrative transportation is another factor at play in relation to the effectiveness of native ads on WOAs. It is an important concept in our understanding of persuasion (Yan and Yang 2013, p. 1126, De Graaf et al. 2012, p. 804). In 2000, Green and Brock conceptualized transportation into a narrative world as a convergent mental process, referring to an integrative melding of attention, imagery, and feelings (p. 701). Narrative transportation is a mechanism whereby narratives can affect belief as to whether a story is real or fictional. A loss of access to real-world facts occurs, and the audience may also experience strong emotions and motivations, although they know the presented scenario is not real (Green and Brock 2000, p. 701).

There are three characteristics of narrative transportation: individuals become less aware of their real-world surroundings, their emotional experience may be strengthened, and their attitudes may be altered when they return to reality (Yan and Yang 2013, p. 1127). Scholars such as Kim et al. (2017) have explained the mechanism of transportation in health communications: messages can enhance the processing of new and/or different information, reduce resistance to change, and enhance the desired change of attitudes and behaviors (p. 286). Based on Green's concept of transportation, scholars in China, such as Li et al. (2015), have explored four processes of how narrative transportation affects individuals' beliefs: reducing negative perception, identifying with the characters in the story, feeling personal involvement in the scenario, and generating a strong emotional response (p. 2002). Identifying with the characters' opinion, purpose, emotion, and behavior enables individuals to create an association with the character, in which they regard themselves as characters in the story, thereby altering their attitudes (Li et al. 2015, p. 2004). Throughout this process, identification with the characters stimulates individuals to model and alter their behavior and to act in a similar manner to the characters in the story.

4 Discourse Analysis of Native Ads on WOAs During the Pandemic

To address the issue of the characteristics of native ads during the pandemic, this study draws on discourse analysis to explore the creative copywriting strategies of native advertising on Tencent's WOAs. We searched the content from 10 WOAs for articles related to the pandemic from December 1, 2019 to April 30, 2020. Then, we selected native ads on WOAs. These ads appear as ordinary editorial content, but, eventually, they are textually disclosed as ads. For example, a WOA dedicated to entertainment news will start a native ad with entertainment news. Toward the end of the news item, there will be an ad for a handbag used by a celebrity mentioned in the news item. Finally, we performed a judgment sampling of six native ads, which had been viewed more than 100,000 times, to generate a detailed qualitative textual analysis that draws upon the theories of identification and transportation outlined above.

This section presents two major sets of findings in relation to Burke's theory of identification and Green's narrative transportation. The first set presents case analyses that interpret the ads in relation to the theory of identification and, to some extent, to narrative transportation. The case analyses are followed by the second set of findings addressing the particular characteristics of the selected native ads on the WOAs.

4.1 Case One: Identification by Sympathy

Identification by sympathy refers to getting close to the audience by presenting similar emotional background and perception from characters in narratives (Chen 2009, p. 135; Yan 2015, p. 237; Zhong 2017, p. 73). During the COVID-19 pandemic, authors of WOA content selected highly relevant topics, organizing the article as a whole as an emotional narrative promoting similar social values to the audience.

Case One: "1.4 Billion Citizens Affected by the COVID-19 Pandemic" is a native ad for an insurance product called Ant Insurance, a product of Alipay, a third-party payment platform belonging to the Alibaba Group, founded by Jack Ma. It was posted by the author known as "Uncle Bu'er." "Er" means insane or abnormal in Chinese, and Bu'er means sane or normal. It may be translated as "Uncle Sanity." The designation "Uncle" here and in the case of other "Uncles" who figure in the native ad we analyze has nothing to do with a biological relationship. In Chinese society, "Uncle" is a common form of address used for a man from his thirties to his fifties. Uncle Bu'er writes for a WOA characterized by articles on emotional matters. Like all the WOAs we chose in this study, Uncle Bu'er's WOA has more than one million active subscribers. The following native ad was posted on January 30, 2020, at a challenging time for China in relation to the pandemic. It told 18 stories from different ordinary people about how they were doing their best to support medical personnel. The article starts with the narrative of the ordinary citizens' daily life (see my translation below):

> Uncle Qin, a 45-year-old man from Hubei province, rode his tricycle 40 kilometers from his hometown to donate 24 boxes of fresh vegetables to frontline doctors. He. said that his vegetables might not look great, but they are very fresh and tasty.
>
> 湖北45岁秦师傅,用三轮车拉24箱新鲜蔬菜,冒风骑行40公里,只为让一线的医生们吃上自己家种的蔬菜。秦师傅说:"菜虽然不好看,但很甜很新鲜"。

At the very beginning, the narrative sets up an emotional context: Uncle Qin is only a farmer, but he donated his produce to people who needed vegetables when there was a shortage in the food supply due to the lockdown. Other brief stories in this native ad tell the stories of inconspicuous ordinary citizens doing their part to help their community (see my translation below):

> Although we are ordinary citizens, who cannot help a lot during the COVID-19 pandemic, we care deeply about the pandemic. Although the fight against the pandemic is very difficult, I believe **we must succeed.**
>
> 虽然我们都是普通人,疫情当前帮不上什么大忙,但也在时时刻刻关心疫情的进展,对抗病毒的路途虽然非常艰辛,但我相信"**此战必胜**"。

Several stories describe challenging moments during the COVID-19 pandemic when everyone co-operated. These accounts continue throughout the entire article. The selection of news items, of stories of daily life, generates emotional value, conveying the message that "it is hard, but we are all willing to fight together" from different groups during the COVID-19 pandemic. Up to this point, the native ad did not reveal any advertising clues, and it consisted of shared emotional values and similar attitudes in the context of the pandemic. In this manner, the native ad easily transports the audience into the narrative and creates identification through an emotional involvement process. However, the emotional context foreshadows the transition to the ad revealed at the end of the article (see my translation below).

> You protect the world. We protect you. We ask medical workers to please spend half a minute to consider **Ant Insurance from Alipay and get 100,000 yuan's worth of insurance for COVID-19**. We hope every medical worker will get this insurance, and we hope none of you will ever use it.
>
> 你们守护世界，我们想守护你。请所有在抗疫一线的医务人员，务必抽出半分钟时间，在支付宝搜索**"蚂蚁保险"**,领取**10**万的确诊保证金。
>
> 希望每一位医生都能够领一下这份保证金,但希望你们永远都用不上。

In the above case, the whole article generates a context of identification to get close to the readers through the emotional context and the similar beliefs and values in relation to the COVID-19 pandemic: "We all believe that we can fight against this terrible virus." This native ad sets up the emotional context throughout the article, and then it transitions into a brief product introduction at the end. The ad information is only in a few sentences, and the brand name only appears once at the end. When the brand is disclosed, it is highlighted in red, clearly separating it from the other surrounding text, making it easy to recognize.

Through this native ad, the brand invites targeted medical personnel to obtain free insurance from Ant Insurance. The ad seems to convey support for medical personnel in the form of insurance. However, it is indirectly addressed to the non-medical audience. The company appears to suggest a parallel between its apparent altruism and that of the characters in the narrative. In essence, by using these more or less emotional responses, the copywriter transports the audience into the ad shown at the end. According to De Graaf et al. (2012), individuals can have similar attitudes to fictional characters. This kind of similarity in attitudes may cause their identification with the characters (p. 804). When reading the article, readers may deem the company as "generous" and "selfless" as the characters in the narrative. This kind of goodwill helps motivate them to identify with the brand's concept, and stimulates purchase intention.

The effectiveness of this native ad needs to be understood in the wider context of how the fight against the pandemic is perceived and experienced in China. When fighting against natural disasters and epidemics, the value of collectivism is strongly upheld in China. Those who sacrifice their own good for the good of the country are heroes. News reports about these heroes abound. An example is one of the most widespread news reports in the early phase of the COVID-19 epidemic in China, when Zhong Nanshan, China's top respiratory disease expert, at the age of 84, leaned back and took a nap in the train to Wuhan, the then epicenter. He had just drafted the investigation plan on the train, having taken on the urgent assignment on January 18, 2020 (Wu 2020). Situations like these are a national issue for Chinese people. Articles about how oridinary individuals help to support frontline medical personnel may work to gain identification. Sympathy is generated through the collectivist sense of sacrifice. Wuhan people sacrificed their freedom of movement during the outbreak of COVID-19. Wuhan was the first city to enter strict lockdown, where people could not travel beyond their own residential area. As Williams (1981) suggests, culture is a structure of feelings, and an element of the feelings of Chinese people during the outbreak of COVID-19 is a sense of conscious or subconscious sacrifice in support of national regulations. In western societies, demonstrations in support of freedom are expressed in an extrovert manner. When the freedom of Chinese people is restricted, they experience the notion of sacrifice in an introverted manner, such as writing diraries. This kind of feeling can be magnified in stories like those of Uncle Qin. The advertised insurance product is offered free to medical personnel, but it is clear that the wider population is being addressed.

4.2 Cases Two to Four: Identification by Sympathy and Identification by Antithesis

Identification by sympathy emphasizes narrowing the emotional gap by sharing similar emotions, while identification by antithesis emphasizes the presence of a common enemy, an urgent problem, or a hazardous situation (Chen 2009, p. 135; Yan 2015; Zhong 2017, p. 73).

After reviewing the selected cases, this study found the following sample native ad presenting identification by sympathy through a long narrative as the introduction to a key context, leading to a core problem. Then identification by antithesis functions as a transition toward the ad that comes at the end. The ad acts as an emotionally satisfying solution to the problem in question.

Case Two is a native ad entitled "The Women Whose Labels Have Been Ripped off by the Pandemic." It is an ad for Ping'an Insurance China. At the beginning of Case Two, the first story is that of a 24-year-old lady who signed up to join the medical team in Wuhan during the COVID-19 pandemic (see my translation below).

> She is not afraid of COVID-19, and two of her reasons really impress me.
>
> *I am young. If I am unlucky enough to be infected, I can recover quicker than the older nurses.
>
> *I am not in a relationship, and I am not married. One of the other nurses shaved her beautiful long hair to avoid infection and save time.
>
> 其中有两条理由让我印象深刻。
>
> *我年龄小，如果不幸被感染了，我恢复的肯定会比年长的护士老师快。
>
> *我没有谈恋爱，也没有结婚。
>
> 还有一个小姑娘，为了避免交叉感染、节约穿防护服的时间，在投入一线工作前剃光了及腰的长发。

The stories in this native ad are all about women using their intelligence and practical skills to create personal value during the pandemic, ripping off the lables of women as being weak or less competent than men. In Case Two, the selection of news stories and the presentation of real moments from daily life create the emotional values of "self-sacrifice" and "being confident in the fight against COVID-19," values designed to resonate with readers who are also enduring hardship and showing resilience. In this way, the narrative paragraph at the start sets up a context that evokes sympathy, and this context lays the groundwork for the ad that follows.

Framed by the emotional context, the article then transitions into the ad by proposing a solution to the problem raised. To support these women, Ping'an Insurance China provides free life insurance. It offers preferential rates on specific insurance products geared toward medical workers, police officers, journalists, volunteers, and people aged 18–65. These groups are at a higher risk of infection due to occupational or age reasons (see the original text below).

> When facing the pandemic, womenmake the common decision, no matter they are mothers or daughters. These women fulfil their maternal duties and feminine duties. Through actions, they tell others that serving the country regardless of gender. **Ping'an Insurance China launched a free life insurance–Ping'an i-Health Insurance, a Public Fight against the pandemic. Aimming to control of the pandemic, the company preferentially offers 200,000 RMB insurance amount for insured death liability of COVID-19 and up-to-one-million RMB insurance amount for insured death liability for traffic accidents.**
>
> **Medical workers, police officers, journalists, and volunteers have priority to receive i-Health Insurance. In addition to the above occupations, oridinary citizens aged 18-65 that are not included in the "High-risk Occupation List" can also receive a preferential rates on this insurance product.**
>
> 疫情面前,女性做出了共同的选择,无论是妈妈还是女儿。她们尽母职、尽女职,却用无声的举动地告诉人们,为国效力,不分性别。平安健康推出免费公益保险——平安i康保.公益战疫, 针对疫情防控, 优先向疫情前线工作人员提供**20**万保额新冠肺炎身故责任+最高**100**万保额交通意外身故责任。
>
> 医护人员、公安民警、媒体记者、志愿者可优先领取**i**康保**.**公益战疫, 除以上职业外, 非《高危职业表》中规定的其他**18-65**周岁的普通群众也可领取。

The central idea of the narrative context is to show how tough the COVID-19 pandemic has been, and how self-sacrificing young women have worked hard to protect the public from the COVID-19 pandemic. Then, the insurance products are presented as a means of responding by supporting those who are making sacrifices for the public good at this difficult time. Here, the antithesis is evident in the problem–solution structure. The context sets up anxiety about a problem, and the advertised product is suggested to be the solution. Hoey and Winter (1983) pointed out that the "problem–solution pattern" is an effective way to uncover the discourse structure (p. 217). The emphasis on the "nuts and bolts" relationship is signaled by sufficient clues on the surface of the discourse (Hoey and Winter 1983). In the selected native ads, the problems and the solutions are narrated directly through interrogative sentences and declarative sentences. There is also the "nervous" emotional context and the setting up of a hazardous state. These factors combine to result in identification by antithesis.

Case Three is a native ad for Quark, a local Chinese search engine. This ad was posted on February 19, 2020. The title of this native ad reads "What the COVID-19 Pandemic has Brought About is beyond Imagination, but Love during the Pandemic is True" (my translation). The text in Case Three is divided into three parts. The first part starts with a video and a moving explanation from the author of the article, apparently recording events in a doctor's life. The doctor is seen sending clean clothes to his wife, who has been working in an isolation ward for COVID-19 patients. The couple can only talk at a distance because the virus is so contagious. The husband is very worried about his wife, who had not been home since the lunar Chinese New Year (from January 25, 2020 to February 19, 2020). They only talk for one minute. When saying goodbye, the wife looks back at her husband several times (see the original text below).

The article narrates how doctors and police officers have been trying their best to serve the public during this terrible period. The second part of the text shows how daily life can move from "everything paused" to "business as usual" (see my translation below).

> So, in this special period, how to protect ourselves comprehensively and efficiently has become the most critical issue. Apart from protection measures like wearing masks and washing hands, **being aware of local prevention measures during the pandemic is quite significant**. This awareness can help you return to work without a hitch.
>
> 所以，在这段特殊的日子里，如何全面高效防护，就成为了大家最关注的问题。除了戴口罩，勤洗手等等卫生方面的防护，**及时了解当地防控措施，**也是重中之重。这样才能助力你，顺顺利利平平安安地复工。

In the third part, the narrative again transitions into advertising. At the end of this article, the author states the problem clearly (see my translation below):

> How do individuals prepare to return to work in daily life? We recommend a good tool for you - **Quark**.
>
> 个人要怎么做好返程复工和日常生活的准备呢?给大家推荐一个好用的工具——夸克
> 。

The article as a whole narrates an emotionally involving scenario with more than 1,800 Chinese characters before the ad appears with the brand name highlighted in red. The advertising section uses 150 Chinese characters. The advertised brand, Quark, is a suggested solution to the problem of maintaining individual awareness of the COVID-19 pandemic. The long introductory stories that take up nearly 90% of the whole article establish an emotional context to get close to the readers. Identification by sympathy is created first through transportation into the narrative without showing ad clues. Step-by-step, the problem of "how to prepare ourselves to go back to work" is gradually introduced as a transition to the ad clues. Then, a solution is presented in the form of the advertised product, Quark.

Similar to Cases Two and Three, Case Four features a problem–solution structure throughout the article as a whole. However, unlike Cases Two and Three, in which ad information appears only at the end of the native ad, in Case Four, ad information runs through the entire article.

Case Four is a native ad for ROEWE, a Chinese car brand. It narrates five stories from ordinary citizens in different occupations. The touching narrative mainly recounts how each of them fight against this hard pandemic. A car is mentioned as an important aspect of the scenario in each of these five stories. In one story, a young nurse tells her father that she is relaxed and well, while, in reality, she is exhausted and vulnerable. Meanwhile, her father is working hard to buy his daughter a car to improve her life.

Each mention of "car" functions as a form of product placement (without revealing the specific brand name) by laying the groundwork for the brand exposure of the specific car. By presenting readers with familiar experiences like "downplaying her difficulties"[1] and similar social values like "contributing to the fight against the virus," the native ad influences readers by mirroring their beliefs. Without being exposed to any ad clues such as specific brand names, specific product names, "advertising" labels, or "sponsored" labels, the audience is transported into the narrative while enjoying the stories. Meanwhile, the emotions and attitudes hidden behind the narrative are making a closer connection with the readers. The scenario turns to a first-person narrative. The character admits feeling anxious and depressed because he feels pressure caused by not returning to work during the COVID-19 pandemic. Since lack of work means a reduced salary, he sees his car as a refuge that protects him from his anxieties: "When I think of the pressures, I stay in my car for a while." (my translation). The car is presented as a charging center where an individual can be "recharged" to get back to work. At the end of the texts, detailed product information is presented as follows (see my translation below).

> Those who are tired of life often stay in their cars and rest.
>
> Tough guys become even braver when they are with their car.
>
> Top quality, born to be perfect.
>
> What you need is a **Roewe MAX or** a **Roewe RX5 Emax**.
>
> 那些被生活钳制的喘不过气的人，偶尔会躲在车里稍作休息。
>
> 那些历经浮沉，坚韧强大的人，也在车的陪伴下愈战愈勇。
>
> 上乘品质，生而极致。
>
> 你需要荣威 **RXS MAX**或**RX5 eMAX**的陪伴。

The copywriter uses five stories to play on emotions that have commonly been experienced during the COVID-19 pandemic: exhaustion, concern for one's elders, and anxiety about the future. Step-by-step, the narratives establish an identifiable set of emotional concerns related to the pandemic. In each story, the concerns are addressed by the presence of the element "car" (but no specific brand is revealed). The climax of the article is the revelation of a brand of automobile that is specifically associated with an escape from the pressures of life in a pandemic—the car is a refuge in which you can relax. The state of exhaustion and anxiety that the stories all portray sets up an antithesis with which readers can identify. Again, the problem–solution structure seeks to persuade readers who identify with this state of exhaustion and anxiety to view the car brand as a means of resolving their issues.

These antithetic ideas demonstrate the concept of identification by antithesis, emphasizing the use of the emotional context throughout a problem–solution structure to develop identification. Identification is targeted to persuade readers.

---

[1] "Downplaying one's difficulties" to parents is a common situation in Chinese culture.

4.3 Identification by Inaccuracy as a Tool in Native Ads

Identification by inaccuracy involves the use of inaccurate cognition, and unconsciously or subconsciously, the mistaken assumption that what happens to others will naturally happen to oneself (Chen 2009, p. 136; Yan 2015, p. 237; Zhong 2017, p. 73). The use of the first-person plural pronoun, "we" is a discourse feature used to negotiate audience involvement. This is a recognized way of establishing solidarity between writers and readers (Philipsen and Huspek 1985, p. 253). De Graff et al. (2012) also proposed that first-person narratives, using "I" are likely to encourage readers to immerse themselves in narratives (De Graff et al. 2012, p. 805). More recently, Zhong (2017) argued that utilizing personal pronouns helps to transport individuals into the narrative and to establish identification (p. 73). In the six case studies, it is clear that personal pronouns "I" and "we" are used for narrative transportation, aiming to draw the readers into the ad. For example, in Case One, the native ad ends with the following statement: "We believe we can overcome the COVID-19 pandemic" (my translation). Sometimes, personal pronouns are used in advertising information to generate identification (see my translation below).

> In the process of fighting against the COVID-19 pandemic, we all need to get accurate information (from Quark) and actively protect ourselves.
> 抗疫路上, 我们都应主动获取信息, 主动保护自己。

Just like the other cases in this study, in Case Five, "How do Couples Spend Their Holidays When They are Temporarily in Different Places?", a native ad for Cartier on Tmall posted on a well-known WOA I Want What You Need on Feburary 8, 2020, we see the use of personal pronoun "we" to call for actions in the advertising part (see my translation below).

> Finally, let us shop together at **Cartier on Tmall**. What if we were to get married one day?
> 最后, 一起在线逛卡地亚吗, 万一以后结婚了呢?

The use of the first-person pronouns "I" and "we" and the adverb "yi qi," which means "together," helps to transport the audience into the narrative. It positions the audience in the role of the characters in the narrative, thereby "misleading" them unconsciously: "What happens to the characters in the narrative may also happen to me." The adverb "yi qi" which is also translated as the third-person plural imperative form, "Let us," an inclusive command for doing something together as a group. This is how the strategy of identification by inaccuracy is used in the selected native ads. What is interesting is that we find this strategy in nearly all the selected cases in this study, along with the strategies of identification by sympathy and identification antithesis.

4.4 Case Six: Narrative Transportation

Case Six, "The First Working Day: Eight-Hour-Crisis," is a native ad for Armani, posted on a popular WOA, GQ Laboratory, on February 10, 2020. The article appears to narrate the working day of a female office worker during the COVID-19 pandemic. The native ad begins with a question "During COVID-19, What's the Difference between their First Day Back to Work and their Usual Working Days?" In this case, the COVID-19 pandemic, which is also regarded as a social background, works as a "cause" throughout the development of the story, while the "effect" is the anxious questions and the emotional narratives related to the pandemic. In Case Five, to transport the audience into the narrative, the cause–effect structure related to the pandemic is set out in chronological order with three main episodes: before going to work, working, and after work.

In Case Six, the advertised product, lip gloss, is mentioned briefly at the beginning of the story, which can be seen as a form of product placement. The appearance of the product name impliedly suggests that Armani lip gloss can be used in different ways (see my translation below).

> 9:00: (Pressing the elevator button)
>
> Fire kills all viruses. (The man uses his cigarette lighter to press the button.)
>
> If I use this toothpick, I will not catch the virus. (The man uses a toothpick to press the button.)
>
> And, I can use my lip gloss. (The woman uses her lip gloss to press the button. The focus moves to a big Armani logo.)
>
> 9:00: (按电梯)
>
> "待会儿出去点个火就等于消毒了。(一名男性正在用打火机按电梯)"
>
> "用牙签撮就不会传染病毒了吧。(一名男性正在用牙签按电梯)"
>
> "早上带的唇釉派上大用场了。"

The story presents several scenes in which people press the elevator button during the pandemic. These are familiar scenes to ordinary citizens in China, and they easily evoke a sense of common purpose. The related emotional response prompts the audience to identify with the characters, especially if the viewers are young urban female professionals. The brand logo becomes an element of the story. The advertised product is mentioned three times in the narrative section, before the explicit promotional stage. After the conclusion of the narrative, the text transitions to the explicit advertising phase (see my translation below).

> Today marks the return to work for many people. Apart from supporting and caring for our doctors, what we can do is to look after our own health and get society working again. Of course, you must not forget to be kind to yourself, for example, by treating yourself to **Armani Lip Gloss**. Although you might not use it in the short term, it represents hope, meaning that one day we will take off our masks and apply lip gloss.
>
> 今天是很多人正式复工的第一天，像我们这样的上班族对待疫情能做的，除了给予一线医护人员尽可能的支持和关注之外，也许就是在保证安全的情况下，让整个社会再次运转起来。当然，别忘了对自己好一点，比如为自己买一支**阿玛尼红管唇釉**。也许现

在暂时还没法涂着出门，但它代表着一种希望，代表着总有一天，我们会脱下口罩，涂上唇膏，安心地出门去。

When viewed in its entirety, this native ad tells a single chronological narrative. The target audience, recognizing the scenario, experiences an emotional response, become immersed in the story, identifies with the characters, experiences emotions of similarity, and shares their feelings about and attitudes toward the product.

It has been suggested that emotional stimulation can make an audience relive the events in an ad and visualize a scenario that includes the advertised products (Kim et al. 2017, p. 284). In this case, emotional stimulation is a progressive process. Compared to traditional advertising copy that appears in magazines, these native ads on WOAs are long. Narratives last for considerably more than half of the length of an article, and pave the way for the advertising information. The Armani Lip Gloss native ad shows pandemic-related issues in chronological order. The step-by-step emotional context is the essential tool used to increase the sense of identification toward the characters in the story. Finally, there is a short product ad, accounting for less than 10% of the article. The most effective emotional strategy here is the presentation of using the product as an act of hope. When people need to wear a mask at work, using lip gloss or not makes no difference, but people hope that the pandemic will be gone before long and their lip gloss will be seen again.

4.5 *Characteristics of Native Ads on WOAs During the COVID-19 Pandemic*

In the previous sections on discourse analysis, we identify several discourse characteristics of the selected native ads on Tencent WOAs during the COVID-19 pandemic. First, as set out in the definition of native advertising, a native ad takes its specific form and appearance of content from the platform where it features (Wojdynski and Evans 2016). Articles on WOAs addressing topical pandemic issues in these challenging times are useful carriers for native ads. Second, concerning the discourse characteristics, the discourse sequence of the selected native ads can be defined as a two-stage inverted pyramid structure: editorial content and advertising information (specific brand or product introduction, see Fig. 1). The selected native ads utilize a relatively long discourse, using most of the article to generate an emotional pandemic resonance. Without revealing specific brands or products, the discourse draws the audience into the narrative and achieves closeness to the audience by presenting similar emotions, similar experiences, or similar values. Then, the narrative transitions to a short product ad, consisting of a brief discourse with a key brand message highlighted in red or bold-type characters (Fig. 1).

In comparison to the length of advertising copy in magazines, Facebook, and Twitter, native ads on WOAs are relatively long, with an average of 1,600 words of narrative, taking up most of their length. The length facilitates the narrative transportation effect. As explained previously, transportation into a narrative world refers

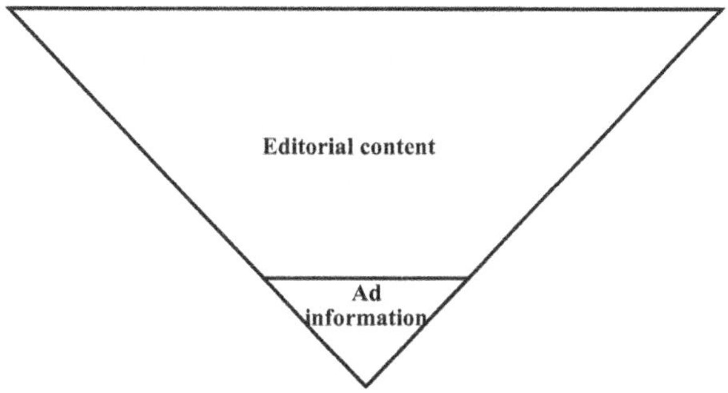

Fig. 1 Inverted pyramid structure of native ad discourse

to an integrative mental process of attention, imagery, and feelings (Green and Brock 2000, p. 701). Transportation is not likely to be achieved by short narratives of a few hundred words. According to previous studies, identification can alter attitudes when these attitudes are related to the same goals as presented in the narratives (De Graaf et al. 2012, p. 818). Essentially, native ads make use of emotional context that is set up by means of three strategies of identification throughout the article. Stories that do not reveal any advertising clues work to transport the audience into the narrative before, finally, the native ads reveals brief product information.

5 Discussion and Conclusion

The transition from emotionally relevant narratives related to the pandemic to an ad may trigger different responses from readers. The disclosure of an ad is unexpected, as the narratives appear to be "ordinary" editorial content. However, toward the end of a piece, readers discover the true intent of the article. Transitions to the product ad can be playful in "normal" times when there is no pandemic. Readers have responded positively to some native ads, responding with comments like "Brilliant" or "This ad took me by surprise, and I am going to buy the advertised product." However, during the pandemic, the copywriter will have to work without the "playful" element. There is a fine line between being offensive and deceptive to being sincere and creative. Without exception, the language used to transition to the ad in the six native ads implied seriousness. For example, although the different ways of pressing the elevator button in the beginning of Case Six are somewhat playful, the ad for Armani lip gloss uses a serious tone to convey the hope that, one day, people can take off their masks and use lipsticks as usual in a serious tone. Case Five, the ad for Cartier on Tmall calls for actions together even though many people are separated by the pandemic, and it also expresses a sense of hope of meeting everyone again. The Ant Insurance ad presents the product as a tribute to frontline medical personnel, as does the Ping'an Insurance ad. The copywriters know that they risk being seen as deceptive. There are no linguistic disclosures like "Branded message" or "Sponsored content," informing readers about the ads. Readers will need to decipher these ads through brand placement and textual cues. Whether readers will respond to this kind of ad calls for an investigation. From the textual perspective, these native ads risk being overshadowed by the pandemic.

Many other factors may affect the effectiveness of native ads. Information utility is one such factor. Information utility theory suggests that when readers perceive the advertising information as useful, they might respond positively (Becker-Olsen 2003). Kirmani and Campbell (2004) argued that, in some cases, consumers recognize a persuasion attempt but still consider it beneficial and, therefore, do not respond negatively to it. Whether the information is useful depends on the audience. According to the use and gratification theory, usefulness can mean emotional gratification (Ruggiero 2000). Researchers have argued that emotional stimulation is the most important element in prompting identification (Kim et al. 2017 p. 298). The products have use values, and the copywriters try to link these use values to emotional resonance.

In general terms, we can identify Burke's strategies of identification behind the discourses, optimizing the structure between the narrative section and the transition to a product ad. The copywriters are not only trying to set up identification between audience and the narrative but are also trying to persuade the audience to transit this identification into product information. In native advertising, the emotional context seems to play a significant role in persuasion, especially during this challenging global pandemic. In previous studies, researchers mentioned that people are more likely to identify with characters holding similar attitudes to themselves (De Graaf et al. 2012). The emotional context throughout the complete duration of native ads plays a vital role in the persuasive mechanism. Kim et al. (2017) also observed that an emotive response to narrative ads positively affects individuals' brand attitudes (p. 293). Cohen argued that "identification" is a process that culminates in one's cognitive and emotional state (2001, p. 252). Further research is needed on the extent of identification that audiences perceive in native ads on WOAs.

Although copywriters might not recognize their use of strategies of identification and narrative transportation when producing native ads, this study shows evidence of the practical significance of guiding the direction of advertising copywriting. When creating native ads on WOAs, advertisers and copywriters tend to focus on daily life stories about topical social issues, such as the COVID-19 pandemic. This focus leads to higher clicking-rates and quickly draws the audience into the narrative. Meanwhile, the two-stage inverted pyramid structure and the three strategies of identification: identification by sympathy, identification by antithesis, and identification by inaccuracy are means of structuring native ads on WOAs. Lastly, native ads are a good way to take advantage of the "emotional context" to optimize the persuasive function of identification brought about by narrative transportation.

This study explores how brands deal with the pandemic and generate identification in the form of native ads. This form of advertising is useful in attracting reader attention by presenting stories that are proximate and relevant to the target audience. However, as previously outlined, the strategic discursive nature of these native ads is intended to generate identification. When consumers recognize the true intention of the article they are reading, there is a risk of the perception of deception and emotional manipulation. It is also noted that the copywriters are aware of the issue and have tried to present the advertising messages in a sincere and serious manner. Advertising is controversial, and native ads during the pandemic are no exception. The main idea behind native ads is to reduce the intrusiveness of an ad, and if possible, to offer some useful information. WOAs provide a vast arena for advertisers to place native ads for the Chinese market. The effectiveness of these ads is undoubtedly influenced not only by the textual performance of these ads, whether they generate identification or succeed in transportation, but also by factors like whether the writer of the WOA is a celebrity, how long has the reader followed the particular WOA, etc. Textually, what other discourse strategies can be identified in these native ads? Will the audiences respond positively or negatively to stories related to the pandemic? These questions call for more empirical studies in the future.

References

Becker-Olsen, K. L. (2003) And Now, a Word from Our Sponsor: A Look at the Effects of Sponsored Content and Banner Advertising. *Journal of Advertising,* 32(2), 17–32.

Brown, W. J. (2015) Examining Four Processes of Audience Involvement with Media Personae: Transportation, Parasocial Interaction, Identification, Worship. *Communication Theory*, 25(2015), pp. 259–283

Burke, K. (1969) *A Rhetoric of Motives.* Berkeley: University of California Press

Chen, L. (2009) A Rhetorical Analysis of Advertisement Discourse from the Perspective of Kenneth Burke's Identification. *Journal of Shaoguan University*, 30(1), pp. 134–137.

Cohen, J. (2001) Defining Identification: A Theoretical Look at the Identification of Audiences with Media Characters: Mass Communication and Society, *Mass Communication & Society*, 4(3), pp. 245–264, https://doi.org/10.1207/S15327825MCS0403_01

Connaughton, S. L. & Jarvis, S. E. (2004) Invitations for Partisan Identification: Attempts to Court Latino Voters Through Televised Latino-Oriented Political Advertisements, 1984–2000. *Journal of Communication*, 54(1), pp. 38–54.

Cook, G. (2001) *The Discourse of Advertising.* London and New York: Routledge.

De Graaf, A. D., Heoken, H., Sanders, J. & Beentjes, J. W. (2012) Identification as a Mechanism of Narrative Persuasion. *Communication Research*, 39(6), pp. 802–823.

Green, M. C., & Brock, T. C. (2000) The Role of Transportation in the Persuasiveness of Public Narratives. *Journal of Personality and Social Psychology*, 79(5), pp. 701–721.

Guttmann, A. (2019) Perception of Targeted Advertising According to Adults in the United States as of May 2019. Statista 11 July [Online]. Available at: https://www.statista.com/statistics/993399/adult-opinion-targeted-ads-us/. (Accessed 1 September 2020).

Hoey, M., & Winter, E. O. (1983) *On the Surface of Discourse.* London: Allen & Unwin.

Ji, Y. (2016) Research on Creative Communication of Microblog Native Advertising. Doctoral dissertation. Northeast Normal University. Available at: http://cdmd.cnki.com.cn/Article/CDMD-10200-1019841839.htm. (Accessed 1 May 2019).

Kim, E., Ratheshwar, S., & Thorson, E. (2017) Why Narrative Ads Work: An Integrated Process Explanation. *Journal of Advertising*, 46(2), pp. 283–296.

Kirmani, A., & Campbell, M. C. (2004) Goal Seeker and Persuasion Sentry: How Consumer Targets Respond to Interpersonal Marketing Persuasion, *Journal of Consumer Research,* 31(3), pp. 573–82.

Li, G., & Liu, X. (2017) A Study on Narrative Structure and Relationship of Native Advertisement. *Marketing and Communication Forum*, 000(005), pp. 22–29.

Li, Q., Hu, Z., Wang, X., & Liu, X. (2015) Narrative Transportation and the Mechanism of Persuasion: Case Study of Narrative Public Service Advertising. *Advances in Psychological Science*, 23(11), pp. 2001–2008.

McCall, V. (2020) How the Pandemic Is Changing Advertising. NPR 29 May [online]. Available at: https://www.npr.org/local/309/2020/05/29/864933302/how-the-pandemic-is-changing-advertising. (Accessed 28 August 2020).

Philipsen, G., & Huspek, M. (1985) A Bibliography of Sociolinguistic Studies of Personal Address. *Anthropological Linguistics, 27*(1), pp. 94–101

Ruggiero, T. E. (2000) Uses and Gratifications Theory in the 21st Century. *Mass Communication and Society, 3*(1). pp. 3–37. https://doi.org/10.1207/S15327825MCS0301_02

Sweetser, K. D., Ahn, S. J., Golan, G. J., & Hochman, A. (2016) Native Advertising as a New Public Relations Tactic. *American Behavioral Scientist*, 60(12), pp. 1–16

Taylor, C. R. (2020) Advertising and COVID-19. *International Journal of Advertising*, 39(5), pp. 587–589

Tencent. (2020a) Tencent Announces 20 Million WeChat Official Accounts Verified by Ministry of Education. QQ 6 July [Online]. Available at: https://new.qq.com/rain/a/20200706A06TFV00. (Accessed 2 September 2020).

Tencent, (2020b) WeChat's Biggest Rival was Born? Accumulate 2 Billion Users, WeChat Becomes the World's First Social Media Platform! [Online]. Available at: https://xw.qq.com/cmsid/202002 27A0FDLR00. (Accessed 13 September 2020).

Wojdynski, B. W., & Evans N. J. (2016) Going Native: Effects of Disclosure Position and Language on the Recognition and Evaluation of Online Native Advertising. *Journal of Advertising*, 0(0), 1–12. https://doi.org/10.1080/00913367.2015.1115380.

Williams, R. (1981) *The sociology of culture*. Chicago: University of Chicago Press.

Wu, B. (September 24, 2020) Zhong Nanshan recalls taking the train to Wuhan. CCTV News. [Online]. Available at: https://new.qq.com/rain/a/20200924a021hw00. (Accessed 8 February 2021).

Xiao, J. (2019) China Mobile Social Report: The User Scale is Expected to Exceed 800 million in 2020, and the Demand for WeChat Product Reform is Increasingly Strong [Online]. Available at: https://www.iimedia.cn/c460/66480.html. (Accessed 13 September 2020)

Yan, Y. (2015) The Application of Kenneth Burke's Identification Theory in Advertisement Discourse. *Overseas English*, 2015(08), pp. 236–237.

Yan, J. & Yang, S. (2013) The Persuasion Mechanism of Narrative Transportation. *Advances in Psychological Science*, 21(6), pp. 1125–1132.

Yang, R. (2018) Research on Native Advertising of Social Media in China. Master Dissertation. Xinjiang University. Available at: http://cdmd.cnki.com.cn/article/cdmd-10755-101883 4582.htm. (Accessed 20 May 2008).

Zhong, J. (2017) Rhetorical Interpretation of Abstracts in Sci-Tech Theses Based on Burke's Identification Theory. *English Language Teaching,* 10(5), pp. 68–75.

Conclusion: COVID-19 Pandemic, Crisis Responses and the Changing World—Perspectives in Humanities and Social Sciences

Charles Lowe

The roots of the term, pandemic, entered into English in the latter stages of a plague in the late seventeenth century and may be traced etymologically to the Greek *pandemos*, an incident or disease pertaining to "all people" (*Oxford English Dictionary*). The present volume has been the product of a proposal to offer topical perspectives on COVID-19: a disease, which by its sweeping character,[1] demonstrates the continued relevance of its etymological roots. However, an endeavor, proposing to offer a reasonable perceptive on a *pandemos*, is hinged on a challenging premise: whether, in the midst of such a crisis that by definition immerses us all, we as scholars have achieved yet the sufficient distance to draw even the most tentative conclusion.

One response to the enquiry may be that topical considerations, such as those featured in the collection, provide a snapshot of an evolving scholarship while contributing to a growing intellectual history of the moment. Furthermore, scholarly work produced in the near future may face a similar objection about prematurity, as pandemics are generally characterized by a propensity to yield benefits and costs that may not surface for generations. The Black Plague, estimated to have killed approximate 1/3 of the population of fourteenth century Europe (*Center for Disease Control*, 2021), is regarded, nevertheless, to have the ironic benefit of contributing to the end of Feudalism, the extensive death of the working-age population leading to a corresponding rise in the price of labor. In the long term, the increased price of labor incentivized the mechanization of production, hence, forming an obscure link between a series of plagues spanning the fourteenth and seventeenth centuries and the industrial revolution of the eighteenth and nineteenth centuries—a revolution that continues to exert force over the present digital transformation.

[1] According to the *Worldometer*, as of February 26, 2021, there has been a total of 113,628,805 COVID-19 cases and 2,521,018 deaths worldwide.

C. Lowe (✉)
Division of Humanities and Social Sciences, Beijing Normal University-Hong Kong Baptist University United International College (BNU-HKBU UIC), Zhuhai, China
e-mail: charleslowe@uic.edu.cn

S.X.B. Zhao et al. (eds.), *COVID-19 Pandemic, Crisis Responses and the Changing World*, https://doi.org/10.1007/978-981-16-2430-8_24

But the unforeseen consequences of the pandemic are not limited to trade and commerce. As Benjamin Barber (2021) notes in "Post-pandemic Literature: Force and Moral Obligation to the Other in Boccaccio's *Decameron* and Camus' *The Plague*", literature has "creative and regenerative capacities" which may be unleashed by the prospect of facing a terrifying contagion, p. 508). A similar observation may be made of a literary criticism and scholarship in general. As an instance, James Shapiro (2020) has presented a powerful analysis on how Shakespeare sourced the bubonic plague—a pandemic causing the death of 30,000 or one in six Londoners leading to the close of London theaters for 14 months–for material for *Romeo and Juliet* (1593): a play where the heroine employs magic potion with medicinal qualities to simulate death and where the Friar is unable to deliver a key message the couple's tragic denouement due to being in an infected home—not to mention Mercutio's last words— "A plague on both your houses" (qtd. in *Octavian Report*, 2020).

A further proof of the power of the pandemic to revitalize scholarly discourse is this volume on the highly topical *COVID-19 Pandemic, Crisis Responses and the Changing World—Perspectives in Humanities and Social Sciences*—a collection containing diverse perspectives from the humanities but linked by a shared set of conclusion reached independently across disciplines that: (1) the pandemic will change permanently the ways individuals and communities interact in business and trade as well as radically altering ways we teach and learn; (2) cooperation, whether on an international or national scale, represents a key factor in mitigating the number of cases and deaths as well as in driving the post-pandemic economy; (3) the leaders in government should take a unified, consistent, and proactive approach in meeting the exigencies of the crisis and should, as a necessity, be honest and open in sharing with their citizens accurate information based on the best available medical expertise. Conversely, if leaders in government, business, medicine, and the academy practice non-transparency, the lay public will replace authorized sources with 'information' retrieved from evidentiary free zones, such as social media, and fail to take reasonable measures such as practicing hygiene and wearing a mask to mitigate the spread of the virus.

Finally, whether overtly and implicitly, the chapters do center on story-telling, each offering an exploration into how the pandemic becomes shaped into a narrative and the ways in which the individual constructs form a crucial part in how we, as a community, address the crisis while also determining the degree to which a society survives and prospers both materially and non-materially during the crisis and afterward.

In Part I of The *COVID-19 Pandemic, Crisis Responses and the Changing World—Perspectives in Humanities and Social Sciences*, "Global Economics, Politics, and Public Health Responses," the authors investigate the causes for and impact of the crisis. In an opening chapter, Zhao Suisheng and Wong Hong Chung critically trace a source to a deficiency in competence on the part of the Trump administration and the limited capacity of China as an emerging power to fill, as of yet, the vacuum in leadership. Further, the studies in the volume share the conclusion that the pandemic will radically alter the ways in which information is disseminated and business is transacted. Zhao Xiaobin and Gong Zekai find one aspect of that transformation will be a localization of the supply chain in countries, such as Vietnam and Mexico—an alteration in the trade patterns that may have as a silver lining a redress to the inadequate distribution of wealth and opportunity worldwide.

There is also a concurrence amongst the scholarship to this volume that cultural and historical background of a society have and will continue to play a fundamental role in determining the effectiveness of a government in responding to the present crisis. Ruan Yong Xin and Charles Leung identify "collectivist" values and a culture ratifying cooperation as critical attributes, predicting positive adaptation to the new conditions imposed by the pandemic (p. 319). Edoardo Monaco, Tang Kwok Cho, Cheng Wah Kwan, Liu Huixin and Pan Bijun add that trust in political leadership and medical expertise serve as a key indicator determining whether a country will adapt to the new conditions and thrive in the post-pandemic period. Ghee Ho centers his analysis on how the attributes of cooperation and cohesion can be enhanced through the skillful deployment of interactive technologies.

The studies on the countries in the East Asian region, though, do suggest that countries, lacking in collectivist values, may face a steep climb in managing the crisis. However, Benjamin Barber and I study how beliefs in individualism and American exceptionalism have not precluded previous drives in the United States to eradicate medical crises unfolding from far-reaching diseases such as polio and chicken pox. Instead, the country reports as a whole support the notion that responsive leadership is characterized by a sensitivity to the specific historical cultural characteristics of a community and a capacity to act on that awareness in inspiring a collective response that transforms a crisis into an opportunity. Further, in the closing chapter of the section, John Corbett asserts powerfully that humanities and social sciences have a vital function in the new dynamic in offering "complementary alternatives" (p. 486) that can foster a sense of connection and community that is in especial need in a period characterized by social distance and the quarantine.

Fittingly, Part III offers a cross-disciplinary approach to the "New Orders and Impacts" of the crisis on business and culture and society. Picking up on a note in Professor Corbett's chapter from the previous section on the growing trend towards the internationalization of education, Edith M. Y. Yan observes the impact of digital technology in altering qualitatively the learning experience in a potentially global classroom.

Likewise, the chapters in the closing third support a finding that the crisis will, by necessity, force a re-envisioning of academic and professional disciplines within the humanities and social sciences. Jiang Mengying perceptively locates the new applications to communicate information on the crisis and the steps to mitigate the spread of COVID-19. Ge Song studies the adaptation strategies of museums in effecting virtual exhibitions that translate one heritage to an "audience that belongs to culturally and linguistically different communities" (p. 419). The chapter draws attention to the possibilities of multimodalities to generate openings for diverse readings. Multimodal translation permits an escape from the translation as a "variety of dichotomies, such as source text and target text" and provokes translation practices that "mediate cultures, languages, perspectives and experiences" (p. 525).

The pandemic and post-pandemic periods will additionally impose the obligation to become conversant in fields which may have previously been perceived to occupy disparate categories. Jesse Owen Hearns-Branaman observes that journalists must, in keeping with a new inclusivity, augment their toolkit with a knowledge of specialized fields, such as virology, as well as attaining a skill to disseminate technical information in chunks accessible to an interested lay public. Failure to exhibit such a cross-disciplinary competence has, indeed, impeded efforts to communicate accurate information that would have mitigated the spread of the virus.

In keeping with the focus on an evolving discipline, Lan Xiaomeng attends to how public relations professionals have come to recognize the import of promoting narratives that distil the significance of a pandemic where uncertainty epitomizes a core feature. Lim Chai Lee similarly remarks that the methods and strategies underpinning media messaging and consumption have been redefined as a consequence of the crisis. Qian Hong and Zhang Jia consider more locally how United International College (UIC) sought to leverage the crisis into an occasion for growth in both the numbers of students served as well as in the quality of learning taking place interactively in the virtual classroom. The analysis serves as an appropriate close to a volume that grew from a conference facilitated by zoom technology, allowing faculty from the Division of Humanities and Social Sciences at UIC to interchange with students and scholars globally during a height of the pandemic.

Each scholar whose work became housed within the volume has suggested the divergent challenges posed by the crisis that, if not fully faced, may yet present an existential risk to the human species. But read in its totality, *COVID-19 Pandemic, Crisis Responses and the Changing World—Perspectives in Humanities and Social Sciences*, offers hope for evolutionary progress should we realize the lessons from the pandemic and most importantly, should we gather the capacity to harness the creative energy released from facing a sweeping crisis. It is that confident determination that we hope is taken away from a collection on a crisis in progress.

* * *

At the close of the massive volume—with the vaccines already becoming distributed—we as editors sincerely express our profound wish for the pandemic to be over and for humanity in the future to be smarter and safer so to avoid the reoccurrence of the vast trauma. This has been an aspiration driving our project—a desire we believe that you as readers share. Thank you.

The manufacturer's authorised representative in the EU is Springer Nature Customer Service Centre GmbH, Europaplatz 3, 69115 Heidelberg, Germany. If you have any concerns regarding our products, please contact ProductSafety@springernature.com

Printed and bound by CPI Group (UK) Ltd, Croydon, CR0 4YY
30/09/2026
02225295-0011